Measurement of Nursing Outcomes

Second Edition

Carolyn F. Waltz, PhD, RN, FANN, is Professor and Associate Dean for Academic Affairs at the University of Maryland School of Nursing. She received her BSN and MS degrees from the University of Maryland and her PhD from the University of Delaware. Dr. Waltz is an expert in the development of outcomes evaluation in clinical and educational settings. She has published numerous books and articles on measurement, nursing outcomes, consultations, and workshops to varied health care audiences nationally and internationally and is widely acknowledged as a pioneer in outcomes evaluation and research.

Louise S. Jenkins, PhD, RN, is Director of Graduate Studies at the University of Maryland School of Nursing. She received a BS degree from Northern Illinois University and MS and PhD degrees from the University of Maryland, Baltimore. Her research program is in the area of individual cardiac recovery and rehabilitation. She has developed and tested various outcome measures for use with self-efficacy theory and the study of quality of life. She serves on a number of editorial and review boards. She is currently principal investigator on a grant to develop an Institute for Teaching and Learning with Technology in Health and Human Services and recently was a collaborator on the development and implementation of a new Clinical Education and Evaluation Laboratory.

Measurement of Nursing Outcomes

Second Edition

Volume 1: Measuring Nursing Performance in Practice, Education, and Research

Carolyn Feher Waltz, PhD, RN, FAAN
Louise Sherman Jenkins, PhD, RN, FAAN

Editors

 Springer Publishing Company

Springer Publishing Company, Inc.
536 Broadway
New York, NY 10012-3955

Acquisitions Editor: Ruth Chasek
Production Editor: Jeanne Libby
Cover design by Susan Hauley

02 03 04 / 5 4 3 2

Library of Congress Cataloging-in-Publication Data

Measurement of nursing outcomes / Carolyn Feher Waltz, Louise Sherman Jenkins, editors,—2nd ed.
      p.   ; cm.
   Includes bibliographical references and index.
   Contents: v.   1. Professional and education focus
   ISBN 0-8261-1417-2 (v. 1)
      1. Nursing—Standards.   2. Nursing audit.   I. Waltz, Carolyn Feher.
   II. Jenkins, Louise Sherman.
      [DNLM: 1. Nursing—methods.   2. Clinical Competence.   3. Nursing—standards.   4. Outcome and Process Assessment (Health Care).   WY 16 M484 2001]
   RT85.5 .M434 2001
   610.73—dc21
                                                                    00-054928

CONTENTS

Part III MEASURING PROFESSIONALISM

Part IV RESEARCH AND EVALUATION

PREFACE

This publication is a compendium of some of the finest tools and methods available to nurses for the measurement of clinical and educational outcomes. It is a second edition of the highly acclaimed series of *Measurement of Nursing Outcomes* books published by Springer Publishing Company:

> Waltz, Carolyn F. and Strickland, Ora L. (1988), *Volume One, Measuring Client Outcomes.*
> Strickland, Ora L. and Waltz, Carolyn F. (1988), *Volume Two, Measuring Nursing Performance: Practice, Education, and Research.*
> Waltz, Carolyn F. and Strickland, Ora L. (1990), *Volume Three, Measuring Clinical Skills and Professional Development in Education and Practice.*
> Strickland, Ora L. and Waltz, Carolyn F. (1990), *Volume Four, Measuring Client Self-Care and Coping Skills.*

A collection of tools and methods is presented with attention given in each chapter to purpose and utility, conceptual basis, development, testing, and the results of reliability and validity assessments.

Many of the tools and methods included are the second generation of tools that were originally developed by participants in the Measurement of Clinical and Educational Outcomes Project. This project, administered by Dr. Carolyn F. Waltz and Dr. Ora L. Strickland and funded by the Division of Nursing, Special Projects Branch, U.S. Dept. of Health, Education, and Welfare (1983–1988), afforded nurse researchers, clinicians, and educators from across the nation the opportunity to refine their skills in measurement through a series of intensive workshops and individualized consultations. The project focused on the development and testing of clinical and educational outcome tools by nurses who participated. Enrollment was limited to those who were actively engaged in research or education, and selection of participants was on a competitive basis. Resulting tools and methods were presented at a conference open to the profession at large that was attended by approximately 250 individuals. Selected tools and methods were subsequently disseminated in the four volumes edited by Drs. Waltz and Strickland and published by the Springer Publishing Company (1988–1990).

Since that time, many of these tools have been widely used, further tested, and revised by the developers and others. Thus, it is time for a second edition. Included here are tools and methods applicable to clinical and educational settings that focus on professional and education outcomes. The collection contains several clusters of topics that address professionalism, clinical decision making, clinical performance, clinical simulation, student outcomes, factors affecting the clusters, and research outcomes. Major topic areas include but are not limited to: effect of language competence and review courses on graduates' NCLEX-RN performance, student leadership characteristics, outcomes of continuing education programs, attitudes toward cost effectiveness, faculty teaching role preparation, diagnostic reasoning, critical thinking, and clinical competence.

Readers will find in this publication not only a collection of tools for measuring clinical and educational outcomes that address a variety of substantive topic areas, but also prototypes of methodologies for the measurement of outcome variables whose utility extends well beyond a given topic area. Other notable features of the tools presented here follow: the tools are conceptually based and resulted from extensive reviews of the literature; tools and methods are well grounded in sound measurement theory and practices; both norm-referenced and criterion-referenced frameworks and varied types of instrumentation are represented; reliability and validity data are provided for all tools and methods, in some cases reflecting more than a decade of further development and testing by the authors and others; and varied methods for determining reliability and validity are presented in an easily understood and replicable manner.

CAROLYN FEHER WALTZ, RN, PHD, FAAN
Professor and Associate Dean for
        Academic Affairs
University of Maryland, School of Nursing

LOUISE SHERMAN JENKINS, RN, PHD
Associate Professor and Director of
        Graduate Studies
University of Maryland, School of Nursing

CONTRIBUTORS

Paulette Freeman Adams, EdD, RN
Assistant Dean, Undergraduate
  Program
School of Nursing
University of Louisville
Louisville, Kentucky

Jean M. Arnold, EdD, RN
Professor, Emerita
College of Nursing
Rutgers, The State University of
  New Jersey
Newark, New Jersey

Eloise M. Balasco, RN, MSN
Division of Education Testing
  Services
Chicago, Illinois

**Elizabeth A. Barrett, PhD, RN,
  FAAN**
Professor and Coordinator
Center for Nursing Research
Hunter College of CUNY
New York, New York

Anne S. Black, RN, MSN
Retired
The Children's Hospital
Boston, Massachusetts

Doris R. Blaney, EdD, RN, FAAN
Professor and Dean Emerita
Indiana University
Northwest School of Nursing
3400 Broadway
Gary, Indiana 46408

Irene M. Bobak, PhD, RN, FAAN
Professor Emerita
Department of Nursing
San Francisco State University
San Francisco, California

Q. Kay Branum, PhD, RN
University of Maryland Medical
  System
Baltimore, Maryland

Janet M. Burge, PhD, RN
Professor
San Antonio, Texas

Barbara Jaffin Cohen, EdD, RN
Director and Professor
Division of Nursing
College of Mount Saint Vincent
Riverdale, New York

Alice Conway, PhD, RN, CRNP
Associate Professor of Nursing
Department of Nursing
Edinboro University of
  Pennsylvania
Edinboro, Pennsylvania

Gretchen Reising Cornell, PhD, RN
Professor of Nursing
Nursing Program
Truman University
Kirksville, Missouri

Felicitas A. dela Cruz, MS, RN
Associate Professor
School of Nursing
Azusa Pacific University
Azusa, California

Mary E. Duffy, PhD, RN, FAAN
Director of Center for Nursing
    Research
and Professor
School of Nursing
Boston College
Chestnut Hill, Massachusetts

Lou Ann Emerson, DNSc, RN
Associate Professor
College of Nursing and Health
University of Cincinnati
Cincinnati, Ohio

Roberta J. Emerson, EdD, RN
Associate Professor
Intercollegiate Center for Nursing
    Education
Spokane, Washington

Linda Finke, PhD, RN
Director of Professional
    Development Services
Sigma Theta Tau International
Indianapolis, Indiana

Linda Holbrook Freeman, RN, MSN
Assistant Dean, Continuing
    Education
School of Nursing
University of Louisville
Louisville, Kentucky

Sara T. Fry, PhD, RN, FAAN
Henry R. Luce Professor of
    Nursing Ethics
School of Nursing
Boston College
Chestnut Hill, Massachusetts

Barbara Gilman, RN, MSN, CS
Assistant Professor
College of Nursing and Health
University of Cincinnati
Cincinnati, Ohio

Janice Giltinan, MSN, RN, CS
Assistant Professor of Nursing
Department of Nursing
Edinboro University of
    Pennsylvania
Edinboro, Pennsylvania

Kathryn S. Hegedus, DNSc, RN
School of Nursing
University of Connecticut
Storrs, Connecticut

Charles J. Hobson, PhD
Associate Professor of
    Management
Division of Business and
    Economics
Indiana University
Gary, Indiana

Elizabeth P. Howard, PhD, RN, CS
Associate Professor of Nursing
Northeastern University
Boston, Massachusetts

Angeline M. Jacobs, MS, RN
Professor Emerita
Azusa Pacific University
Azusa, California

Helen M. Jenkins, PhD, RN
Longwood, Florida

Joan M. Johnson, PhD, RN
Assistant Professor Emerita
College of Nursing
University of Wisconsin-Oshkosh
Oshkosh, Wisconsin

Joan Gittins Johnston, EdD, RN
Associate Professor of Nursing
Lehman College
Bronx, New York

Barbara A. Kakta, EdD, RN
Professor and Director of
    Undergraduate Studies
College of Nursing
Lewis University
Romeoville, Illinois

Karen Kelly, EdD, RN
Director of Clinical Services
Special Care Hospital
    Management Corp.
St. Louis, Missouri

**Margaret R. Kostopoulos, RN,
    MSN, CNA**
Director of Outcomes
    Management
Doctor's Community Hospital
Lanham, Maryland

Muriel W. Lessner, PhD, RN
Assistant Professor Emeritus
University of Connecticut
Farmington, Connecticut

Katherine N. McDannel, MSN, RN
Instructor
Lewis University
Romeoville, Illinois

Pamela A. Martyn, MS, RN
Instructor
Lewis University
Romeoville, Illinois

**Patricia R. Messmer, PhD, RN,
    FAAN**
Associate for Nursing Research
Mount Sinai Medical Center/
Miami Heart Institute
Miami Beach, Florida

**Barbara Clark Mims, PhD, RN,
    MSN**
Assistant Professor
School of Nursing
Kent State University
Kent, Ohio

Peggy R. Rice, MS, RN
Assistant Professor
Lewis University
Romeoville, Illinois

Carol L. Rossel, EdD, RN, CS
Professor and Coordinator
Lewis University
Romeoville, Illinois

Nelda Samarel, EdD, RN
Professor (Retired) and Visiting
    Research Prof.
William Paterson University
Wayne, New Jersey

Linda J. Scheetz, EdD, RN
Chairperson and Professor
Division of Nursing
Mount Saint Mary College
Newburgh, New York

E. Ann Sheridan, EdD, RN
University of Massachusetts
School of Health Sciences
Division of Nursing
Amherst, Massachusetts

Bonnie Ketchum Smola, PhD, RN
Professor, Nursing
University of Dubuque
Dubuque, Iowa

Marie Spruck, EdD, RN
Professor
College of Nursing and Health
University of Cincinnati
Cincinnati, Ohio

Jacqueline Stemple, EdD, RN
Associate Professor of Nursing
Department of Health Systems
Morgantown, West Virginia

Anna B. Stepniewski
Graduate Research Assistant
Division of Business and
    Economics
Indiana University
Gary, Indiana

Cheryl B. Stetler, PhD, RN
Amherst, Massachusetts

Donna Ketchum Story, PhD, RN
Associate Professor
Luther College
Decorah, Iowa

Kathy Stroh, MSN, MA, RN
Assistant Professor of Nursing
Department of Nursing
Edinboro University of
    Pennsylvania
Edinboro, Pennsylvania

Barbara S. Thomas, PhD
Professor
College of Nursing
University of Iowa
Iowa City, Iowa

**Sandra Millon Underwood, PhD,
    RN**
Professor
University of Wisconsin-Milwaukee
Milwaukee, Wisconsin

Gail A. Vitale, MS, RN
Assistant Professor
Lewis University
Romeoville, Illinois

Elizabeth Weiner, PhD, RN
Associate Professor
College of Nursing and Health
University of Cincinnati
Cincinnati, Ohio

DeAnn M. Young, RN, MS
California State University
Los Angeles, California

PART I

Measuring Clinical Decision Making and Performance in Education and Practice

1

Diagnostic Reasoning Simulations and Instruments

Jean M. Arnold

PURPOSE

This chapter describes the U-Diagnosis(tm) instrument, which is used to measure diagnostic reasoning process. Its development as a tool for gerontological nursing is described, and the Gerontological Nursing U-Diagnosis(tm) Instrument is provided at the end of this chapter. Six simulations written in accord with the diagnostic reasoning model were tested using six expert panels. Identification of nursing diagnoses unique to gerontological nursing derived from these six case studies and validation by an expert panel led to evolution of a gerontological nursing U-Diagnosis(tm) instrument. This chapter discusses further validation of the diagnostic reasoning instrument and how it led to development of the gerontological nursing U-Diagnose(tm) instrument.

Specific objectives were to:

1. Further validate the diagnostic reasoning instrument by using six gerontological simulations with six different expert panels;
2. Develop an instrument to collect nursing care data from a gerontological care record;
3. Determine nursing diagnoses with related interventions and outcomes representing the gerontological nursing specialty; and
4. Link nursing diagnoses with interventions and outcomes.

INSTRUMENT DESCRIPTION

Diagnostic reasoning refers to the decisions made during the problem identification assessment of a situation and development of intervention strategies. It is based on the problem-solving approach that humans use to handle everyday activities and professional situations. It is not unique to a single discipline. However, each individual views a situation based on his or her education and experience. The author believes that diagnostic reasoning is a component of critical thinking. The U-Diagnosis(tm) instrument is used to measure the diagnostic reasoning process only, not all cognitive processes inherent in critical thinking.

Diagnostic reasoning in clinical fields was first described in medicine and subsequently in nursing. The diagnostic process is performed in the context of a clinical situation in this model. The diagnostician examines a situation by gathering data; the next step is to sort relevant data from inaccurate and irrelevant data. The data sorting either results in data that supports or does not support the diagnosis. A tentative listing of diagnoses emerges, and as more data are collected, the major diagnoses are selected from the diagnosis listing. These determine the here-and-now intervention strategies, meaning they could change as the situation changes. An intervention plan is developed for each major diagnosis. The clinician has a stated or written objective, and takes action based on her or his expertise. If asked, the clinician would cite a reason for the written and observable behavior. Criteria for evaluation of the clinician's actions are actual client outcomes compared with the standard client outcomes. The diagnostic process is iterative, although it appears as linear when described in a step-by-step manner. The diagnostic process as conceived by the author is illustrated in Figure 1.1, and the components of an intervention plan are illustrated in Figure 1.2. The intervention plan of each major diagnosis consists of objectives, actions, rationale, and outcomes. The diagnostic reasoning protocols are based on previous research by the author (Arnold, 1988, 1990).

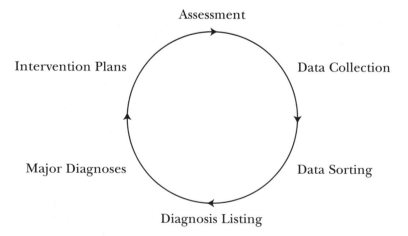

FIGURE 1.1 Diagnostic process.

Literature reviews on diagnostic reasoning are published elsewhere (Arnold, 1988, 1990). The four components or stages of the reasoning process as applied to medicine are cue acquisition, hypothesis generation, cue interpretation, and hypothesis evaluation (Elstein, Shulman, & Sprafka, 1978). These stages describe the process physicians use in arriving at a medical diagnosis. Carnevali (1984) described diagnostic reasoning in greater detail by incorporating these components in steps called pre-encounter data, data gathering and shaping, formation of clusters using cues, hypothesis development, and testing resulting in diagnosis. Problem solving became known as the "nursing process" in the nursing literature. Nursing process was described as the steps of assessment, planning, implementation, and evaluation; nursing diagnosis was added later as a step occurring at the end of assessment (Wilkinson, 1996). The diagnostic process consists of collecting information, interpreting the information, clustering the information, and naming the cluster (Gordon, 1987). This description is similar to that developed by Elstein et al. (1978) when describing problem solving and the diagnostic process in medicine. The diagnostic reasoning component was necessary to incorporate the first nursing taxonomy, nursing diagnosis. The diagnostic reasoning model in medicine is similar to those of other professions. A recent review of nursing decision-making studies (Harmer, Abu-Saad, & Halfrens, 1994) demonstrated that this model has broad-based support. Thus, the nursing process is another way of describing problem solving and the diagnostic reasoning process.

Pesut and Herman (1998) have described the evolution of nursing process as generational. The first generation (1950–1970) was focused on problems and process, and the second generation (1970–1990) on diagnosis and reasoning. The third generation (1990–2010) of nursing process

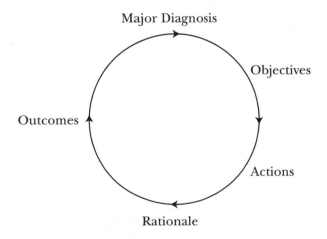

FIGURE 1.2 Intervention plan.

is characterized by a focus on outcome specification. The outcome-present-state-test (OPT) model of clinical reasoning is an example of the third generation of nursing process. "Clinical judgements are conclusions drawn from tests that compare present state data to specified outcome state criteria" (Pesut & Herman, 1998). Today's health care environment focuses on evaluation of the health team's interventions as measurable outcomes. Evaluation itself is not new, but stating the standard patient outcome at the initiation of care as a means for comparison with client outcomes is a new approach to evaluation. The OPT model focuses on outcomes in the context of a particular situation, similar to the diagnostic reasoning model proposed by the author, but its major emphasis is on outcomes. The role of diagnosis is not explicit in the OPT model, whereas diagnosis is central to the author's model and outcomes are related to each major diagnosis and actions (interventions) identified for a given clinical situation.

Nursing process is problem solving that involves critical thinking; critical thinking focuses on deciding what to believe or do (Wilkinson, 1996). Diagnostic reasoning, critical thinking, and nursing process are interrelated.

In 1926, nursing diagnosis was defined as "what the immediate problem seems to be" (Hamer, 1926). Another definition was published nearly 40 years later: "Nursing diagnosis involves discriminative judgment, is based on a body of scientific knowledge and is a process which provides nursing with a systematic way of assessing patient problems and needs" (Komorita, 1963, p. 86). Collective efforts to classify nursing information began in 1973 at the first national conference on the classification of nursing diagnosis and continue to the present (e.g., Aydelotte & Peterson, 1987). Nursing actions or ministrations appeared in the nursing literature in the 1950s. A consensus-based definition of nursing actions emerged as part of nursing data elements at the Nursing Minimum Data Set Conference in 1985. Nursing intervention was described as an action intended to benefit the patient or client and for which nurses are responsible (Werley & Lang, 1988).

Nurse educators began teaching the four steps of the nursing process in the 1970s, which included assessment (diagnosis), planning, implementation (action), and evaluation. Nurses were encouraged to use nursing diagnosis by the development and publication of the nursing diagnosis taxonomy by the North American Nursing Diagnosis Association (NANDA). At the ninth NANDA biennial nursing conference, nursing diagnosis was defined as a clinical judgment about individual, family, or community response to actual or potential health problems/life processes (Carroll-Johnson, 1990).

Research is needed to identify the client problems unique to nursing. The initial step in developing diagnosis-intervention links is to identify common diagnoses. Case study research that interrelates nursing diagnosis with nursing care planning, using case study simulation such as those developed by NANDA in defining a common taxonomy for accepted nursing language is one means to accomplish this task. Empirically developed relationships between nursing diagnoses and interventions are part of nursing theory development (Woolridge, Brown, & Herman, 1993). Nursing diagnosis provides the basis for selection of nursing interventions to achieve outcomes for which the nurse is accountable (Carroll-Johnson, 1990). This working definition unequivocally links nursing diagnosis with interventions and outcomes.

Simulations (case studies) have been used to identify the accuracy of nursing diagnosis (Lunney, 1992). Case studies have been used by several researchers, but few have used them to evaluate diagnostic reasoning, and even fewer have used them to evaluate the accuracy of nursing diagnoses. Lunney concluded that the outcomes or diagnostic statements to explain the data in case studies can be evaluated in relation to those of clinical experts, and used to promote accuracy of nursing diagnoses.

A few researchers have examined the use of nursing diagnosis with specific population groups. There are parallel studies on the identification of diagnoses for client populations using expert panels and RN pairing. These client populations include home health, critical care, rehabilitation, public health and long-term care, and schools (Gordon, 1995a, 1995b; Gordon & Butler-Schmidt, 1997; Fielding et al., 1997; Lesh, 1997; Lunney, Cavendish, Kraynyk-Luise, & Richardson, 1997). Listings of 10 to 20 diagnoses with the highest frequency resulted from these investigations of population groups. This delimitation of nursing diagnoses within the 100-plus of the NANDA taxonomy provides the foundation for further development of the essential characteristics of each nursing specialty. Once common nursing diagnoses are identified, related intervention plans can be formulated.

The theoretical basis of the author's diagnostic reasoning model is information theory, which describes how decisions are made. The individual making the decision processes information using short- and long-term memory. Humans' short-term memory capability is used to view the current situation and long-term memory is called upon for retrieval of knowledge and experiential information. Further description of this theory can be found in a previous study (Arnold, 1990).

The U-Diagnosis(tm) simulations are based on four components or stages in the problem-solving process described by Elstein et al. (1978) as follows: (a) cue acquisition, (b) hypothesis generation, (c) cue interpretation, and (d) hypothesis evaluation. The author's diagnostic reasoning model is comparable: (a) data collection, (b) data sorting, (c) diagnosis listing (problem identification), and (d) major diagnoses (problem listing). Problem solving was adapted to the nursing discipline as the nursing process. The four steps of this process are assessment, planning, implementation, and evaluation. In the author's diagnostic reasoning model, problem identification and data sorting constitute assessment, which concludes with a diagnosis. Planning encompasses objectives, rationale, and outcomes. Further detail of the conceptual framework for the diagnostic reasoning model can be found in previous research (Arnold, 1988, 1990).

Definitions of terms used in this study follow:

Actions are nurse behaviors that resolve client problems.

Assessment is the determination of NANDA diagnoses for a given U-Diagnose(tm) simulation including supporting data.

Criteria are measurable behaviors indicating the outcome of a goal.

Critical thinking is reasonable reflective thinking focused on deciding what to believe and do (Norris, 1989). Diagnostic reasoning is one component of critical thinking.

Data are descriptions and observations of client behaviors.

The diagnostic reasoning model describes the process the clinician uses to analyze a situation, which includes data collection and sorting to identify all relevant client problems and then to develop a care plan for major problems that encompasses objectives, criteria, actions, and rationale.

The Gerontological Nursing U-Diagnose(tm) Instrument (GNUDI) is an instrument designed to measure gerontological diagnoses and related intervention plans for a gerontological population.

Intervention plans are the nursing measures for a client diagnosis.

The objective is goal related to resolution of a client problem.

The problem is the problem component of a North American Nursing Diagnosis (excepting altered metabolism).

The rationale is the reason chosen by a nurse for a specific nursing action.

U-Diagnose(tm) simulations are written simulations designed in accord with the diagnostic reasoning model.

This methodological study required four phases: (a) development of the six simulations, (b) testing of the six simulations, (c) refinement of derived data to identify common nursing diagnoses and intervention plans, and (d) development of the GNUDI.

The author has described how a simulation could be written using her diagnostic reasoning protocols elsewhere (Arnold, 1990, 1995). A review of this development process follows. Lunney (1992) recommends the use of two groups of experts; one for creation of case studies because experts are the primary source of nursing diagnoses and another group for validation. This procedure was followed in the current study.

Three simulations related to acute gerontological nursing and three simulations related to community nursing were developed over a period of two years. First, a practicing gerontological clinical specialist was selected to write the initial scenario with the relevant nursing diagnoses. A gerontological nursing clinical specialist served as consultant for all six simulations. Her role was to critique and maintain uniformity for the six simulations. The assessment and intervention plan sections were created using the U-Diagnose(tm) reasoning protocols of diagnoses, objectives, criteria, action, rationale, and outcomes. The content of the scenario determined the number of problems. The major difficulties encountered centered on the writing of the intervention plans. The existing nursing care planning texts did not include objectives, criteria, actions, and rationale. The author and consultant provided a training session and then assisted the clinical specialist with the development of intervention plans incorporating the diagnostic reasoning protocols.

A nursing diagnosis taxonomy was in existence at the time of case study development, but this was not the case for the other diagnostic reasoning protocols. The specific nursing diagnosis (problem component) affected the number of actions and the rationale. The problem listing included 12 to 15 items. Each problem had supporting data ranging from four to nine phrases within the clinical scenario. Each intervention plan included five to nine problems with one to two objectives with related criteria as well as five to eight sets of actions and rationales. About 20% of the items within the simulation were incorrect to determine the discrimination ability of the expert rater. This procedure was in accord with recommendations by the consulting statistician.

Next, an expert panel of clinical specialists was formed. Criteria for selection included the following: (a) minimum of a master's degree, (b) experience in the specialty area related to the content of the simulation (e.g., care of a stroke client), and (c) current employment involved clinical practice. A gerontological clinical specialist consultant composed the six expert panels of approximately 36 specialists. Due to content differences within the simulations it was not possible to use the same expert panel more than once. These experts were employed by educational and health care agencies in the mid-Atlantic region. All panel members used nursing diagnosis in their respective gerontological practice settings.

Human subject procedures were followed. The institutional review board of a university approved the study. Each expert panel member signed a consent form. The author assigned a numerical identification number to each respondent to maintain anonymity.

The expert panels were directed to rate each item within the simulation using a four-point rating system. This rating system was a modified version of a relevance rating scale used previously with other U-Diagnose(tm) simulations (Arnold, 1990). The rating system follows: primary importance—very relevant to situation presented (1); secondary importance—relevant to situation provided (2); inaccurate or incorrect—not accurate for situation presented (3); and not applicable for situation presented or irrelevant for the situation presented (4). The rating code was placed at the beginning of each problem throughout the simulation.

The written case studies were mailed to the expert panel members upon completion of the simulation. The data collection time period was one to two months for each case study. Reminder letters were sent after a two-week period and follow-up telephone calls were placed every few weeks until the rating was returned. There was a 100% return rate because the raters were colleagues of the consultant and interested in the study.

Limitations of this study follow: (a) all respondents resided in the same geographical area; (b) client perspectives were not included due to the use of simulations; and (c) the richness and dynamics of an actual clinical situation were not present. Strengths of the research include: (a) the use of a standardized format for all simulations; (b) use of the uniform diagnostic reasoning model; and (c) use of content experts for each simulation.

RELIABILITY AND VALIDITY ASSESSMENTS

Two-way analysis of variance was used to calculate interrater reliability for each nursing diagnosis and intervention plan within each simulation (Winer, 1971). A content validity index (CVI) was calculated using the ratings by expert panels for items within each nursing diagnosis (Waltz, Strickland, & Lenz, 1991). The occurrence of a nursing diagnosis within a simulation was dependent on the nature of the scenario.

All interrater reliability results across the six case studies were examined to compile a listing of common nursing diagnoses. A nursing diagnosis had to occur in one or more simulations to be selected for inclusion in the master listing. This procedure resulted in 32 nursing diagnoses. The incidence of a given nursing diagnosis ranged from one to six. Table 1.1 provides the interrater reliability results for nursing diagnoses. The mean interrater reliability results for nursing diagnoses and intervention plans were .736 and .762, respectively.

The expert panels varied in their degree of agreement for specific nursing diagnoses. Interrater reliability results ranged from .807 to .961 for the following nursing diagnoses: ineffective airway clearance; decreased cardiac output; potential for infection; knowledge deficit; medication use; impaired physical mobility; self-esteem disturbance, situational; impaired skin integrity; social isolation; altered thought processes; altered cerebral tissue perfusion; and peripheral tissue perfusion. This listing comprised 34% of nursing diagnoses. Interrater reliability results for another 25% of the nursing diagnoses ranged from .530 to .667. These diagnoses included impaired communication; ineffective family coping; diarrhea; impaired gas exchange; grieving; home maintenance; impaired noncompliance; prescribed medication; and self-care deficit; toileting.

Four intervention plans could not be computed. The highest intervention plan interrater reliability results, ranging from .817 to .937, pertained to 38% of the diagnoses. These diagnosis included ineffective airway

TABLE 1.1 Nursing diagnoses interrater reliability across six case studies

Nursing Diagnosis	Frequency	Diagnosis Interrater Reliability	Frequency	Plan Interrater Reliability
Airway clearance, ineffective	1	.865 to .934	1	.817 to .874
Cardiac output, decreased	2	.940		
Communication, impaired	2	.429 to .530		
Constipation, colonic	3	.770 to .884	3	.720
Coping, ineffective, individual	4	.739 to .771	4	.858 to .937
Coping, family, ineffective: compromised	2	.618		
Diarrhea	1	.633	1	.637
Diversional activity deficit	4	.705 to .790	2	.859 to .877
Fluid volume deficit	1	.777	1	.924
Gas exchange, impaired	1	.556	1	.764
Grieving	1	.530	1	.745
Home maintenance management, impaired	2	.558 to .732	1	
Hyperthermia	1	.711	1	.727
Injury, potential for	4	.785 to .929	4	.777 to .815
Infection, potential for	2	.893 to .946	1	.735

TABLE 1.1 *(continued)*

Nursing Diagnosis	Frequency	Diagnosis Interrater Reliability	Frequency	Plan Interrater Reliability
Knowledge deficit, medication use	5	.807 to .915	2	.936
Metabolism	3	.647 to .724	3	.605 to .670
Mobility, impaired physical	5	.923 to .961	4	.666 to .837
Noncompliance, prescribed medication	3	.662 to .666	1	.574 to .845
Nutrition, altered, more than body requirements	6	.608 to .957	5	.630 to .892
Pain	5	.713 to .938	3	.831
Self-care deficit, hygiene	3	.685 to .890		.919
Self-care deficit, toileting	3	.570 to .653	2	.803
Self-esteem disturbance, situational	2	.867		.766
Sensory/ perceptual alteration: visual, auditory	5	.685 to .976	1	.867
Skin integrity, impaired	2	.820 to .913	2	
Sleep pattern disturbance	2	.766	1	
Social isolation	2	.850 to .909	2	.904
Thought processes, altered	3	.925 to .970	2	.813 to .817
Tissue perfusion, altered cerebral	1	.879	1	.671 to .769

TABLE 1.1 *(continued)*

Nursing Diagnosis	Frequency	Diagnosis Interrater Reliability	Frequency	Plan Interrater
Tissue perfusion, peripheral	1	.951	1	.719
Urinary elimination, altered	1	.667	1	.474
Violence	1	.715 to .813	1	.838 to .905

clearance; ineffective individual coping; diversional activity deficit; fluid volume deficit; knowledge deficit; medication use; pain; self-care deficit, hygiene; self-care deficit, toileting; sensory/perceptual alteration; social isolation; altered thought processes; and violence. High interrater reliability results, ranging from .807 to .970, for both diagnosis and intervention plans were reported for knowledge deficit, medication use; social isolation; and altered thought processes.

Nursing diagnoses with CVIs of 1.0 included decreased cardiac output; grieving; impaired gas exchange; impaired home management; knowledge deficit; medication use; impaired skin integrity; and altered urinary elimination. Nursing diagnoses with the next highest CVIs ranging from .917 to .958 were ineffective family coping; fluid volume deficit; self-care deficit; hygiene; and altered cerebral tissue perfusion. The lowest nursing diagnosis CVI was .50 for violence. The highest intervention plan CVIs of 1.0 occurred for ineffective individual coping; grieving; noncompliance; prescribed medication; and altered urinary elimination. Intervention plan CVIs for sleep pattern disturbance, decreased cardiac output, impaired communication, ineffective family coping, and home maintenance management were not computed. Considering both diagnoses and intervention plans, the highest CVIs were for impaired gas exchange, grieving, fluid volume deficit, impaired skin integrity, and altered urinary elimination.

The mean content validity indices for nursing diagnoses and intervention plans were 77.7 and 79.2, respectively. The content within the simulations and the items within the diagnoses may have affected the results.

There was a moderate degree of agreement among the expert panels on the 32 NANDA problems used within the six U-Diagnose(tm) simulations. The diagnostic reasoning model facilitated the identification and validation of nursing diagnoses for gerontological clients. The use of six gerontological client simulations demonstrated the existence of a unique

TABLE 1.2 Nursing Diagnoses Content Validity Across Six Case Studies

Nursing diagnosis	Diagnosis content validity index	Plan content validity index
Airway clearance, ineffective	.714	.720
Cardiac output, decreased	1.0	1.0
Communication, impaired	.625 to .660	
Constipation, colonic	.750 to .917	.688 to 1.0
Coping, ineffective, individual	.832 to .958	1.0
Coping, family, ineffective: compromised	.958	
Diarrhea	.666	.583
Diversional activity deficit	.857 to 1.0	.80 to .857
Fluid volume deficit	.917	.979
Gas exchange, impaired	1.0	.950
Grieving	1.0	1.0
Home maintenance management, impaired	1.0	
Hyperthermia	.625	.714
Injury, potential for	.875	.786 to .923
Infection, potential for	.875 to .917	.854 to .875
Knowledge deficit, medication use	1.0	.750
Metabolism	.889	.667 to 1.0

grouping of nursing diagnoses representing this population. However, further validation testing of these 32 diagnoses is recommended.

The next step in the author's research program was the validation of 32 common gerontological nursing diagnoses through the use of another expert panel and development of an instrument. The purpose of this research was to develop reliability and validity for the Gerontological Nursing U-Diagnose(tm) Instrument (GNUDI). An expert panel of gerontological advanced practice nurses was used to establish the reliability and validity of the GNUDI. A complete description of this research is available

TABLE 1.2 *(continued)*

Nursing diagnosis	Diagnosis content validity index	Plan content validity index
Mobility, impaired physical	.833 to 1.0	.750 to .875
Noncompliance, prescribed	.833 to .875	1.0
Nutrition, altered, more than body requirements	.571 to 1.0	.833 to .941
Pain	.625 to .958	.750
Self-care deficit, hygiene	.945 to 1.0	.917
Self-care deficit, toileting	.833 to 1.0	.858
Self-esteem disturbance, situational	.857	.857
Sensory/perceptual alteration visual, auditory	.667 to .917	.889
Skin integrity, impaired	1.0	.955 to .986
Sleep pattern disturbance	.889	
Social isolation	.857	.857
Thought processes, altered	.667 to 1.0	.929 to .962
Tissue perfusion, altered cerebral	.917	.833
Tissue perfusion, peripheral	.800	.857
Urinary elimination, altered	1.0	1.0
Violence	.50	.833

elsewhere (Arnold, 1997). The sample consisted of 15 gerontological nurse specialists in the same state.

The GNUDI contains demographic data (Part I), and categorizations of nursing diagnoses (Part II), and ratings of nursing diagnoses, interventions, and outcomes (Part III). The demographic variables include educational preparation, age, employment status, years in practice as a registered nurse, years in practice as a gerontological nurse, and position title. In Part II the expert panels indicated their degree of agreement regarding the placement of 32 nursing diagnoses in five categories (Reitz, 1985):

1. Emotional response
2. Social system, cognitive responses, and health management pattern
3. Nutrition and elimination
4. Sensory function and structural integrity
5. Neurological/cerebral function respiratory and circulatory

The Reitz (1985) nursing intensity index was chosen for use as a nursing diagnosis classification scheme, because it is based on research and the patient is the unit of analysis rather than the discrete nursing intervention. The 4-point scale ranged from strongly agree to strongly disagree. The rating of the 32 diagnoses and interventions plans is in Part III. A 5-point rating relevance scale ranging from essential to not applicable is used. Two-way analysis of variance and CVIs were used as described in previous sections of this report.

Table 1.3 illustrates interrater reliability regarding agreement by the expert panel for the placement of 32 gerontology nursing diagnoses within the five categories described. The raters' agreement results of .55 to .91 indicate moderate to high consensus. The highest reliability figure was for the social, cognitive and health category at .91, and the lowest was for the nutrition and elimination category. Significant differences occurred for physiological diagnoses in categories 3 and 5 at a probability level of .05. Interrater reliability for the combination of categories 1 and 2 was .86; for categories 3, 4, and 5, .55; and for categories through 5, .74. The author noted that the experts suggested that some psychosocial diagnoses be moved from one category to another. One recommendation was to move self-esteem disturbance diagnosis from category 2 to category 1.

Table 1.4 illustrates GNUDI category 2 social, cognitive, and health management diagnoses. The raters' agreement ranged from .92 to .97, and all six intervention groupings were significant at a probability of .05. The social isolation and health management interrater reliability agreement could not be computed because items numbered only one to two. The interrater reliability agreement results for these outcomes ranged from .75 to .94. The outcomes grouping for these diagnoses contained a small number of items, which may have affected results. The CVIs for category 2 ranged from .80 to .96. The highest was for the social isolation diagnosis.

The three other categories of diagnoses results do not appear in table format due to space limitations. The interventions for GNUDI category 3 ranged from .90 to .97 and all were significant at a probability of .05. The exception was the diarrhea diagnosis at .80 with five items. Outcomes agreements ranged from .76 to .98, and all were significant except one containing four items.

GNUDI category 4 interrater reliability agreements regarding interventions ranged from .88 to .97 and all were significant. Four outcomes

TABLE 1.3 Interrater Reliability for Five Nursing Diagnosis Categories

Diagnosis category	Items	Interrater reliability
Emotional (1)	6	.87
Social, cognitive, and health (2)	6	.91
Nutrition and elimination (3)	8	.55*
Sensory and structural (4)	5	.61
Neurological, respiratory, and circulatory (5)	7	.60*
1 & 2	12	.86
3, 4, & 5	20	.55*
1, 2, 3, 4, & 5	32	.74*

*$p = .05$.

agreements ranged from .76 to .89, with three of the five diagnoses significant.

GNUDI category 5 interventions interrater reliability agreement ranged from .73 to .95, and all were significant at a probability of .05. The outcomes agreements had a larger range at .53 to .92, with four of seven significant at the .05 probability level.

The CVI for remaining categories ranged from .75 to 1.0. For category 3 diagnoses, the CVI of only one was below .80, at .79 for urinary elimination outcomes. The combined total of six interventions and outcomes in categories 4 and 5 were .80 or above.

Interrater reliability was generally above .80 for psychosocial diagnoses, with two exceptions: ineffective individual coping and noncompliance, prescribed medications outcomes. Most interrater reliability and CVIs were acceptable, leading to the conclusion that GNUDI reliability was evident.

The original diagnostic reasoning model is operational as a measurement tool that can be scored. The GNUDI is usable as a paper-based data collection tool in clinical settings to monitor documentation of nursing practice. The author used it in two sub-acute settings to organize data scattered throughout client records (Arnold, 1999). Data collection time required is 1 hour per client record. This appears to be time consuming, but once data are collected they can and have been converted to a database format. A coding system can be assigned to each diagnostic reasoning protocol. However, the author has used diagnoses, interventions, and outcomes protocols with standardized classification systems: NANDA for diagnoses, the Nursing Intervention Classification, and the Nursing

TABLE 1.4 Interrater Reliability for Social, Cognitive, and Health Management Diagnoses

Variable	Items	Interrater reliability
Social isolation interventions	4	.97*
Social isolation outcomes	2	Not done
Self-esteem disturbance interventions	4	.92*
Self-esteem disturbance outcomes	6	.94*
Knowledge deficit for medication interventions	12	.97
Knowledge deficit for medication outcomes	4	.81*
Diversional activity deficit interventions	7	.94
Diversional activity deficit outcomes	4	.93*
Home maintenance management interventions	5	.94*
Home maintenance management outcomes	1	Not done
Noncompliance with prescribed medication interventions	7	.94*
Noncompliance with prescribed medication outcomes	3	.75 with rater 15 eliminated

Outcome Classification. The GNUDI database is a prototype that has been used with nursing students to teach coding of standardized nursing languages. It provides data about the effect of nursing interventions on patient outcomes by nursing diagnoses. It allows for use of clinical vocabulary coding systems. Increased availability of technology has enabled the development of national data sets that employ a common nursing taxonomy. The American Nurses' Association has a committee devoted to development of a unified nursing language (Warren, 1997). The author's research is a part of the profession's efforts to represent nursing practice in measurable terms using a commonly accepted language.

REFERENCES

Arnold, J. M. (1988). Diagnostic reasoning protocols for clinical simulations in nursing. In O. L. Strickland & C. F. Waltz (Eds.), *Measurement of nursing outcomes: Vol. 2. Measuring nursing performance: Practice, education and research* (pp. 53–75). New York: Springer Publishing Company.

Arnold, J. M. (1990). Development and testing of a diagnostic reasoning simulation. In C. F. Waltz & O. L. Strickland (Eds.), *Measurement of nursing outcomes: Vol. 3. Measuring clinical skills and professional development in education and practice* (pp. 85–101). New York: Springer Publishing Company.

Arnold, J. M. (1995). Validation of nursing diagnoses across six gerontological U-Diagnose(tm) case studies. In M. J. Rantz & P. LeMone (Eds.), *Classification of nursing diagnoses: Proceedings of the eleventh conference, North American Nursing Diagnosis Association* (p. 239). Glendale, CA: CINAHL Information Systems.

Arnold J. M. (1997). A gerontological nursing instrument for coding nursing U-Diagnoses(tm), interventions and outcomes. In M. J. Rantz & P. LeMone (Eds.), *Classification of nursing diagnoses: Proceedings of the twelfth conference, North American Nursing Diagnosis Association* (pp. 222–227). Glendale, CA: CINAHL Information Systems.

Arnold, J. M. (1999). Comparison of use of nursing language in documentation of rehabilitation nursing. In M. J. Rantz & P. LeMone (Eds.), *Classification of nursing diagnoses: Proceedings of the thirteenth conference, North American Nursing Diagnosis Association* (pp. 285–290). Glendale, CA: CINAHL Information Systems.

Aydelotte, M., & Peterson, K. (1987). Nursing taxonomies—state of the art. In A. McLane (Ed.), *Classification of nursing diagnoses: Proceedings of the seventh conference*, North American Nursing Diagnosis Association (pp. 1–15). St. Louis, MO: Mosby.

Carnevali, D. L., Mitchel, P. H., Woods, N. F., & Tanner, C. A. (1984). Diagnostic reasoning in nursing. Philadelphia: J. B. Lippincott.

Carroll-Johnson, R. M. (1990). Reflections on the ninth biennial conference. *Nursing Diagnosis, 1,* 50.

Elstein, A. S., Shulman, L. S., & S. A. Sprafka (1978). *Medical problem solving: an analysis of clinical reasoning.* Cambridge, MA: Harvard University Press.

Fielding, J., Beaton, S. Baier, L. Rallis, D. Ryan, R. M., & Siripornsawan, D. (1997). In M. J. Rantz & P. LeMone (Eds.), *Classification of nursing diagnoses: Proceedings of the twelfth conference, North American Nursing Diagnosis Association* (pp. 182–188). Glendale, CA: CINAHL Information Systems.

Gordon, M. (1987). *Nursing diagnosis: Process and application.* New York: McGraw-Hill.

Gordon, M., & Butler-Schmidt, B. (1997). In M. J. Rantz & P. LeMone (Eds.), *Classification of nursing diagnoses: Proceedings of the twelfth conference, North American Nursing Diagnosis Association* (pp. 145–158). Glendale, CA: CINAHL Information Systems.

Gordon, M. (1995a). Report of an RNF study to determine which nursing diagnoses have high frequency and high treatment priority in rehabilitation nursing, Part I. *Rehabilitation Nursing Research, 4*(3), 1–10; Part II. *Rehabilitation Nursing Research, 4,* 38–46.

Gordon, M. (1995b). High frequency-high treatment priority nursing diagnoses in critical care. *Nursing Diagnosis, 6,* 143–154.

Hamer, B. (1926). *Methods and principles of teaching the practice of nursing.* New York: Macmillan.

Harmer, J., Abu-Saad H., & Halfrens, R. (1994). Diagnostic process and decision making in nursing: a literature review. *Journal of Professional Nursing, 10*(3), 154–163.

Komorita, N. I. (1963). Nursing diagnosis: What is a nursing diagnosis? How is it arrived at? What does it accomplish? *American Journal of Nursing, 63,* pp. 83–86.

Lesh, K. (1997). Use of nursing diagnosis in public health nursing. In M. J. Rantz & P. LeMone (Eds.), *Classification of nursing diagnoses: Proceedings of the twelfth conference, North American Nursing Diagnosis Association* (pp. 161–172). Glendale, CA: CINAHL Information Systems.

Lunney, M., Cavendish, R., Kraynyk-Luise, B., & Richardson, K. (1997). Relevance of NANDA diagnoses and wellness diagnoses to school nursing. In M. J. Rantz & P. LeMone (Eds.), *Classification of nursing diagnoses: Proceedings of the twelfth conference, North American Nursing Diagnosis Association* (pp. 173–174). Glendale, CA: CINAHL Information Systems.

Lunney, M. (1992). Development of written case studies as simulations of diagnosis in nursing. *Nursing Diagnosis, 5*(4), 165–171.

Norris, S. P. (1989). Can we test validly for critical thinking? *Educational Researcher, 18*(9), 21–26.

Pesut, D., & Herman, J. (1998). OPT: Transformation of nursing process for contemporary practice. *Nursing Outlook, 46*(1), 29–36.

Reitz, J. A. (1985). Toward a comprehensive nursing intensity index: Part I, Development, *Nursing Management, 16*(8), 21–30.

Waltz, C. F., Strickland, O. L., & Lenz, E. R. (1991). *Measurement in nursing research.* (2nd ed.). Philadelphia: F. A. Davis.

Warren, J. J. (1997). Developing the unified nursing language system: The American Nurses Association perspective. In M. J. Rantz & P. LeMone (Eds.), *Classification of nursing diagnoses: Proceedings of the twelfth conference, North American Nursing Diagnosis Association* (pp. 3–7). Glendale, CA: CINAHL Information Systems.

Werley, H. H., & Lang, N. M. (1988). *Identification of the nursing minimum data set.* New York: Springer Publishing Company.

Wilkinson, J. M. (1996). *Nursing process in action: A critical thinking approach* (2nd ed.). Menlo Park, CA: Addison-Wesley Nursing.

Winer, B. J. (1971). *Statistical principles in experimental design* (2nd ed.). New York: McGraw-Hill.

Woolridge, J. B., Brown, J. F., & Herman, J. (1993). Nursing diagnosis: The central theme in nursing knowledge. *Nursing Diagnosis, 4*(2), 50–55.

GERONTOLOGICAL NURSING U-DIAGNOSE(tm) INSTRUMENT

Directions: You have been selected as a nurse expert in gerontological nursing. There are three parts to this questionnaire. First, rate a listing of gerontological nursing diagnoses. Second, rate selected nursing diagnoses with related interventions and outcomes.

COMPLETION OF THIS QUESTIONNAIRE IMPLIES CONSENT TO PARTICIPATE IN THE GERONTOLOGICAL U-DIAGNOSE STUDY. THERE IS NO OBLIGATION TO PARTICIPATE. REFUSAL TO PARTICIPATE WILL NOT JEOPARDIZE MY EMPLOYMENT AT THIS INSTITUTION. THE IDENTIFICATION CODE YOU INDICATE WILL BE USED TO TRACK RESPONSE. THE IDENTITY CODES WILL NOT BE MATCHED WITH NAMES OR ADDRESSES OF RESPONDENTS.

ID. # _____

PART I. DEMOGRAPHIC DATA

1. Your educational background (check all that apply)

_____ Bachelor's degree
      a. _____ Nursing
      b. _____ Other (please describe)

_____ Master's degree
      a. _____ Nursing
      b. _____ Other (please describe)

_____ Doctorate
      a. _____ Nursing
      b. _____ Other (please describe)
      c. _____ Doctoral student/candidate

2. Age _____

3. Employment status

_____ full-time

_____ part-time

4. Years in practice

_____ < 1 year

_____ 1–5

_____ 6–10

5. Position title

_____ staff nurse level 1

_____ staff nurse level 2

_____ gerontological nurse specialist

6. _____ Number of years in geriatric nursing

_____ 16–20

_____ > 20

Definitions:

Nursing Diagnosis—problem component of a NANDA diagnosis

Outcome—measurable behavior related to given nursing diagnosis

Intervention—actions to be taken by nurse for specific nursing diagnosis

PART II. Gerontological Nursing Categories with Diagnoses

Note the definitions for each category and then indicate the degree of agreement with placement of the nursing diagnoses within the categories using the following scale:

4 = *Strongly Agree*

3 = *Agree*

2 = *Disagree*

1 = *Strongly Disagree*

GROUP 1
EMOTIONAL RESPONSE

EMOTIONAL RESPONSE—expression of feelings and behavioral outcomes which arise from an individual's perception of self (mind, body) as it interfaces with a change in health status.*

_____ Coping, ineffective, family

_____ Coping, ineffective, individual

_____ Grieving

_____ Sexuality patterns, altered

_____ Sleep pattern disturbance

_____ Violence

Comments:

GROUP 2
SOCIAL SYSTEM, COGNITIVE RESPONSE &
HEALTH MANAGEMENT PATTERN

SOCIAL SYSTEM—those interpersonal relationships with family and community which determine the use of resources and services available to maintain health status.*

_____ Social isolation
_____ Self-esteem disturbance, situational

Comments:

COGNITIVE RESPONSE—those intellectual processes which enable an individual to receive, process and transmit (feedback) information, influenced by the individual's physiological, educational, and developmental capabilities.*

_____ Knowledge deficit regarding medication use
_____ Diversional activity deficit

Comments:

HEALTH MANAGEMENT PATTERN—motivation to manage personal health related activities. This pattern includes a person's perception of his own health status and his motivation to strive for an optimal level of wellness, as demonstrated by follow through with therapeutic treatment plan.*

_____ Home maintenance management, impaired
_____ Noncompliance with prescribed medications

Comments:

GROUP 3
NUTRITION AND ELIMINATION

NUTRITION—intake of nutrients and metabolic processes.

_____ Fluid volume deficit
_____ Metabolism, alteration in
_____ Nutrition alteration, less than body requirements
_____ Nutrition alteration, more than body requirements

Comments:

ELIMINATION—excretions of waste products from the body.

_____ Constipation, colonic
_____ Diarrhea
_____ Self-care deficit, toileting
_____ Urinary elimination, altered

Comments:

GROUP 4
SENSORY FUNCTION AND STRUCTURAL INTEGRITY

SENSORY FUNCTION—use of senses to include proprioception, taste, smell, hearing, vision and an individual's perception of pain.*

_____ Injury, potential for
_____ Pain
_____ Sensory perceptual alterations

Comments:

GROUP 5
NEUROLOGICAL/CEREBRAL FUNCTION,
RESPIRATORY & CIRCULATORY

NEUROLOGICAL/CEREBRAL FUNCTION—integration and direction of body regulatory processes related to reception of and response to stimuli.*

_____ Hyperthermia
_____ Mobility, impaired physical
_____ Thought processes, altered

Comments:

RESPIRATORY—transfer of gases to meet ventilatory needs.*

_____ Airway clearance, ineffective
_____ Gas exchange, impaired

Comments:

CIRCULATORY—supply of blood to body tissues through the cardiovascular system.*

_____ Tissue perfusion, altered, cerebral
_____ Tissue perfusion, altered, peripheral

Comments:

---

* Source: Reitz, J. A. (1985). Toward a comprehensive nursing intensity index: Part I, development. *Nursing Management, 16*(8), p. 24.

Rate the relevance of the following emotional nursing diagnoses with related outcomes and interventions. Rate each item using a 1–5 rating scale. Note the definitions for each rating:

5 = Essential   outcome or intervention that is always related to the diagnosis presented

4 = Very relevant   outcome or intervention that is often used with the diagnosis presented

3 = Relevant   outcome or intervention

2 = Not relevant   outcome or intervention that is rarely used in your nursing practice

1 = Not applicable   outcome or intervention that does not apply to the diagnosis presented

GROUP 1   ID. # _____
EMOTIONAL RESPONSE

EMOTIONAL RESPONSE

1. _____ COPING, FAMILY INEFFECTIVE

Outcomes

_____ Family will share their feelings with nurse or client.

_____ Family will assist client with activities of daily living.

_____ Client will accept help from family members.

_____ Client will take an active part in rehabilitative treatment and ADL.

Interventions

_____ Refer client to psychiatrist.

_____ Request tranquilizer from client's physician.

_____ Request physician's assessment for tranquilizer.

_____ Request family to set limits on client's demands.

_____ Assess client's attitudes toward participation in activities of daily living.

_____ Instruct significant others regarding client's care requirements.

_____ Encourage client to verbalize concerns and to express feelings with family members.

_____ Provide opportunities for significant others to talk with client and/ or staff.

_____ Refer family member to support group(s).

Comments:

2. _____ COPING, INDIVIDUAL INEFFECTIVE

Outcomes

_____ Client will cope with stress of illness.

_____ Client will perform activities of daily living independently.

_____ Client will share feelings with nurse or family members within three visits.

_____ Client will accept help from others in coping with life's problems.

_____ Client will agree to join support group.

_____ Client will be able to discuss his concerns with health care workers.

_____ Client will perform activities of daily living with assistance.

Interventions

_____ Refer patient to psychiatrist.

_____ Request tranquilizer for client.

_____ Request physician's assessment.

_____ Explain procedures simply and calmly.

_____ Assess client's attitudes toward participation in activities of daily living.

_____ Instruct significant others regarding client's care requirements.

_____ Relate to client in a positive, warm manner.

_____ Encourage client to verbalize concerns and to express feelings.

_____ Provide opportunities for significant others to talk with client and/or staff.

_____ Refer client to support group(s).

_____ Teach client means of stress reduction.

Comments:

GROUP 2   ID. # _____

SOCIAL SYSTEM, COGNITIVE RESPONSE & HEALTH MANAGEMENT PATTERN

SOCIAL SYSTEM

1. _____ SOCIAL ISOLATION

Outcomes

_____ Client will leave apartment 3 times weekly to perform errands.

_____ Client will engage in social activities once a week.

Interventions

_____ Assess client's social activities.

_____ Advise client to share apartment with companion.

_____ Refer client to senior citizen center.

_____ Explore with client the importance of contact with significant others.

COGNITIVE RESPONSE

2. _____ KNOWLEDGE DEFICIT REGARDING MEDICATION USE

Outcomes

_____ Client will take prescribed medications as ordered.

_____ Client will read labels of all medications prior to their administration.

_____ Client will have physician approve use of all non-prescription drugs.

_____ Client will cite one example of an interaction of a non-prescription drug with a prescribed medication.

Interventions

_____ Instruct client to report all experienced drug side effects to the health care provider.

_____ Instruct regarding effects of all drugs taken.

_____ Encourage use of analgesic medications.

HEALTH MANAGEMENT PATTERN

3. _____ HOME MAINTENANCE MANAGEMENT, IMPAIRED

Outcomes

_____ Client will function safely and healthfully in home environment.

Interventions

_____ Obtain homemaker assistance three times weekly.

_____ Refer client to meals-on-wheels program.

_____ Discuss rearrangements of furniture and removal of clutter.

_____ Teach homemaker to support client's independence in home maintenance.

_____ Monitor ability to continue to live safely in present environment.

Comments:

GROUP 3   ID. # _____

NUTRITION & ELIMINATION

NUTRITION

1. _____ **FLUID VOLUME DEFICIT**

Outcomes

_____ Total fluid intake (IV and Oral) will be 2000cc/24 hours.

_____ Related laboratory values will be within normal limits.

Interventions

_____ Measure intake and output.

_____ Monitor intravenous fluids.

_____ Check skin turgor.

_____ Offer coffee and/or low caloric beverages as supplements to meals.

_____ Monitor laboratory results for Hematocrit, Hemoglobin and electrolytes.

Comments:

ELIMINATION

4. _____ **CONSTIPATION, COLONIC**

Outcomes

_____ Client will have a bowel movement q 1–2 days without medication.

_____ Dietary intake will be higher in bulk and fiber.

_____ Use of laxatives and enemas will be gradually tapered within 1–2 months.

_____ Client will use mineral oil for laxative purposes.

Interventions

_____ Perform rectal examination.

_____ Administer fleets enema prn.

_____ Place on bedside commode for 20 to 30 minutes.

_____ Place client on bedpan according to toileting schedule.

_____ Record frequency and characteristics of BM.

_____ Instruct in dangers associated with overuse of laxatives.

_____ Give mineral oil, one ounce @ HS.

_____ Establish a regular time for bowel movement according to client's past routine.

_____ Increase daily fluid intake to 1–2 qts. daily.

_____ Provide nutritional meals which are high in fiber.

_____ Encourage gradual increase in use of fresh cooked vegetables, bran and other whole grain products along with prunes/prune juice daily.

Comments:

GROUP 4

SENSORY FUNCTION & STRUCTURAL INTEGRITY

1. _____ INJURY, POTENTIAL FOR

Outcomes

_____ Client will describe the importance of exercise and nutrition in maintaining mobility.

_____ Client will identify factors in environment that increase potential for injury.

_____ Client will not fall during hospitalization.

_____ Safety measures to prevent injury will be utilized.

_____ Less stiffness and improved mobility will be reported.

Interventions

_____ Keep bed elevated and lock brakes on wheels.

_____ Maintain side rails up in bed.

_____ Apply posey vest restraint prn for agitation.

_____ Check restraints q 4 hours and take off for 30 minutes.

_____ Make arrangements for friend/family member to telephone in am or pm at a specified time to check status.

_____ Allow client to maintain habitat as she wishes.

_____ Teach basic safety measures in living environment.

_____ Encourage client to wear glasses.

_____ Instruct to wear properly fitted shoes with non-skid soles.

_____ Offer food, fluids and toileting assistance frequently.

_____ Monitor side effects of medication.

_____ Place client in a room near nurse's station.

_____ Keep call button within client's reach.

_____ Encourage client to consider move to senior housing.

_____ Monitor ability to continue to live safely in home environment.

Comments:

GROUP 5

NEUROLOGICAL/CEREBRAL FUNCTION

1. _____ HYPERTHERMIA

Outcomes

_____ Vital signs will return to normal limits within 3–4 hours following intervention.

Interventions

_____ Administer alcohol sponge bath q hour for 15 minutes.

_____ Monitor intravenous intake.

_____ Encourage oral fluid intake of $2^1/2$ to 3 quarts per 24-hour time period.

_____ Monitor vital signs q 4 hours.

_____ Contact MD regarding order for antibiotics.

_____ Encourage patient to stay in bed covered with blankets.

_____ Administer aspirin gr. × q 4 hours prn for elevated temperature over 101 rectally.

_____ Monitor hypothermia equipment.

2

Clinical Decision Making in Nursing Scale

Helen M. Jenkins

PURPOSE

The **Clinical Decision Making in Nursing Scale** (CDMNS) can be used to assess and evaluate clinical decision making in nursing (Jenkins, 1988). The author's aim was to examine decision making as an element of the curricular process by developing a self-report measure to assess how students perceived themselves making clinical decisions.

INSTRUMENT DESCRIPTION

Proficiency in thinking skills is an essential requirement of today's nurse who is faced with making knowledgeable, confident, and effective decisions regarding health in a complex and changing environment. Thus, nurse educators are challenged to design strategies that prepare nursing students to think critically in varied health care settings (Frye, Alfred, & Campbell, 1999).

The conceptual basis for the CDMNS was derived from Janis and Mann's *Decision Making: A Psychological Analysis of Conflict, Choice, and Commitment* (1977). To develop a decision-making theory about conflict situations, they examined at normative structures and arrived at seven criteria assumed to be ideal for making decisions. Janis and Mann have stated that when an individual meets all criteria adequately, a state of "vigilant information processing" has occurred, and the decision maker's objectives have an excellent change of being implemented. Their criteria, summarized below, derived from an extensive review of the literature on effective decision making.

To the best of his or her ability and within his or her information processing capabilities, the decision maker:

1. thoroughly canvases a wide range of alternative courses of action;
2. surveys the full range of objectives to be fulfilled and the values implicated by the choice;
3. carefully weighs whatever he or she knows about the costs and risks of negative consequences, as well as the positive consequences, that could flow from each alternative;
4. intensively searches for new information relevant to further evaluation of the alternatives;
5. correctly assimilates and takes account of any new information or expert judgment to which he or she is exposed, even when the information or judgment does not support the course of action he or she initially prefers;
6. reexamines the positive and negative consequences of all known alternatives, including those regarded as unacceptable, before making a final choice;
7. makes detailed provisions for implementing or executing the chosen course of action, with special attention to contingency plans that might be required if various know risks were to materialize (Janis & Mann, 1977, p. 11).

These seven criteria were examined critically to determine how they could provide the basis for a tool to measure clinical decision making.

Janis and Mann's (1977) seven criteria were condensed to simplify their procedural ordering. Criteria 1 and 2 remained stable. Criteria 3, 6, and 7 refer to risks and benefits and thus were combined into a single catergory. Criteria 4 and 5, which concern information search and acquisition, were considered together. The process produced four categories of decision making: (a) search for alternatives or options, (b) canvassing of objectives and values, (c) evaluation and reevaluation of consequences, and (d) search for information and unbiased assimilation of new information.

Items that applied to each of the four categories were obtained from decision-making and nursing decision-making literature; these items eventually became subscales for the CDMNS. Grouping items together was important, as it allowed rationales to be developed for each category. For example, in the Search for Alternatives or Options subscale, one factor influencing decision making is past experiences, especially in the way humans search for options. Most authors, including those in nursing (e.g., Holle & Blatchley, 1982; Marriner, 1977) agree that humans use habitual patterns to approach this task and tend to use the same set of actions to make similar decisions. As items were developed, rationales from the literature were written for the other three categories in like manner.

Representative items were written in simple terms, avoiding qualifiers or words likely to be misunderstood. Both negative and positive items were included and, insofar as possible, items were constructed to be applicable to clinical decision making.

A preliminary test was administered to 32 senior nursing students in order to clarify directions and format and to isolate misunderstood material. Following this administration a debriefing session was conducted with the students. That process yielded suggestions for correction of overlaps and options for refinement and improvement. A total of 23 items were discarded, and the resultant 44 items then comprised the tool.

A pilot test of the tool was carried out with 10 additional baccalaureate nursing students from each level (sophomore, junior, and senior) who were actively involved in clinical experiences. No student taking the preliminary or pilot test was involved in the final testing. Scores were coded and computed. Four items with low item-to-total coefficients were discarded.

Items on the CDMNS are rated from 5 (always) to 1 (never) by the nurse or nursing student to reflect perceptions of his/her own behavior while caring for clients. Item ratings are summed to obtain a total score. The final tool consists of 40 items. Therefore, the potential score range is 40 to 200, with higher scores indicating higher perceived decision making. A copy of the tool appears at the end of the chapter.

RELIABILITY AND VALIDITY ASSESSMENTS

Content validity (Isaac & Michael, 1995) was established in several ways:

1. Items were based on the literature of normative decision making and nursing decision making (initially 67 items).
2. A preliminary test of the tool improved clarity and congruity within each item and subscale.
3. A panel of five nurse experts in baccalaureate education rated each item with a specification matrix and gave each item several scores, based on representativeness, sense, appropriateness, and degree of independence from other items. The matrix yielded a total score for each item. All items that received a total score of 77% or greater were rated good and were retained. Items scoring 70% to 75% were rated as fair and evaluated critically for inclusion or exclusion. Items scoring less than 70% were excluded.

Formal testing of the tool took place near the end of the semester with generic students who were engaged in clinical experiences. The available population consisted of about 250 students. Of these, 111 students chose to participate (27 sophomores, 43 juniors, and 41 seniors).

Using the Statistical Package for the Social Sciences (SPSS) subprograms, reliability was assessed throughout the testing phases by means of

Cronbach's alpha. These procedures measure internal consistency and can be considered the mean of all split-half coefficients (O'Muircheartaigh & Payne, 1978). When pilot scores were calculated, the resulting Cronbach's alpha was 0.79 for 44 items. Four items having the lowest coefficients were dropped, and Cronbach's alpha for the remaining 40 items was 0.83 ($N= 111$).

No significant differences in results were found among levels of students except for Subscale A, Search for Alternatives or Options. The multiple range Scheffe test was used to determine statistical significance between means. It was found that seniors differed from juniors, with the greatest differences between means, and that sophomores did not differ significantly from either group, having a mean higher than that of the juniors but lower than that of seniors. Using analysis of covariance procedures, no effects related to age or full-time work experience were noted.

The results of no differences in total scores were not as expected because if decision making was being effectively taught, then there should be some perceptions that would vary from sophomore to senior. It is likely that students in general do not perceive themselves as decision makers in the fairly restricted environment in which they are placed. Perhaps the opportunities to make decisions are unknowingly being restricted. Stress seems to play a large part in students' ability to make and to be responsible for decisions. It is also possible that students do not have accurate perceptions of their decision-making processes or that social desirability may have influenced students' responses on the tool to the extent that differences were not noted.

Using a normative model raises certain issues. For instance, some basis exists for the presumption that totally rational decision making is not possible in the real world, that is, we can never gather enough information, calculate outcomes with certainty, or predict all variables that impact on a decision (Steinbruner, 1974). Consequently, nurses may be limited in using a purely rational approach because of situational and temporal influences.

Tool construction focused on decision subprocesses, because the literature emphasized that they are separate constructs. This separation is artificial, and in real life one does not proceed through decision phases in this fashion. The mental processes involved in making decisions are complex, multifaceted, and almost simultaneous.

There are also several important implications (Jenkins, 1985, 1988). Nurse educators need to help students become aware of broad curricular aims and objectives. If decision making is a desired thread in the framework of the curriculum, it should be emphasized. Decision-making patterns for student nurses should be used early and consistently throughout the curriculum so that effective decision making is truly an outcome of the process. Nursing programs must provide students with opportunities and contexts in which decision making can occur.

REFERENCES

Frye, B., Alfred, N., & Campbell, M. (1999). Use of Watson-Glaser critical thinking appraisal with BSN students. *Nursing and Health Care Perspectives, 20*(5), 253–255.

Holle, M., & Blatchley, M. (1982). *Introduction to leadership and management in nursing.* Monterey, CA: Wadsworth.

Isaac, S., & Michael, W. B. (1995). *Handbook in research and evaluation* (3rd ed.). San Diego, CA: EdITS.

Janis, I. C., & Mann, L. (1977). *Decision making: A psychological analysis of conflict, choice, and commitment.* New York: Free Press.

Jenkins, H. M. (1985). Improving clinical decision making in nursing. *Journal of Nursing Education, 24,* 242–243.

Jenkins, H. M. (1988). Measuring clinical decision making in nursing. In O. L. Strickland & C. F. Waltz (Eds.), *Measurement of nursing outcomes: Vol. 2. Measuring nursing performance: Practice, education and research* (pp. 191–200). New York: Springer Publishing Company.

Marriner, A. (1977). The decision making process. *Supervisor Nurse, 8,* 58–67.

O'Muircheartaigh, C. A., & Payne, C. (Eds.) (1978). *The analysis of survey data: Vol. 1. Exploring data structures.* New York: Wiley.

Steinbruner, J. D. (1974). *The sybernetic theory of decision.* Princeton, NJ: Princeton University Press.

THE CLINICAL DECISION MAKING IN NURSING SCALE*

Directions: For each of the following statements, think of your behavior while caring for clients. Answer on the basis of what *you are doing now in the clinical setting.* There are no "right" or "wrong" answers. What is important is your assessment of how you ordinarily operate as a decision maker in the clinical setting. None of the statements cover emergency situations.

Do not dwell on responses. Circle the answer that comes closest to the way you ordinarily behave.

Answer all items. About 20 minutes should be required to complete this exercise, but if it must be taken from the classroom, a 24-hour time limit will be imposed for its return.

Scale for the CDMNS

Circle whether you would likely behave in the described way:

A — Always: What you consistently do every time.
F — Frequently: What you usually do most of the time.
O — Occasionally: What you sometimes do on occasion.
S — Seldom: What you rarely do.
N — Never: What you never do at any time.

Sample statement: I mentally list options before making a decision.

Key: A   (F)   O   S   N

The circle around response F means that you usually mentally list options before making a decision.

Note: Be sure you respond in terms of what you are doing in the clinical setting *at the present time.*

1. If the clinical decision is vital and there is time, I conduct a thorough search for alternatives.
2. When a person is ill, his or her cultural values and beliefs are secondary to the implementation of health services.
3. The situational factors at the time determine the number of options that I explore before making a decision.
4. Looking for new information in making a decision is more trouble than it's worth.
5. I use books or professional literature to look up things I don't understand.

---

* Copyright 1983, Helen Jenkins.

6. A random approach for looking at options works best for me.
7. Brainstorming is a method I use when thinking of ideas for options.
8. I go out of my way to get as much information as possible to make decisions.
9. I assist clients in exercising their rights to make decisions about their own care.
10. When my values conflict with those of the client, I am objective enough to handle the decision making required for the situation.
11. I listen to or consider expert advice or judgment, even though it may not be the choice I would make.
12. I solve a problem or make a decision without consulting anyone, using information available to me at the time.
13. I don't always take time to examine all the possible consequences of a decision I must make.
14. I consider the future welfare of the family when I make a clinical decision which involves the individual.
15. I have little time or energy available to search for information.
16. I mentally list options before making a decision.
17. When examining consequences of options I might choose, I generally think through "If I did this, then. . .".
18. I consider even the remotest consequences before making a choice.
19. Consensus among my peer group is important to me in making a decision.
20. I include clients as sources of information.
21. I consider what my peers will say when I think about possible choices I could make.
22. If an instructor recommends an option to a clinical decision making situation, I adopt it rather than searching for other options.
23. If a benefit is really great, I will favor it without looking at all the risks.
24. I search for new information randomly.
25. My past experiences have little to do with how actively I look at risks and benefits for decisions about clients.
26. When examining consequences of options I might choose, I am aware of the positive outcomes for my client.
27. I select options that I have used successfully in similar circumstances in the past.
28. If the risks are serious enough to cause problems, I reject the option.
29. I write out a list of positive and negative consequences when I am evaluating an important clinical decision.
30. I do not ask my peers to suggest options for my clinical decisions.
31. My professional values are inconsistent with my personal values.
32. My finding of alternatives seems to be largely a matter of luck.
33. In the clinical setting I keep in mind the course objectives for the day's experience.

34. The risks and benefits are the farthest thing from my mind when I have to make a decision.
35. When I have a clinical decision to make, I consider the institutional priorities and standards.
36. I involve others in my decision making only if the situation calls for it.
37. In my search for options, I include even those that might be thought of as "far out" or not feasible.
38. Finding out about the client's objectives is a regular part of my clinical decision making.
39. I examine the risks and benefits only for consequences that have serious implications.
40. The client's values have to be consistent with my own in order for me to make a good decision.

Thank you for being a participant in this study. Do you have any ideas about decision making in nursing that were not covered by the scale that you would like to share? You can speak to specific items or give any general comments you would like to. Feel free to use this last page or the back of the answer sheet.

3

Creativity in the Application of the Nursing Process Tool

Roberta J. Emerson

PURPOSE

The **Creativity in the Application of the Nursing Process Tool** (CNPT) is a norm-referenced, projective instrument designed to assess the ability of nurses, or nursing students at the conclusion of their education program, to apply the nursing process in a creative manner (Emerson, 1990).

INSTRUMENT DESCRIPTION

The work of Guilford (1950, 1954, 1959, 1967) has served to provide a conceptual framework for a large proportion of the most promising research into the creative process. His structure-of-intellect (SI) model, while designed to provide a basis for "a unified theory of human intellect, which organizes the known, unique or primary intellectual abilities into a single system" (Guilford, 1959, p. 469), has within it the specific factors characteristic of creativity. The component of the model that deals with creativity is termed "divergent thinking." Guilford's description of creativity as divergent thinking was used as the operational definition of creativity for this study. Divergent thinking involves a process of grazing through data, searching broadly for information that, when applied to a given situation, results in a variety of potentially right alternatives. He devised and tested many existing instruments to tap this mode of thinking and is widely recognized within the field of creative research (Guilford, 1950, 1959, 1967). His conceptual framework of creativity, derived from the SI model, has served as the basis for much of the subsequent research into creativity involving a wide variety of populations. The three dimensions of the model are *operations, content categories, and product categories.*

Each dimension is further broken down into smaller, discrete components.

Operations are the intellectual activity factors of cognition (knowledge), memory, divergent production, convergent production, and evaluation (Guilford, 1967). Cognition is listed first in the model, since it is felt to be basic to all the other operations.

Convergent production is described as the ability to zero in one's thought processes on only those factors that are relevant to a given problem, culminating in the one right answer. Guilford felt that to be truly creative, divergent thinking skills need to be present to a well-developed degree and combined with convergent thinking. Convergent production has been termed "logical necessity," while divergent production has been labeled "logical possibility" (Guilford, 1950, 1954, 1959, 1967).

Content categories are the intellectual process factors. The components of this dimension are described as figural (spatial), symbolic (numbers/letters), semantic (verbal), and behavioral (actions of others).

Another dimension of the SI model is composed of the product categories resulting from the interaction of the operations with the content categories. This final aspect of the model is what makes it truly unique.

The term "product" refers specifically to the "way or form in which any information occurs. An appropriate synonym for the term 'product' could be the term 'conception,' which also pertains to ways of knowing or understanding" (p. 63). The product categories are as follows:

1. *Units*—things, segregated wholes, figures on grounds, "chunks"; nouns.
2. *Classes*—set of objects with one or more common properties.
3. *Relations*—a connection between two things, a connection having its own character; prepositions alone or with other terms ("married to").
4. *Systems*—complexes, patterns, or organizations of independent or interacting parts (an outline, a plan).
5. *Transformations*—changes, revisions, redefinitions, modifications by which there is a change from one state to another by an informational product (participle or verb in noun form, e.g., "softening," "coloring").
6. *Implications*—a prediction or anticipation from available information.

Again, the order in which the product categories are presented in the model has significance because it is reflective of a progressive complexity.

The steps of the nursing process (Marriner, 1983; Leonard & George, 1995; Meleis, 1997) were used to provide a consistent operationalization of the nursing process. These definitions are:

1. *Assessment*—the collection of data about the health status of the patient; analysis of data, formulation of a nursing diagnosis.

2. *Planning*—prioritizing problems, establishing goals, preparation of individualized plans of care.
3. *Implementation*—continuous and ongoing assessment, planning and evaluation of the plan during the provision of the care, communication of the plan.
4. *Evaluation*—comparison of the outcome of care with the desired outcome, identification of problems solved and those that need to be reassessed and replanned.

Guilford provided a wide variety of tests in *The Nature of Human Intelligence* (1967), assessing all aspects of the SI model. Since the tool attends to creativity, only those tests of divergent production were utilized. By virtue of their educational experience, nurses, as well as nursing students at the conclusion of their educational program, were felt to already have sufficient cognition and memory of the field of nursing to be adequately prepared for testing in their divergent production skills.

Since the applied science of nursing attends primarily to the semantic (verbal) products, figural and symbolic products were not tested. Guilford himself has no tests in the divergent production category of behavioral products. The few existing tests of this product category are in other operational categories.

Tests chosen for modification demonstrated clear factor loading according to the work of Guilford. This was a major strength of the resulting tool and one indicator of its validity.

The content validity evaluation of the relationship of Marriner's (1983) definitions of the steps of the nursing process to Guilford's (1967) definitions of the product categories resulted in a content validity index of .83.

Therefore, as tests of divergent production of units, classes, or relations were rewritten and placed in a nursing context, the resulting new instrument tested the creative application of the assessment portion of the nursing process. The step of the nursing process devoted to planning was addressed by tests of divergent production of systems. Transformation tests of divergent production reflected the implementation portion of the nursing process. Finally, evaluation was tapped by tests of divergent production of implications. This approach was followed, yielding a new instrument composed of previously designed tests that were modified as little as possible when placed in a nursing context, to measure all components of the nursing process.

The resulting instrument is composed of a guide for the test administrator and the CNPT itself, both presented at the end of this chapter. The tool is composed of eight parts, some of which are scored more than once in different fashions to reflect more than one product.

The first and second tests in the CNPT are reflective of the product categories of units and transformations, depending on how they are scored. As a measurement of *units*, only the more direct or obvious responses are scored as frequency counts. As a measurement of *transformations* (the originality factor), frequency counts of unusual responses are made. During the pilot study of the original test by Guilford and of the new nursing test, it was discovered that the first 1 to 2 minutes elicited obvious responses; after that, remote associations were produced. Maximum productivity was attained at the 4-minute mark.

The third test is a measurement of transformations. It is a test of unusualness derived from rare responses to stimulus words. For adaptation to nursing, a list of words was developed, drawn from the index of a nursing fundamentals textbook (Wolff, Weitzel, Zornow, & Zsohar, 1983). The list was confined to 25 stimulus words to reduce the length of the total testing time.

Sentence construction tests have been the mainstay of divergent production in semantic *systems*, a reflection of expressional fluency. A noun, verb, adjective, and adverb were given, and subjects were directed to write as many sentences as possible using all four words. Sentence generation decreased for the majority of subjects who piloted this test at $3^1/2$ minutes. Four minutes was the administration time of this test.

The divergent production of semantic *relations* mirrors the factor identified as "associational fluency." To identify another correlate given one correlate and the relationship between them would test convergent production. To tap divergent production, multiple relations are requested. The respondent is directed to write as many words as possible that are similar in meaning to eight stimulus words; a 2-minute maximum is provided for each word. Eight words were again chosen from a nursing fundamentals textbook (Wolff et al., 1983).

Spontaneous flexibility was the factor Guilford identified with the divergent production of semantic *classes*. One of the most consistent markers of this quality was a test called "Alternate Uses." Guilford indicated that by directing the respondent to focus on unusual uses, repetitious responses were excluded and a change of use category was essentially demanded for each response.

Implications have been identified as the factor of elaboration ability. In divergent production of semantic implications, tests calling for expanding and modifying a plan based on a given amount of data have been developed and analyzed. Two of these tests were modified to conform to a nursing context. Test 7, adapted from "Unusual Methods," asks the respondent to suggest two different and unusual methods for dealing with a problem. The eighth test is a modification of "Effects." In this test, the subject is given several current events or trends and directed to forecast different future events.

Administration guidelines should be followed meticulously in order to enhance reliability and validity. Tests should be placed facedown on tables or desks. A general introduction is read aloud. Each individual test in the tool is printed on a separate page. Directions for the individual test are printed above it and read aloud by the test administrator. Tests 1 to 5 are timed, and the administrator announces the time frame after reading the instructions. The administrator should monitor the time with a stopwatch. The respondents are instructed not to return to any of the timed tests as they move into the final three untimed tests. When they complete the last test, they are to return the test to the administrator. Total administration time is approximately 1 hour.

The responses elicited by the CNPT are qualitative in nature. This format was necessitated by the need to access divergent thinking, which is characterized by the spontaneous generation of an answer or several potential answers. The CNPT provides only cue words or ideas that stimulate the respondents' divergent responses. The subjects' responses must be submitted to content analysis. The process of content analysis includes the identification of categories (subject matter), response units (words and themes) that are placed into the categories, and coding by systems of enumeration (frequency, weighting for rarity) (Holsti, 1969).

Scoring CNPT 1 and 2

Instructions by Guilford (1967) directed that the responses for these tests be scored in two fashions. First, frequency counts are to be made of the obvious or direct responses. Second, responses identified as being unusual are to be subjected to frequency counts.

Each response is examined for keywords and themes, which are used to create subcategories, and the number of responses are listed for each of the subcategories, producing frequency counts. The following rules are used in analyzing the subjects' responses:

1. Responses that contain more than one theme are divided; the respondent receives credit for the different response units (themes) represented.
2. Incomplete thoughts are eliminated.
3. Responses that begin with a direct/obvious theme (one that occurs frequently) but takes an unusual turn are coded as unusual.

The scoring of frequency of response units (themes) is as follows: more than 10% of N (number of respondents) = "1 Direct"; equal to or less than 10% of N = "1 Unusual." A respondent then received a score reflecting a combination of direct and unusual responses (e.g., "3 Direct/2 Unusual") for CNPT 1 and 2.

Scoring of CNPT 3

Guidelines presented by Guilford were scant; this test was to be scored in terms of rare responses, which implied analysis by frequency. Responses to each cue word are listed, and the following rules are presented for clustering the responses:

1. Forms of the same word, such as "walk" and "walking," are grouped together as one response unit (theme).
2. Root words or phrases ("unable to move" and "without movement") are grouped as a single response unit (theme).
3. The presence or absence of the same state or condition is grouped as a single response unit (theme) if it employs the identical word (e.g., "air"/"no air" and "infection"/"no infection").
4. Two words, where one serves to amplify the other, such as "clean out," are grouped with the same root word.
5. If two words are given by the respondent and represent two isolated concepts ("nurse/Mom"), the response is recognized as a separate response unit (theme).

The resulting response units for each cue word are then recorded by their frequency of occurrence.

Ten percent of the total number of respondents is used as the cut point to differentiate rare from common responses. The response units for each of the 25 stimulus words are then weighted for rarity according to the following scale:

More than 10% of N (Number of respondents) = 0
10% of $N = 1$
3 responses alike = 2
2 responses alike = 3
Unduplicated response = 4

A respondent's score is obtained by summing the scores given for all of the stimuli words. The maximum possible score a respondent could receive for this test would be a score of 4 for each of the 25 cue words, or $4 \times 25 = 100$.

Scoring of CNPT 4

Guilford's (1967) instructions for scoring directed that frequency counts of the number of sentences written be performed. Guidelines for what constitutes an acceptable sentence follow:

1. Incomplete sentences are eliminated.
2. Each sentence must use all four words.
3. Respondents are permitted to change the tense of the verb ("assess" to "assessed") but not to change the verb to noun form ("assessment").
4. "Health" is still accepted as a noun when joined with another word for elaboration ("health care").

Each respondent receives a score reflecting a frequency count of the number of written accepted sentences; there is no maximum score.

Scoring of CNPT 5

Guilford's (1967) directions for the scoring of his test were again on the basis of frequency counts of responses. The response units (words) are then totaled for each respondent, and the frequency count of the total number of acceptable words written is recorded as the score for this test. There is no maximum possible score for this test.

Scoring of CNPT 6

Guilford's (1967) test was to be scored by eliminating the consistent and frequent response units (themes). The remaining response units were to be weighted for rarity and frequency counts of the weighted response units performed.

Each of the four items becomes a separate category for content analysis. All responses are listed under the appropriate category and assessed for thematic content. The following rules govern the acceptability of responses:

1. Responses in which the item is used in a fashion ascribed to it in common usage are eliminated.
2. Responses felt to be too general (e.g., using the newspaper for protection) are eliminated.
3. Responses that do not imply an action or use (e.g., using the medicine cup to look at) are eliminated.
4. Responses in which the usage for the item is not felt to be a part of a health care setting (e.g., using the medicine cup as a shot glass or jigger) are eliminated.

The resulting acceptable response units (themes) are arranged according to the frequency of their occurrence under each of the categories (items). The system of enumeration for this test is the frequency of rare responses, according to a weighting system. The same scoring system devised for CNPT 3 is applied in this test. To review, that system is:

More than 10% of N (number of respondents) = 0
10% of $N = 1$
3 responses alike = 2
2 responses alike = 3
Unduplicated response = 4

Once all responses are scored, the scores for each category are summed and become the total score for the respondent for this test. The maximum potential score for a respondent is 4 times 6 responses = 24 points for one item, and 24 times 4 items = 96 points for the entire CNPT 6.

Scoring of CNPT 7

Guilford (1967) instructed that the responses to this test be weighted for rarity for the purpose of scoring. The two rules established for the content analysis of the responses were:

1. Responses must relate to the problem given in the cue.
2. Answers that begin in a common fashion but take an unusual turn are listed as discrete, unusual response units (themes).

Fewer responses are available for content analysis in CNPT 7. Therefore, the following scoring system is used:

More than 2 response units (themes) alike = 0
2 responses alike = 1
Unduplicated response = 2

Scoring of CNPT 8

Guilford's (1967) instructions for scoring his test were again based on weighting for rarity. Rules established for content analysis of CNPT 8 are as follows:

1. Responses that can be assumed by the cue are eliminated from consideration.
2. Responses that are a potential *cause* of the trend rather than a future event due to the trend are eliminated.
3. Responses that initially appear to represent a more common response unit but take an unusual direction or use unique vocabulary are isolated as unique response units.

The scoring system established for CNPT 3 and used again for CNPT 6 is applied here as well:

More than 10% of N (number of respondents) = 0
10% of N = 1
3 responses alike = 2
2 responses alike = 3
Unduplicated responses = 4

The maximum potential score for this test is a 4 for all four responses to the three cue trends, or 4 times 4 times 3 = 48.

In order to make the weighting of the scores for all tests as similar in scale as possible, the scores were modified slightly. This facilitated computer analysis of test results, reliability, and validity. Each test was examined in turn.

CNPT 1 and 2: The total number of direct and unusual responses for both tests are summed. Then the percentage of total responses that have been scored as "unusual" is calculated. This figure is multiplied by 10 in order to obtain numbers more similar in size to those obtained in the other tests. This figure is then recorded for analysis and represents a combined score for both CNPT 1 and 2.

CNPT 3: In order to produce a more even scale, each respondent's score for CNPT 3 is divided by 25 (the total number of cues) to yield an average score.

CNPT 4: The number of sentences is summed. The resulting number of sentences produced is used as the score for each respondent.

CNPT 5: For computer analysis, an average score for CNPT 5 is obtained by dividing the respondent score by 8, for the eight cue words.

CNPT 6: Scores for this test represent the rarity weight of all responses given by each respondent. Dividing the scores by 24 produces a number reflecting the average rarity score for each individual respondent.

CNPT 7: An average score is obtained for analysis by dividing each respondent's score by 4, for the total number of responses provided by the test.

CNPT 8: By dividing each respondent's score by 12, an average score is obtained, which is used for statistical analysis.

RELIABILITY AND VALIDITY ASSESSMENT

The Cronbach's alpha coefficient for the CNPT was found to be .57. Intercorrelations between tests ranged from .03 between Tests 1 and 2 and 4 to .42 between Tests 5 and 8. Four intercorrelations were negative: Tests 1 and 2 with 6 (–.07), Test 3 with 6 (–.11), Tests 1 and 2 with 8 (–.01), and Test 6 with 7 (–.04). When tests were correlated with total CNPT scores, the resulting coefficients ranged from .30 for Test 6 to .67 for Test 5.

As an evaluation of the content validity of the CNPT, the content validity index was used to examine the agreement of experts in the field regarding the congruency of Guilford's (1967) definitions of product categories and Marriner's (1983) definitions of the steps of the nursing process. This was found to be equal to .83, indicating a highly acceptable level of content validity in the conceptual base of the instrument. In addition, Guilford's tests selected for modification had previously scored well in his factor analysis, reflecting their validity as measures of that product category of divergent thinking.

Construct validity was determined using contrasted groups. This was performed in two separate ways, producing two different assessments of construct validity.

Forty senior generic baccalaureate nursing students in their final semester of the program agreed to participate in the reliability and validity testing of the CNPT. Prior to taking the test, the students were asked to assess their creativity according to a visual analogue scale in terms of their perceptions of their creativity in general and their creativity in applying the nursing process to their practice. The correlation between the two creativity self-perceptions was calculated. The Pearson product-moment correlation coefficient was found to be .66. Therefore, the two scores were averaged, yielding a new student self-perception variable, total creativity. This new variable was then correlated with the students' scores on the CNPT. The resulting Pearson product-moment correlation coefficient of .30 indicated minimal positive correlation between the students' scores on the CNPT and their total self-perceptions of their creativity at $p = .05$.

Faculty members who had observed the work of the students in a clinical setting during the term prior to the study were identified. They were asked to rank their former students' clinical practice according to Guilford's (1967) definition of divergent thinking along a 4-point Likert scale. Students who were assigned a score of 1 or 2 on the scale were placed in the low-creativity group. The high-creativity group encompassed students who were scored as a 3 or 4 by the faculty members. A t test of these two groups and their scores on the CNPT was performed. The mean score for the high-creativity group was 10.7061, with a standard deviation of 2.482. The low-creativity group had a mean score of 11.8545, with a standard deviation of 4.059. The calculated t value of -1.05 was not significant (at an alpha level of 0.05 and df of 38). There was no significant difference in creativity scores between the student groups identified by faculty members as being highly creative and the group identified as being less creative.

The methods designed to assess the content validity of the CNPT indicate minimal support that the instrument actually measures the creative application of the nursing process. This is a statistical fact, supported by the analyses performed. However, it is possible that the instrument is valid and that other measures would substantiate its validity. As validity is never proved once and for all, neither is it necessarily disproved. The strength of the conceptual basis for the instrument and the relationship among product categories and steps of the nursing process add validity to the instrument. Unfortunately, no other measure exists of the construct being studied; testing with another measure could not be used to infer validity. It is also possible that there was sufficient error in the content analysis and scoring to invalidate the instrument.

The Cronbach's alpha of .57 indicates moderate reliability for the instrument. Most of the tests had little, if any, correlation to one another, implying that the tests were measuring unique attributes of creativity. Correlations between tests that measure the same product category and step of the nursing process were higher. All tests had positive correlations with the total score on the CNPT. Most of the tests had moderate to high correlation coefficients.

The issue of reliability and validity of projective measures as a whole is open to question. Uniqueness may not go hand-in-hand with proficiency. It may be that the score on a paper-and-pencil test has nothing to do with performing in a highly creative manner in clinical practice. This study does not deal with this issue.

It appears that the CNPT has not been shown to be a valid measure of the creative application of the nursing process. Reliability appears to be adequate but open to doubt regarding some components of the instrument. Yet the need for creativity in all spheres of the nursing profession seems significant in the literature review. The issue is an important one; this study provides a starting point, and the problem will certainly receive more attention in the future.

The author has a few specific suggestions for modifications of the CNPT. CNPT 5 requested that respondents provide as many words as possible similar in meaning to the cue word, within a timed interval. In order to reduce the number of unacceptable dissimilar word associations produced, it is suggested that an example of both an acceptable and an unacceptable response to another sample cue be verbally presented to the respondents prior to providing the first cue word during the period when the directions are read. For CNPT 4, it might be advisable to show the parts of speech in parentheses following the four words used to construct the sentences. It should be emphasized in the directions that the words are to be used *only* as the part of speech shown and that all four words *must* be used in each sentence. This latter information is provided at the time of testing, but failure to follow directions reduced the number of acceptable sentences. In CNPT 3, the cue word "adventitious" seemed to be confused with the word "advantageous." This problem could be eliminated by selecting a different cue word since the two words sound quite similar when spoken aloud. Finally, there was confusion in the interpretation of the cue in Test 1. It might be helpful to emphasize the visual nature of the cue when reading the directions to the respondents.

Once these changes are made in the instrument, alternative methods of establishing validity should be explored. The visual analogue scale provides a large amount of variance regarding student perceptions of their creativity. It is possible that the broad variance was eliminated when the two student creativity scores were averaged. A low positive correlation was found between the students' scores for the CNPT and their total creativity score. A higher correlation might be found if the general creativity and creativity in the application of the nursing process scores were correlated separately with the scores on the CNPT. If more than one clinical faculty member were to assess students' creativity, interrater reliability could be examined and the validity of the contrasted groups enhanced. In addition, the use of larger samples would be helpful in adding credence to findings regarding the instrument's reliability and validity.

REFERENCES

Emerson, R. J. (1990). Measuring creativity in the application of the nursing process. In O. L. Strickland & C. F. Waltz (Eds.), *Measurement of nursing outcomes: Vol. 3. Measuring clinical skills and professional development in education and practice* (pp. 102–124). New York: Springer Publishing Company.

Guilford, J. P. (1950). *American Psychologist, 5,* 444–454.

Guilford, J. P. (1954). *A factor-analytic study of creative thinking* (Psychological Laboratory Rep. No. 11). Los Angeles: University of Southern California.

Guilford, J. P. (1959). Three faces of intellect. *American Psychologist, 14,* 469–479.

Guilford, J. P. (1967). *The nature of human intelligence.* New York: McGraw-Hill.

Leonard, M. K., & George, J. B. (1995). *Ida Jean Orlando.* In J. B. George (Ed.), *Nursing theories: The base for professional nursing practice* (4th ed.) (pp. 145–164). Norwalk, CT: Appleton & Lange.

Marriner, A. (1983). *The nursing process: A scientific approach to nursing care* (3rd ed.). St. Louis: Mosby.

Meleis, A. I. (1997). *Theoretical nursing: Development and progress* (3rd ed.). New York: J. B. Lippincott.

Wolff, L., Weitzel, M. H., Zornow, R. A., & Zsohar, H. (1983). *Fundamentals of nursing* (7th ed.). Philadelphia: Lippincott.

INSTRUCTIONS TO THE ADMINISTRATOR OF THE CREATIVITY IN THE APPLICATION OF THE NURSING PROCESS TOOL (CNPT)

General: For purposes of validity and reliability, instructions must be followed precisely. The tool is composed of eight separate tests. The first five tests must be timed with a stopwatch, and instructions are to be read aloud. Do not repeat any portions of the instructions, return to any portion of the test, or repeat any stimulus word that is part of the test.

Tests should be face down on the desks in front of the participants. Pencils or pens may be used to respond to the questions.

Read Aloud: Turn the tool over, please.

On the first page, you are given a creativity continuum line.
I will read the instructions to you:

> On the following line, draw a vertical mark that corresponds to how creative you perceive yourself to be, *in general.*

(Pause. When the group is finished, read the following):
Next:

> On the following line, draw a vertical mark that corresponds to how creative you perceive yourself to be in the application of the nursing process theory to your practice.

When you are finished, do not turn the page.
(When all respondents are finished, read the following):
As we proceed, please turn only one page at a time, folding the last page back (demonstrate this). Most of the activities are timed. Do not return to any timed activity. No portion will be repeated. I will read the instructions, which are also printed on the page, and tell you when to begin and stop. If you are in the middle of a word or sentence, do not finish it.
Turn the page.

> #1. List all the consequences to health care if people had only black and white vision.

You have four minutes. Begin.
(After four minutes): Stop.
Turn the page.

> #2. List all the consequences to health care if people no longer wanted or needed sleep.

You have four minutes. Begin.
(After four minutes): Stop.
Turn the page.

#3. As each of the following words is given, write the first word that comes to mind. You will have five seconds to respond to each word.

(Allow five seconds after giving the word before giving the next word.)

Ambulation	Asepsis	Turgor
Hypoxia	Somatic	Necrosis
Infusion	Incontinence	Circadian
Caregiver	Empathy	Excoriation
Immobility	Communication	Developmental
Membrane	Accountability	Stress
Adventitious	Debridement	Electrocardiogram
Footdrop	Pernicious	Compression Discharge

Turn the page.

#4 Write as many sentences as possible, within any nursing context, using these four words in each sentence:

Health
Assess
Carefully
Moderate (as an adjective)

You will have four minutes. Begin.

(After four minutes): Stop.

Turn the page.

#5. Write as many words as possible, similar in meaning to each of the following eight words.

You will have two minutes between words. Do not return to any previous word, please.

(Read each word, allowing two minutes between each word.)

Cyanosis	Restriction
Incision	Reference
Medication	Monitor
Dressing	Massage

The remaining activities are not timed. They ask for a specific number of responses. You may take as much time as you wish for these three activities. Do not return to any of the timed activities. When you are finished, bring the tool to me.

CREATIVITY IN THE APPLICATION OF THE
NURSING PROCESS TOOL (CNPT)

_____Code

On the following line, draw a vertical mark that corresponds to how creative you perceive yourself to be, *in general.*

Highly   Not at all
Creative   Creative

_____

On the following line, draw a vertical mark that corresponds to how creative you perceive yourself to be in the application of the nursing process theory to your practice.

Highly   Not at all
Creative   Creative

_____

For administration, each test should be on a separate page.

#1. List of the consequences to health care if people had only black and white vision.

#2. List of all consequences to health care if people no longer wanted or needed sleep.

#3. As each of the following words is given, write the first word that comes to mind. You will have five seconds to respond to each word.

1.	6.	11.	16.	21.
2.	7.	12.	17.	22.
3.	8.	13.	18.	23.
4.	9.	14.	19.	24.
5.	10.	15.	20.	25.

#4. Write as many sentences as possible, within any nursing context, using these four words in each sentence.

Health
Assess
Carefully
Moderate (used as an adjective)

#5. Write as many words as possible, similar in meaning, to each of the following eight words.

1.   5.
2.   6.
3.   7.
4.   8.

#6. State six (6) possible uses (other than the common ones) in any nursing setting, for each of the following:

1. A two (2) foot square of plastic

    1.   4.
    2.   5.
    3.   6.

2. A plastic medicine cup

    1.   4.
    2.   5.
    3.   6.

3. A pillowcase

    1.   4.
    2.   5.
    3.   6.

4. A newspaper

    1.   4.
    2.   5.
    3.   6.

#7. Give two different and unusual ways of dealing with a problem.

1. Staff complain of too much paperwork.
    1.
    2.
2. Gross motor skills have been slow to develop in an 18-month-old with a congenital hip dislocation.
    1.
    2.

#8. Given a trend, forecast four (4) different future events.

1. Hospital personnel will be required to participate in a formal exercise program.
    1.
    2.
    3.
    4.

2. The number of admissions for acute COPD increase from November through February.
    1.
    2.
    3.
    4.
3. More parents are caring for their handicapped infants in the home.
    1.
    2.
    3.
    4.

4

Measuring Clinical Judgment in Home Health Nursing*

Angeline M. Jacobs and Felicitas A. dela Cruz

PURPOSE

This chapter presents a clinical nursing judgment test to measure the clinical judgment of home health care nurses, using written simulated patient care situations. The development of the instrument (Jacobs & dela Cruz, 1990) was undertaken in an effort to obtain a pre- and post-program measure of clinical judgment in the program evaluation of a federally funded continuing education program in home health nursing. When no instrument specific to home health nursing and no general instrument that might be adapted to home health nursing were found, the project staff decided to develop an individualized instrument specifically for this project.

INSTRUMENT DESCRIPTION

The measurement of clinical decision making in public health and home care settings and the development of models for describing nurses' decision making are global concerns (Lauri, et al., 1997).

Various theoretical perspectives regarding clinical decision making and the equivocal and contradictory nature of findings from studies of clinical decision making within practice settings have resulted in methodological dilemmas for those seeking to conceptualize and measure this important outcome (Schnell & Cervero, 1993; dela Cruz, 1994). Adding to the challenge in this regard is the fact that while trends in the delivery of health care have shifted from hospitals to community-based set-

*Funded by Grant D 10 NU 29182, Division of Nursing, U.S. Department of Health and Human Services.

tings, especially to home care, nursing studies of clinical decision making have focused primarily on hospital nurses (dela Cruz, 1994). Information processing theory (Newell & Simon, 1972; Simon, 1979) has served as the conceptual basis for the development of the measure of nursing clinical judgment. Two postulates underlying information processing theory are: (a) human beings are information processing systems operating in complex task environments, and (b) the human mind has limits in its capacity to process information because of the nature of short- and long-term memory.

Applying information processing theory to studies on the clinical judgment of physicians, Elstein, Shulman, and Sprafka (1978) delineated the following dimensions of the diagnostic process: (a) attending to initial data, (b) hypothesis generation, (c) information gathering relative to the identified hypotheses, (d) evaluation of each hypothesis based on acquired data, and (e) formulation of the diagnosis. The diagnostic process as outlined embodies the dimensions of the concept of clinical judgment in this study.

The first element of the diagnostic process is the availability of cues— the bits of data about the patient that come to the attention of the nurse and guide or direct the diagnosis of the patient's problems. Cues include signs and symptoms manifested, as well as psychosocial information about the patient. Based on information processing theory, a nurse selects relevant cues and, using just a few cues, generates from experience several hypotheses that would probably explain the state of the patient. The generated hypotheses are the tentative impressions about the patient's problems. With several hypotheses in mind, the nurse gathers or acquires more information to rule in or out each of the hypotheses. In other words, the hypotheses that are generated direct a further search for cues. Data obtained from or about the patient prompt the nurse to consider new hypotheses and to test or discard others. In this sense, the search for further cues enables the nurse to evaluate the generated hypotheses. Once a cluster of critical cues is available to explain or account for the clinical findings, then the nurse chooses a specific hypothesis that will be the diagnostic conclusion.

An important characteristic of the diagnostic process is its uncertain or probabilistic nature. The diagnostic process underscores the uncertainty involved in linking patient cues with the internal state of the patient (Tanner, 1984). See Figure 4.1 for a schematic representation of the diagnostic process.

Clinical judgment was defined as the series of decisions made by the home health nurse in arriving at the diagnosis of the patient's actual and potential health problems. It entails deciding: (a) what initial data to attend to, (b) which hypotheses to generate, (c) and what further data to acquire to confirm or reject the generated hypotheses. The diagnosis of the patient's actual or potential problems follows from these steps.

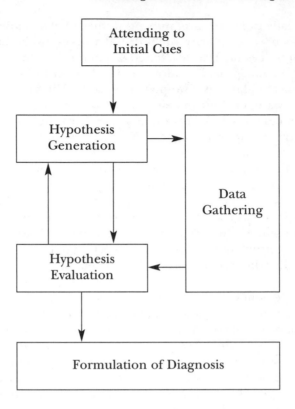

FIGURE 4.1 Schematic representation of the diagnostic process.

The methodology of the development of the clinical nursing judgment test followed standard test development procedures, including review of the literature; drafting of the instrument by a team of content experts and test experts; content analysis by home health nursing experts; field testing on a sample of nurses equivalent to the targeted group but not part of the group; and reliability and validity studies.

The instrument focuses only on the diagnostic phase of clinical judgment. Following information processing theory precepts, it assesses these four dimensions of the diagnostic phase: (a) problem sensing/cue utilization, (b) hypothesis generation, (c) data gathering, and (d) priority setting of the patient's problems. Three written patient care simulations are used.

Two formats of the instrument were developed and tested in order to determine their relative worth: an objective version and an open-ended version. The objective version uses two patient care simulations. It provides lists of patient problems, supporting data or "cues" from the case, and additional data to be collected to verify the patient's problems. The examinees make selections of the correct answers from these lists. After the examinees read the patient care situation, they are asked to respond to the following questions:

1. What are the patient's possible problems? This question taps the dimension of hypothesis generation.
2. What information from the patient care situation did you use to suspect the presence of these problems? This question assesses the problem-sensing/cue-utilization dimension.
3. What further information would you obtain to verify that the problem(s) actually exist? This question measures the hypothesis-driven, data-gathering dimension.
4. Of the problems listed in Question 1 above, which is the patient's priority problem? This last question, which measures priority setting, has been added to the most recent version of the instrument, after problems with test administration and scoring were resolved by the implementation of the in-basket/out-basket procedure.

The test procedure employed an in-basket/out-basket approach, in which the correct answers are given to the examinees after they have selected and submitted their answers to the first question. The correct answers provide essential feedback that gives each examinee an equal opportunity to achieve the maximum score on each of the three subsequent questions. Obviously, if the examinee chose the wrong set of problems in answer to the first question, all subsequent answers would be wrong, even though the answers might be relevant for the set of problems chosen. This in-basket/out-basket technique allows the provision of feedback in a way that prevents examinees from changing incorrect answers. Thus, examinees were instructed to hand in the first answer sheet after selecting the two patients' problems from the list. Figure 4.2 shows the "correct" answers for Mrs. Sussex and Mr. Kaiser, the two patients. The vignettes presented to the students for the two cases follow.

> *CASE A:* Mrs. Sussex is 69 years old and has chronic obstructive pulmonary disease (COPD). She had maintained a position as an executive in a large corporation until several months ago when her condition worsened. She has expressed being upset over "chronic fatigue" and inability to bathe herself.

> *CASE B:* Mr. Kaiser, a retired contractor, recently had a cerebrovascular accident (CVA). He is paralyzed on his left side and has aphasia. A very dependent wife is taking care of him at home. She has expressed her frustration at his crying episodes and his inability to care for himself.

FIGURE 4.2 Answer Sheet 1 for objective version of instrument.

What are the possible patient problems for each case? Place a check mark under the "Case" column for each relevant problem. Note that you must check 4 problems for Sussex, and 7 for Kaiser.

Problems	CASES	
	A Sussex	B Kaiser
	Check 4	*Check 7*
1. Potential for infection		
2. Impaired physical mobility		✓
3. Alteration in comfort		
4. Alteration in nutrition		
5. Self-care deficit	✓	✓
6. Activity intolerance	✓	
7. Decreased cardiac output		
8. Ineffective ventilation and perfusion	✓	
9. Sexual dysfunction		
10. Impaired verbal communication		✓
11. Knowledge deficit of spouse		✓
12. Grieving		✓
13. Ineffective coping of spouse related to patient's illness		✓
14. Ineffective coping of patient related to loss of control	✓	✓
15. Noncompliance		
TOTAL SCORE	4	7
TOTAL POSSIBLE SCORE = 11		

When the examinees turn in Answer Sheet 1, they pick up from the "out" box Answer Sheet 2, which lists the "correct" patient problems (see Figure 4.3). On this answer sheet, they are instructed to select from the data lists: (a) the cues they used from the case to derive their hypotheses about the patient's problems, and (b) additional historical, physical, or laboratory data they would collect in order to confirm or reject their hypotheses. In

Figure 4.3 the numbers in the cells refer to numbered items on Data Lists 1 and 2 (the continuation of Figure 4.3). Copies of the data lists are at the end of the chapter. These answers were judged to be critical or priority answers by a panel of four content experts (practitioners and teachers of home health nursing). The scoring also is indicated in Figure 4.3.

The open-ended version of the instrument uses one written patient care simulation. Examinees are asked to read the case to reply to the same four questions asked in the objective format. The "correct" answers, as determined by consensus of four content experts, are shown in Figure 4.4.

On the pretest, scorers accepted diagnoses not stated according to the North American Nursing Diagnosis Association (NANDA) diagnostic categories. On the posttest, following instruction on the nursing diagnostic process, the scorers were stricter about the wording of the patient problems.

Use of the in-basket/out-basket technique for the administration of this instrument enhanced scoring ability. The final version of the open-ended instrument incorporates two answer sheets, as did the objective format. The first answer sheet for the open-ended format presents the examinees only with the written case and the first question asking them to list the patient's possible problems. They then turn in the answer sheet and receive a second answer sheet, which lists the "correct" problems delineated by the panel of content experts. Then the examinees complete the remainder of the test.

The instrument is administered to a group of examinees, with one proctor. There are four baskets located in a central place in the room, labeled "In," "Out—Answer Sheet #2," "Out—Answer Sheet #3," and "Out—Answer Sheet #4." Part of the instrument, including the two cases, the data lists, and Answer Sheet 1, are distributed to the examinees, and verbal instructions are given. To prevent cueing from feedback, examinees completed Answer Sheets 1, 2, 3, and 4 in sequence as described earlier, placing their completed sheets in the "In" box and taking the next answer sheet in sequence.

Scoring of the objective format is straightforward and can be done manually or by computer using the key shown in Figures 4.2 and 4.3. Scoring of the open-ended responses is best accomplished by two independent judges reaching a consensus score. The scoring criteria are depicted in Figure 4.4. Interrater reliabilities were acceptable, indicating that careful adherence to the criteria for scoring will yield a reliable score (see Table 4.1).

The maximum possible total scores and subscale scores for both versions of the instrument are shown in Table 4.2. The total score is 33 for the open-ended format and 105 for the objective version. Both versions contain subscales that are discrete and uncontaminated by effects from any of the other subscales because of the control of cueing by the test procedure.

FIGURE 4.3 Answer Sheet 2 for objective version of instrument.

Column 1 Patient problem	Column 2 Data from case	Column 3 Additional information	Scoring for column 3
	Enter as many #s as you wish from Data List #1.	For each problem, enter up to 5 numbers from Data List #2. No more than 5.	
Case A: Sussex			
#5: Self-care deficit	1, 2, 3	1, 2, 4, 6, 30, 32	Any 5
#6: Activity intolerance	1, 2, 3	1, 2, 3, 29, 30, 40	Any 5
	1	2, 25, 26, 27, 32, 42	Any 5
#8: Ineffective ventilation	3, 4, 1*	8, 9, 10, 14, 35, 36	Any 5
#14: Ineffective coping-loss of control	10		20
Total possible score: Sussex			
Case B: Kaiser			
#2: Impaired physical mobility	5, 6	1, 12, 23, 30	All 4
#5: Self-Care deficit	5, 6, 3*	1, 6, 19, 23,29, 30	Any 5
#10: Impaired communication	5, 7, 11*	7, 24, 31	All 3
#11: Knowledge deficit-spouse	9, 10, 5*, 6*, 7*	15, 37, 38	All 3
#12: Grieving	5, 6, 7, 11, 12*	8, 9, 10, 11, 18, 20, 35	Any 5
#13: Ineffective coping-spouse	8, 9, 10	8, 9, 10, 11, 33, 35, 36	Any 5
#14: Ineffective coping-patient	11, 12, 8*	8, 9, 10, 11, 14, 20	Any 5
Total possible score: Kaiser	24		30

Priority problem for Sussex: #6 Activity intolerance (5 points)
Priority problem for Kaiser: #5 Self-care deficit (5 points)
*Optional, not critical answers.

RELIABILITY AND VALIDITY ASSESSMENTS

The population on which the first drafts of the instrument were field tested was a convenience sample of 36 home health nurses employed in four home health agencies in southern California. The revised instrument was administered to 19 students as a pretest in the 220-hour, post-RN continuing education program in home health nursing. Postprogram data were available on 11 students who had graduated to date. The sample was augmented by another group of eight students who were entering the program. The nurses in both groups were similar in terms of age, marital status, basic nursing preparation, and highest degree attained. The field-test sample of 36 home health nurses, of course, had more experience in home health nursing than the student group.

The properties of the instrument assessed in the testing of the instrument were: sensitivity to measurement of pre-post educational gains, reliability, content validity, criterion validity, construct validity, ease and accuracy of scoring, and examinee acceptability. The results indicated that the two versions complement each other. Students preferred the open-ended format, but it was more difficult to score than the objective format, and the reliability of scoring was lower. The interrater reliability for the objective format was 1.00 (perfect reliability); for the open-ended format, it ranged from .55 to .88 (Pearson r, $p < .01$) over four independent judges.

The reliability of the instrument, as measured by Cronbach's alpha coefficient, was .79 for the objective format and .74 for the open-ended format, based on a sample of 25. The objective and open-ended formats were highly correlated with each other (Pearson $r = .44$, $p < .01$).

Both versions of the test were sensitive to pre-post measurement of gains, the open-ended version being slightly more sensitive than the objective format. There were gains in all four of the subscales. However, significant differences, as measured by paired t tests, were found only for the cue-utilization and hypothesis-generation subscales ($p < .001$ to .02). The gain in the total score (the sum of the four subscale scores) was significant ($p < .01$) for the open-ended version and not significant for the objective format.

Content validity was assessed by the ratings of four content experts on a 4-point scale. The experts rated the validity of the following dimensions: the patient care situation, the patient's age as related to health conditions presented, the patient's ethnic background relative to health conditions, the situation as being within the scope of nursing practice, and the likelihood that a registered nurse could make a correct diagnosis of the problems. The rating scale points were as follows: not valid, slightly valid, moderately valid, and totally valid. All three patient vignettes were rated, and a mean score was derived for each dimension assessed. A content validity index (CVI) was derived by dividing the sum of the mean ratings

FIGURE 4.4 Answer Sheet 4 for open-ended version of instrument.

ANSWER SHEET #4 Form 08 (Key)

Student Name _____ Student ID _____

Read the case below and answer the four questions about it on this answer sheet.

CASE D: Mrs. Marchese is 73 years old and a new diabetic. She was discharged from the hospital two days ago and has been referred to your Home Health Agency for diabetic teaching, especially diet and food exchange. She is widowed and lives alone. While she is literate in Italian, she speaks very little English and cannot read or write English. Upon arrival at her home, Mrs. Marchese tells you her eyes are "blurry."

1. In the case above what are the possible patient problems? Name all you can think of. State them in nursing diagnosis terms. (10 points)

   The preferred answers are circled, but credit can be given for any 3 answers.

   1. *Knowledge deficit related to diabetic management (4 points)*
   2. *Potential self-care deficit secondary to vision deficit (3 points)*
   3. *Alteration in nutrition related to potential hypo/hyperglycemia (3 points)*
   4. *Impaired communication secondary to language problem (3 points)*
   5. *Visual alterations secondary to diabetes mellitus (3 points)*
   6. *Potential for social isolation (3 points)*

2. What information did you use from the case as a basis for suspecting each of the patient's problems? List below. (9 points)

PROBLEM NUMBER	FOR EACH PROBLEM, STATE BRIEFLY THE CUES YOU USED FROM THE CASE:
#1	Referral for diabetic teaching
#2	Blurry vision
#3	Needs diet teaching

3. What additional information would you obtain to determine whether each of the problems you listed is an actual problem for this patient? (9 points)

PROBLEM NUMBER	FOR EACH PROBLEM, STATE BRIEFLY THE ADDITIONAL INFORMATION YOU WOULD SEEK:
	Only the broad categories of information are indicated. Judge whether the specific statement or question fits the Broad categories.
#1	*Asking patient questions*
#2	*Observation, interview questions*
#3	*Observation, interview questions, urinalysis, blood sugar*

3. Of the problems you listed in 1 above, which one is the patient's priority problem? (5 points)

   #1 *Knowledge deficit related to diabetic management*

TOTAL NUMBER OF POINTS (MAXIMUM = 33)
Use back of page for more space as needed.

TABLE 4.1 Construct and Criterion Validity: Actual Results Compared to Expected Results

	Clinical judgment test (objective)		Clinical judgment test (open ended)		Clinical instructor ratings	
	Actual	Expected	Actual	Expected	Actual	Expected
Knowledge score	(.32)	NS	(−.03)	NS	(.00)	NS
Clinical judgment Test (objective)	—		(.44*)	sig	(.16)	sig
Clinical judgment Test (open-ended)	(.44*)	sig	—		(.11)	sig

Note. Numbers in parentheses are Pearson correlation coefficients.
* *p* < .01.

TABLE 4.2 Maximum Possible Scores on Clinical Judgment Instrument

	Sussex	Kaiser	Total
Objective			
Hypothesis generation	4	7	11
Cue utilization	10	24	34
Data gathering	20	30	50
Priority setting	5	5	10
Total	39	66	105
Open-ended			
Hypothesis generation			10
Cuc utilization			9
Data gathering			9
Priority setting			5
Total			33

obtained by the sum of the highest possible mean ratings (5 dimensions times 4 = 20). The CVI was .995, almost perfect.

Criterion validity was assessed by comparison (Pearson *r*) of the simulation scores with ratings by clinical instructors of the same four dimensions of the diagnostic process, plus an overall rating of clinical decision-making ability. The rating scale consisted of 6 points, ranging from *not competent* to *outstanding*. The five questions asked were:

1. *Problem sensing.* How competent is the student in sensing, from an initial brief observation of the patient, that the patient has a problem or problems?
2. *Hypothesis generation.* How competent is the student in utilizing the cues from the initial assessment to formulate hypotheses about the patient's problems?
3. *Information gathering.* How competent is the student in gathering relevant data precisely targeted to confirming the hypotheses regarding the patient's problems?
4. *Priority setting.* How competent is the student in recognizing which of the patient's multiple problems should have intervention priority?
5. *Overall rating.* Please indicate your general opinion of the student's level of competency in clinical decision making in the home health situations you have observed.

Although both versions of the instrument were positively correlated with the clinical instructor ratings, they were not significant (see Table 4.1).

Construct validity was assessed via a discrimination analysis. Assuming that the construct being measured by the instrument truly is clinical judgment, scores on the instrument should be more highly correlated with ratings of clinical judgment in the actual practice setting than with a paper-and-pencil test measuring knowledge about the health problems reflected in the simulations. Students took a 43-item, multiple-choice knowledge test about the care of patients with diabetes mellitus, chronic obstructive pulmonary disease, and cerebrovascular accident during the postprogram testing session. They were rated during the same period by their clinical instructors, using the rating scale described above for criterion validity. Scores were compared by means of Pearson correlations. The analyses were inclusive, in part because of the small sample of 11 students. In the optimum paradigm (expected results), the clinical judgment scores should not be related to the knowledge test scores, but should be significantly related to the clinical ratings. In Table 4.1, the actual results are superimposed on expected results. The knowledge test scores were *not* related to the clinical instructor ratings, indicating that they were *not* measuring the same construct. In addition, the knowledge scores were not significantly related to either the open-ended or objective format total scores of the clinical judgment test. The clinical judgment scores were positively, but not significantly, related to the clinical instructor ratings ($r = .16$ for the objective format and .11 for the open-ended format). These findings are very encouraging, but the validity studies should be repeated over a period of time and with a larger sample.

DISCUSSION AND CONCLUSIONS

A paper-and-pencil simulation test of clinical nursing judgment has been developed for use in the program evaluation of a 220-hour, post-RN continuing education program in home health nursing. Two versions of the instrument were tested: an objective and an open-ended format. The two versions complement each other and will continue to be used together to obtain a complete picture of the student's competency in clinical judgment.

This research is an early pioneering effort and a first step in a series of refinements planned for this instrument. To date, only the hypotheses generation, cue utilization, and data gathering subscales have been studied with any degree of thoroughness. More feedback to the examinees is planned for the instrument, specifically feedback about the additional patient data they have selected. Then the priority setting of patient problems and subsequent interventions can be studied. In addition, greater realism has been achieved by transforming these written case descriptions into videotaped simulations. The videotaped version was well accepted by the first group of students tested. Finally, a computer-interactive mode with video discs will resolve the feedback problem and at the same time will allow more examinee-generated answers and fewer list-generated selection options.

Reliability of the instruments has been demonstrated and there is high interrater reliability of scoring the open-ended version of the instrument, using the scoring criteria. Content validity has been demonstrated. There is some small evidence for criterion and construct validity, but larger numbers of subjects are required to conclusively assess these characteristics. Validity studies should be repeated with successive groups of students, as well as with practicing home health nurses, until a total number of 100 is achieved. Reliability and validity studies also should be conducted on the videotaped simulations. Comparisons should be made between the scores of students and those of incumbent home health nurses. If the clinical judgment instrument proves to discriminate between nurses who make accurate clinical diagnoses and those who do not, it would have widespread applicability for selection and hiring of nurses, as well as for evaluation in education programs.

REFERENCES

dela Cruz, F. A. (1994). Clinical decision-making styles of home health nurses. *Image—The Journal of Nursing Scholarship, 26*(3), 222–226.

Elstein, A. S., Shulman, L. S., & Sprafka, S. A. (1978). *Medical problem solving: An analysis of clinical reasoning.* Cambridge, MA: Harvard University Press.

Jacobs, A. M., & dela Cruz, F. A. (1990). Measuring clinical judgment in home health nursing. In O. L. Strickland & C. F. Waltz (Eds.), *Measurement of nursing outcomes: Vol. 3. Measuring clinical skills and professional development in education and practice* (pp. 125–141). New York: Springer Publishing Company.

Lauri, S., Salantera, S., Bild, H., Chalmers, K., Duffy, M., & Kim, H. S. (1997). Public health nurses' decision making in Canada, Finland, Norway, and the United States. *Western Journal of Nursing Research, 19*(2), 143–165.

Newell, A., & Simon, H. A. (1972). *Human problem solving.* Englewood Cliffs, NJ: Prentice-Hall.

Schnell, B. A., & Cervero, R. M. (1993). Clinical reasoning in occupational therapy: An integrative review. *The American Journal of Occupational Therapy, 47*(7), 605–610.

Simon, H. (1979). Information processing models of cognition. *Annual Review of Psychology*, (pp. 363–396).

Tanner, C. (1984). Factors influencing the diagnostic process. In D. L. Carnevali, P. H. Mitchel, N. F. Woods, & C. A. Tanner (Eds.), *Diagnostic reasoning in nursing* (pp. 61–81). Philadelphia: J. B. Lippincott.

DATA LIST #1
SUPPORTING DATA FROM THE CASES
USED TO DERIVE HYPOTHESES ABOUT PATIENT PROBLEMS

Need to Derive Hypotheses about patient problems
1. Diagnosis of chronic obstructive pulmonary disease (COPD)
2. Complaint of chronic fatigue
3. Inability to bathe self
4. Recently retired from executive job in large corporation
5. Diagnosis of cerebrovascular accident (CVA)
6. Left hemiplegia
7. Aphasia
8. History of caretaker wife's dependence on husband
9. Expression of frustration by wife about patient's crying
10. Expression of frustration by wife about patient's inability to bathe self
11. Patient's crying episodes
12. Patient is a retired contractor

DATA LIST #2
ADDITIONAL HISTORICAL, PHYSICAL OR LABORATORY
DATA TO COLLECT TO CONFIRM OR REJECT
HYPOTHESES ABOUT PATIENT'S PROBLEM

A. HISTORY/INTERVIEW QUESTIONS
   1. Take history of functional abilities
   2. Take history of activities that cause shortness of breath
   3. Take history of endurance time or level for activities such as walking, climbing steps, doing housechores, etc.
   4. Ask patient how bathing is performed
   5. Ask about recent chills or sweating episodes
   6. Ask about any problems experienced with care procedures
   7. Ask about communication techniques used
   8. Assess current support system
   9. Assess usual coping mechanisms
   10. Assess life situation before and after illness
   11. Assess patient and spouse's feelings about the illness
   12. Assess for paresthesia
   13. Determine how family decisions are made
   14. Determine how patient gains or maintains control
   15. Determine how much the spouse knows about the illness or about care procedures
   16. Assess sexual dysfunction
   17. Do complete history of family illness

18. Assess symptoms of stress (headache, nervousness, cardiac and pulmonary symptoms, illnesses, etc.)

B. PHYSICAL ASSESSMENT/OBSERVATION
   19. Observe general appearance, facial expression, grooming
   20. Observe for tearfulness
   21. Take vital signs
   22. Examine skin characteristics, conjunctiva
   23. Perform neuromusculoskeletal assessment
   24. Assess mental status
   25. Assess respiratory rate, rhythm and pattern
   26. Observe thoracic expansion of tactile fremitus
   27. Auscultate for breath sounds, adventitious sounds, voice sounds
   28. Percuss for thoracic dullness
   29. Observe how patient bathes self
   30. Assess functional abilities by actual observation
   31. Assess pace, clarity and appropriateness of speech
   32. Observe for dyspnea on exertion
   33. Observe for bradycardia, tachypnea and other indicators of stress
   34. Check urinary output for color, amount, odor, etc.
   35. Listen for verbalization of stress or reports of maladaptive coping mechanisms
   36. Listen for verbalization about feelings, control, decision-making, loss, frustration
   37. Observe for verbal or behavioral indications of lack of knowledge about illness
   38. Observe return demonstration of procedures
   39. Have patient keep a 24-hour food diary
   40. Have patient keep an activity log with endurance times

C. LABORATORY STUDIES
   41. Hemoglobin, Hematocrit
   42. Skull X-ray
   43. Blood chemistries
   44. Urinalysis

5

Postpartum Caseload Priority-Setting Instrument

Irene M. Bobak

PURPOSE

The chapter describes the **Postpartum Caseload Priority Setting Instrument**, which is used to measure nurses' postpartum caseload priority-setting effectiveness (Bobak, 1990). The instrument is designed to assess critical elements that experienced nurses use in managing their client assignment. Other uses include as a teaching tool in basic nursing curricula, to assist new graduates and RNs reentering the workforce to adapt more quickly to the demands of the workplace.

INSTRUMENT DESCRIPTION

Nursing process (Leonard & George, 1995), inherent in planning and delivering care to a group of patients (caseload assignment), serves as the conceptual basis for this measure. The nurse assesses, makes nursing a diagnosis for each patient in the caseload, and then plans, intervenes, and evaluates from the perspective of the entire caseload. The relationship between the time involved to perform interventions, the type of intervention performed, and the importance of the intervention to the welfare of individual patients affects the nurse's decision-making process for the whole. Because priority setting is a dynamic process, clinical emergency cannot be overlooked as a possible intervening variable. The nurse's skills and the values attributed to an intervention affect the process of priority setting.

Caseload priority setting is defined as the decision-making process for determining the delivery of nursing care to a group of patients. Modes of intervention are the nurturant, generative, and protective characteristics of nursing that meet the health needs of individuals as integrated persons, rather than as biological systems (American Nurses' Association, 1982). Nurturant or nurturing behaviors provide comfort and therapy in the presence of illness or disease and foster personal development. Generative behaviors are oriented to development of new behaviors and modification of environments or systems to promote health-conducive adaptive responses of the individuals to health care crises or problems. Protective behaviors involve surveillance, assessment, and intervention in support of adaptive capabilities and developmental functions of persons. Time is the projected amount of time in minutes to perform a nursing intervention. Ordering interventions means ordering nursing care behaviors based on judgments regarding each behavior's importance or necessity for providing optimal care to a group of clients/patients. Clinical emergency is a clinical situation that demands immediate attention from the nurse. Caregiver attributes are defined as the skill levels and values of the nurses who provide nursing care to a patient caseload.

The Postpartum Caseload Priority-Setting Instrument, a criterion-referenced measure, is comprised of a simulated caseload and 17 questions with a total of 143 items employing nominal, ordinal, and ratio scales for ranking and rating and multiple-choice items. Four background questions deal with job title, years worked as an obstetric nurse, work status, and educational levels. The patient care assignment of a nurse working on the day shift at a university hospital postpartum unit served as the basis for developing the instrument. Information obtained at morning report, data from the Kardex, and a brief description of each of five patients was compiled. This combined information was used to list nursing care activities for each patient.

Brief descriptions of the five women in the caseload are listed below.

1. Althea is a gravida 3, para 3. Her baby is normal and is bottle fed. She had an uneventful labor, delivery, and postpartum period. She is being discharged today.
2. Cho-Ling is a gravida 1, para 1. Her baby is normal. She had a cesarean delivery for cephalopelvic disproportion at 0100.
3. Dora is a 32-week gestational diabetic. She is gravida 1, para 0.
4. Betty is a 16-year-old gravida 1, para 1. She is unmarried, with no family member or friend accompanying her. Her baby is in the intensive care unit (premature and small for gestational age). The baby is to be adopted. Betty delivered 30 minutes ago.
5. Esther is a gravida 2, para 2. She is 1 day postpartum, has a third-degree laceration, and has been evaluated as slow normal intelligence. She has a 13-year-old daughter.

The description of the caseload and a list of 41 identified patient care activities were given to 4 maternity nurse clinical specialists to review for relevance and completeness. To determine how the 41 interventions identified for the five-patient caseload related to the three major domains in the conceptual model, a sample of 10 experts who were clinical specialists from a university hospital postpartum unit undertook three activities: (a) identified anticipated time by writing the number of minutes it would take to perform each intervention; (b) read the interventions and identified each as either nurturant, generative, or protective behaviors; (c) ranked patients according to how they would be cared for and rank ordered the interventions for each of the five women. Items were then developed to measure (a) caseload and intervention ordering, and (b) the effect of a clinical emergency on caseload and intervention ordering.

The measure was designed to be administered to practicing obstetrical nurses, in-service educators in hospital orientation programs, preceptorships, and intern programs for new graduates and RNs reentering the work force. Respondents are to complete the tool independently and then return it by mail or in person to the investigator. Items for each of five subcategories—mode of intervention, time for intervention, ordering of intervention, clinical emergency, and caregiver attributes—are summed using the following scoring system:

1. Ranking data are scored 1 through 5.
2. Ratio data (time) are scored as written.
3. Rating data are scored according to the number of levels in the Likert scales.
4. Responses for multiple choice items are scored 1 for a correct response and 0 for an incorrect response.
5. Nominal data are scored 1 if checked and 0 if not checked.

Sample items can be found at the end of the chapter.

RELIABILITY AND VALIDITY ASSESSMENT

Interrater agreement of the panel of experts who assessed the time, mode, and ordering of the nursing interventions for the five-patient caseload was determined. Modifications were made until there was 70% or higher agreement among the experts for all interventions. The interrater reliability of the judges' rankings for the caseload as a whole and for each of the five patients was assessed using the interclass correlation within the context of the variance-component model of the analysis of variance (ANOVA) (Winer, 1971; Nunnally and Bernstein, 1994). Resulting interclass coefficients ranged from a low of .46 to a high of .93, with all but one .66 or higher. Additional assessments to be undertaken include internal consistency reliability and stability estimates when administered to subjects to determine homogeneity of the constructs; and time for interventions, mode of interventions, and ordering of interventions. Validity assessment will employ a variety of nonparametric and parametric procedures including cross tabulations, ANOVA, step-wise multiple regression, and step-wise discriminate analysis to determine criterion-related and construct validity.

REFERENCES

American Nurses' Association. (1982). *Nursing: A social policy statement.* Kansas City, MO: Author.

Bobak, I. M. (1990). Postpartum caseload priority-setting instrument: Development and testing. In O. L. Strickland & C. F. Waltz (Eds.), *Measurement of nursing outcomes: Vol. 3. Measuring clinical skills and professional development in education and practice* (pp. 142–153). New York: Springer Publishing Company.

Leonard, M. K. & George, J. B. (1995). Ida Jean Orlando. In J. B. George (Ed.). *Nursing theories: The base for professional nursing practice* (4th ed.).

Nunnally, J. C. & Bernstein, I. H. (1994). *Psychometric theory* (3rd ed.). New York: McGraw-Hill.

Winer, B. J. (1971). *Statistical principles in experimental design* (2nd ed.). New York: McGraw-Hill.

SAMPLE ITEMS
POSTPARTUM CASELOAD PRIORITY-SETTING INSTRUMENT

A total of five multiple-choice questions were used to measure Objective 2, "group (combine) interventions for the 5 women in the caseload." An example follows:

NURSES MAY COMBINE ONE OR MORE INTERVENTIONS WHICH THEY PERFORM SIMULTANEOUSLY. IN THE NEXT 5 QUESTIONS INDICATE THE *BEST* COMBINATION OF INTERVENTIONS THAT CAN BE DONE SIMULTANEOUSLY.

Althea (check one)

_____ 1. Discuss family planning and assess plans for coping with sibling rivalry.

_____ 2. Perform final OB assessment and reconfirm that baby has approved car seat for discharge home.

_____ 3. Review care of normal newborn and call nursery regarding discharge orders.

Ranking questions were used to measure Objective 3, "order patients in the caseload according to priority of care." An example follows:

Rank the five patients according to how you would care for them. You will award #1 to the patient you will care for first, #2 to the patient you will care for second, #3 to the patient you will care for third, and so on.

_____ Althea
_____ Cho-Ling
_____ Dora
_____ Betty
_____ Esther

SAMPLE RATING SCALE*

Rating scales were used to measure a number of the objectives. An example of how Objective 6—"demonstrate how the skill levels and values of the nurse (caregiver) affects priority setting"—was operationalized is shown below.

LISTED BELOW ARE STATEMENTS RELEVANT TO CARE OF POSTPARTUM WOMEN. PLEASE RATE EACH STATEMENT ON A SCALE OF 1 TO 4 FOR ITS LEVEL OF IMPORTANCE TO YOU AS A CAREGIVER. FOUR (4) HAS HIGHEST PRIORITY AND ONE (1) HAS LOWEST PRIORITY.

	HIGHEST PRIORITY		LOWEST PRIORITY	
	4	3	2	1
Teaching is heart of nursing				
Hands-on nursing				
Teenage mothers				
Women who are alone				
Women having 1st baby				
Adopting out baby				
Physically ill mothers				
Mothers with prematures				
Mothers with many questions				
Professional women				
Mothers with minimal questions				

*Used with permission: Bobak, Irene M. Additional information regarding the Postpartum Priority-Setting Instrument can be obtained by contacting Irene M. Bobak, RN, PhD, 1284 Laurel Hill Drive, San Mateo, CA 94402.

6

Performance Appraisal Tool

Margaret R. Kostopoulos

PURPOSE

This chapter describes the **Performance Appraisal Tool**, which is used to measure nursing job performance in medical surgical nursing. It is designed to be used for both probationary and annual evaluation of the medical surgical registered nurse.

INSTRUMENT DESCRIPTION

An important contemporary and corporate issue is the clinical competence of newly graduated nurses during their first year of employment and the difficulty in evaluating their performance in an objective, reliable, and valid manner (O'Connor, Pearse, Smith, Vogeli, & Walton, 1999). The significance of the need for developing and implementing measures of job performance is underscored by the requirement of accrediting groups such as the Joint Commission on Accreditation of Health Care Organizations (1999) that institutional leaders be held accountable for ensuring that clinical competence is assessed, maintained, demonstrated, and continually improved for all nursing staff. Orem's (1980, 1995; Alligood & Marriner-Tomey, 1997) self-care framework served as the conceptual basis for the tool's development. The focus throughout the tool is on those activities of the nurse that facilitate the meeting of identified holistic self-care needs that the patient cannot meet independently. Specifically, the five sections of the tool address: (a) nursing activities that demonstrate the utilization of the nursing process, such as initial and ongoing assessment, an initial plan of care with revisions as necessary, the implementation of that plan, and evaluation of the effectiveness of the interventions; (b) evaluation of the supportive-educative role of the professional nurse, defined by Orem as a valid way of assisting the patient and/or family to

achieve self-care including assessment of learning needs, the use of appropriate teaching methods and resources, and evaluation of learning that
has taken place; (c) ability to meet patient needs in an organized manner
including activities and characteristics of the professional nurse that fulfill the other roles defined by Orem, doing for another, or providing a
helping environment; (d) the professional nurse's responsibility for self-
development; and (e) the professional nurse's responsibility and accountability for quality care including contributions to increase the effectiveness
of nursing practice.

The original measure, The Nurse Performance Evaluation Tool
(Kostopoulos, 1988) is a criterion-referenced measure. Criteria reflect
major concepts of Orem's self-care framework, standards of performance
established by nursing service, and the role of the registered nurse as
defined by the nurse practice act within the state it was developed. Nursing
managers and nursing staff participated in the original tool's development
and subsequent revision. The original tool contains a total of 35 items (10
items in Section 1, 7 items in Section 2, 9 items in Section 3, 4 items in
Section 4, and 5 items in Section 5). Each of the items is rated on a Likert
scale ranging from 1 (below standard performance) to 4 (outstanding
performance) by an individual familiar with the nurse's performance in
the work setting, such as a supervisor or head nurse. Scores for each item
are summed and divided by the number of items scored for an average
overall rating. Each criterion is given equal weight in the scoring. Copies
of the position description on which the performance appraisal tool was
based and the original tool can be found at the end of the chapter.

RELIABILITY AND VALIDITY ASSESSMENT

Content validity was determined by having four content specialists—two
nursing educators teaching in a graduate program in nursing and two
clinical specialists familiar with self-care theory—rate the congruence of
each item relative to its measurability, reflection of expected performance
for an RN on a medical/surgical unit, relevance to the domain, fit with
the rating scale; and representation of the performance expectation for
the domain. Congruence scores follow: +1, congruence; 0, undecided;
and –1, incongruence. The percentage of agreement among the content
specialists was 100% for 28 of the 42 criteria. There were only four criteria for which there was less than 75% agreement with one or more of the
five areas of congruency assessed: criterion C3d, establishes priorities
appropriately and identifies stress-producing situations; criterion C6,
accessible and approachable; criterion C7, participates in group process
and facilitates communication; and criterion E5, demonstrates responsibility for maintaining certification in CPR and for reviews in isolation
and fire safety.

To further determine evidence for content validity, a questionnaire was distributed to all RNs employed on a medical/surgical unit who had been evaluated using the study tool ($N = 58$). This questionnaire was designed to measure employee acceptance of the evaluation tool as applicable for evaluating performance using a four-point rating scale ranging from strongly agree (1) to strongly disagree (4). Resulting scores ranged from 10 to 40 (10 being the highest agreement) with the mean score for all respondents, 22.33, and the mode, 21. Over 75% of the respondents agreed that the statements on the tool related to their respective objective and 63.8% felt that the performance evaluation described the expectations for an RN and that the tool helped them to know what is expected of them. Only 51.7% agreed that the tool was useful in helping them identify the need for professional growth, and 48.3% agreed that it was useful in identifying areas of strength.

Interrater reliability was evaluated by having four nursing managers of a medical/surgical nursing unit, a clinical supervisor, and three assistant clinical supervisors independently rate the performance of 10 RNs. The results were compared using percentage of agreement with 75% agreement determined acceptable a priori. Reliability was examined in two ways: (a) percentage of agreement about each RN, and (b) percentage of agreement about each item for all RNs. Average percentage of items for which there was at least 75% agreement between raters for a specific nurse was 59%, with a range of 42.9% to 81.0%. Nineteen of the items were found to be reliable. Interrater reliability for the entire tool ranged from .10 to 1.00 for the evaluations of the RNs.

Although results indicated a basically useful tool for the performance evaluation of the medical/surgical RN, the tool's reliability and validity would be improved by critically examining and modifying items for each criterion for which there was less than 75% agreement by either the content specialists or nursing managers and by training raters and providing clearer explanations of item meanings and related behaviors.

On the basis of this testing and subsequent use, the original tool was modified and renamed Performance Appraisal. The modified tool contains 48 items that are rated from 0 (does not meet performance standards) to 4 (routinely exceeds performance standards). Items on the tool are more specific than those in the original version and reflect more emphasis on service excellence (e.g., communication, teamwork, and accountability); accountability; ongoing evaluation; administering health care needs, and meeting health care education needs of clients and families. Unlike the scoring for the original tool, the Performance Appraisal sections are differentially weighted and provision was made for an improvement/development plan. Reliability and validity testing of the revised tool should be undertaken prior to its use.

REFERENCES

Alligood, M. R., & Marriner-Tomey, A. (1997). *Nursing theory: Utilization and application.* St. Louis: Mosby, Inc.

Joint Commission on Accreditation of Health Care Organizations. (1999). *Comprehensive accreditation manual for hospitals: The official handbook.* Oak Park, IL: Author.

Kostopoulos, M. R. (1988). Reliability and validity of a nurse performance evaluation tool. In O. L. Strickland & C. F. Waltz (Eds.), *Measurement of nursing outcomes: Vol. 2. Measuring nursing performance: Practice, education, and research* (pp. 77–95). New York: Springer Publishing Company.

O'Connor, S. E., Pearse, J., Smith, R. L., Vogeli, D., & Walton, P. (1999). Monitoring the quality of pre-registration education: Development, validation and piloting of competency based performance indicators for newly qualified nurses. *Nurse Education Today, 19*(4) 334–341.

Orem, D. E. (1980). *Nursing: Concepts of practice.* New York: McGraw-Hill.

Orem, D. E. (1995). *Nursing Concepts of practice* (5th ed.). St. Louis: Mosby Year Books.

PERFORMANCE EVALUATION TOOL
(REGISTERED NURSE, MEDICAL/SURGICAL UNIT)
(ORIGINAL TOOL)

Position Description*

The following is a description of the position for which the following Performance Evaluation Tool was developed.

Title: Registered Nurse
Supervisor: Clinical Supervisor

I.   Summary of Responsibilities:
     The Registered Nurse is responsible for assessing the self-care needs of each patient in his/her care and for planning with the patient/family the actions of both nurse and patient necessary to meet those self-care needs which may be physiological, psychological, social, or spiritual. Once planned, the Registered Nurse is responsible for implementing the plan of care directly and/or through leadership of unit personnel. The Registered Nurse utilizes principles of teaching and learning to assist patients, staff, and self in the identification of the need for new knowledge and skills.

II. Qualifications:
     A.   Graduate from an accredited school of nursing.
     B.   Current registration as a professional nurse in the State of Maryland.
     C.   One year of previous experience in medical/surgical nursing within the past five years.
     D.   Ability to assess, plan, direct and/or implement, and evaluate the activities necessary to meet the self-care needs of the patients in his/her care.
     E.   Ability to communicate effectively.

III. Job relationships:
     A.   Responsible to:
          1.   The patient for whom care is provided.
          2.   Self and peers as professional nurses.
          3.   Clinical Supervisor or Assistant Clinical Supervisor.
          4.   Evening Assistant Clinical Supervisor or Administrative Nursing Supervisor when working the evening shift.
          5.   Charge Nurse or Administrative Nursing Supervisor when working the night shift.
     B.   Employees supervised:
          1.   Licensed Practical Nurses and unlicensed patient care givers.
          2.   As preceptor, orientees and nursing graduates.

C. Interdisciplinary relationships:
 1. Works effectively toward collaborative relationships with the Medical Staff, other members of the health team and administrative personnel.
 2. Maintains a cooperative working relationship with ancillary departments.

IV. Responsibilities:
 A. Adheres to the purpose and objectives of nursing practice of the department of nursing services, utilizing the nursing process to assist patients in meeting their self-care needs.
  1. Assesses the patient on admission and documents appropriate data.
  2. Initiates and maintains an individualized patient care plan which includes nursing diagnosis, patient and nurse goals, nursing system to be utilized, patient and nurse actions, and evaluation of plan using outcomes.
  3. Implements the medical and nursing plan of care and revises plan according to ongoing evaluation.
  4. Identifies, documents, and reports appropriately changes in patient's status.
  5. Coordinates the plan of care in preparation for discharge.
 B. Organizes and carries out a plan for teaching the self-care required to patient and/or family.
  1. Utilizes principles of teaching and learning.
  2. Identifies barriers to learning.
  3. Displays the attitudes, knowledge, and skills necessary to stimulate motivation in patients to achieve results appropriate to the patient's condition and circumstances.
  4. Evaluates learning and modifies teaching plan as necessary.
  5. Contacts other hospital departments/services and community resources to assist with self-care.
 C. Synchronizes the nursing activities toward achievement of patient and nurse goals safely, efficiently, and effectively.
  1. Formulates a plan of care based on priority self-care needs.
  2. Utilizes resources and other nursing personnel commensurate with their educational preparation and experience.
  3. Instructs, supervises, and evaluates activities of other members of the nursing team.
  4. Contributes to the promotion of a climate that fosters supportive communication and problem solving.
 D. Identifies and pursues his/her professional self-development plan.
  1. Utilizes the current literature and pertinent workshops in nursing and related fields to enhance his/her professional development.

    2. Continually evaluates own practice and outcome of care in light of emerging knowledge.

E. Participates in programs designed to increase the effectiveness of nursing practice.

    1. Demonstrates awareness of the value and relevance of research in nursing.

    2. Suggests need for and participates in quality assurance measures.

PERFORMANCE EVALUATION TOOL
(REGISTERED NURSE, MEDICAL/SURGICAL UNIT)
(ORIGINAL)

_____

(Employee Name)

_____

(Reason for Review)

_____

(Department—Unit)

From _____ To _____

Ranking Guidelines:

Below standard (1) — Fulfills defined expectation inconsistently, requiring repeated assistance and follow-up.

Meets standard (2) — Fulfills defined expectation consistently (90% of the time) in routine situations, requiring assistance initially and/or with difficult or unusual situations.

Above standard (3) — Fulfills defined expectation consistently (90% of the time) in routine situations, requiring assistance some of the time with difficult or unusual situations.

Outstanding (4) — Fulfills defined expectation independently and consistently in almost all situations.

A. Adheres to the "Purpose and Objectives of Nursing Practice" of the Department of Nursing Services, utilizing the nursing process to assist patients in meeting their self-care needs.

   1. Identifies in the admission nursing assessment progress note the relationship among data collected from the nursing history, systems assessment, and self-care needs within 24 hours of admission.   1   2   3   4

_____

_____

   2. Documents nursing diagnoses in the nursing progress notes and on the master problem list within 24 hours of admission.   1   2   3   4

_____

_____

3.   Initiates a written plan of care within 24
     hours of admission collaborating with
     the physician, patient, and family, utilizing:
     a.   Nursing diagnosis   1   2   3   4

     _____

     _____

     b.   Long- and short-term goals   1   2   3   4

     _____

     _____

     c.   Nursing systems   1   2   3   4

     _____

     _____

     d.   Specific patient/nurse actions   1   2   3   4

     _____

     _____

     e.   Measurable outcome criteria   1   2   3   4

     _____

     _____

4.   Documents implementation of the
     medical/nursing plan of care in the
     nursing progress notes.   1   2   3   4

     _____

     _____

5.   Documents an evaluation of the patient's
     compliance and response to the
     therapeutic regimen.   1   2   3   4

     _____

     _____

6.   Reviews/revises and updates patient care
     plan at least every 48 hours to reflect
     resolution of problems, new nursing
     diagnoses, and/or revisions in patient/
     nurse actions.   1   2   3   4

     _____

     _____

7.   Documents the reason for changes in
     patient care plan in nursing progress notes.   1   2   3   4

     _____

     _____

8. Revises master problem list as status of
    active and inactive problems change.   1   2   3   4
    _____
    _____

9. Identifies need for and includes preparation
    for discharge on the patient care plan as
    appropriate.   1   2   3   4
    _____
    _____

10. Documents progress of patient/family in
    preparation for discharge in nursing
    progress notes.   1   2   3   4

B. Organizes and carries out a plan for teaching
    the self-care required to patient and/or family.

    1. Documents learning needs, readiness to
        learn and motivation of patient and family
        in the nursing progress notes.   1   2   3   4
        _____
        _____

    2. Includes patient and family while developing
        goals for the teaching/learning plans.   1   2   3   4
        _____
        _____

    3. Documents the teaching/learning plans on
        the patient care plan.   1   2   3   4
        _____
        _____

    4. Selects teaching tools consistent with the
        patient's ability to learn.   1   2   3   4
        _____
        _____

    5. Documents use of community resources in
        teaching more complex self-care activities. 1   2   3   4
        _____
        _____

    6. Documents patient's behavioral response
        to teaching.   1   2   3   4
        _____
        _____

7. Revises teaching/learning plans in response to patient need.　　　　1　2　3　4

C. Synchronizes the nursing activities toward achievement of patient and nurse goals safely, efficiently, and effectively.

1. Completes nursing activities within established time frame and with consideration to patient desires.　　　1　2　3　4

_____

_____

2. Collaborates with other members of the health team to establish priorities of patient care.　1　2　3　4

_____

_____

3. Establishes priorities appropriately.

a. Gives immediate priority to emergency situations.　　　　　1　2　3　4

_____

_____

b. Identifies time sequences for completion of procedures.　　　　1　2　3　4

_____

_____

c. Seeks assistance, if necessary, in order to accomplish immediate priorities without loss of control.　　　　1　2　3　4

_____

_____

d. Identifies stress-producing situations.　1　2　3　4

_____

_____

4. Assigns nursing activities to those qualified to perform them.　　　　1　2　3　4

_____

_____

5. Assesses learning needs of nursing personnel
    and makes recommendations for and/or
    provides instruction.   1   2   3   4

    _____

    _____

6. Is accessible and approachable.   1   2   3   4

    _____

    _____

7. Participates in group process and facilitates
    communication.   1   2   3   4

    _____

    _____

8. Organizes nursing activities and uses
    equipment and supplies as intended,
    resulting in cost containment.   1   2   3   4

    _____

    _____

9. Demonstrates knowledge and skill while
    performing technical skills indicated on skill
    inventory checklist.   1   2   3   4

    _____

    _____

D. Identifies and pursues his/her professional
    self-development plan.

    1. Incorporates new concepts, procedures,
        and skills obtained from continuing
        education into clinical practice.   1   2   3   4

        _____

        _____

    2. With assistance of unit supervisor, identifies
        areas of strength and those needing further
        development at appropriate intervals.   1   2   3   4

        _____

        _____

    3. Conducts patient care conference.   1   2   3   4

        _____

        _____

4. Makes suggestions for topics for investigation to unit representatives of appropriate nursing/hospital committees. 1 2 3 4

_____

_____

5. Demonstrates responsibility for maintaining certification in CPR and for reviews in isolation and fire/safety as designated in nursing policy. 1 2 3 4

_____

_____

SIGNATURES OF REPORTING OFFICERS:
This report is based on my observation and/or knowledge. It represents my best judgment of the employee's performance.

RATED BY _____ DATE _____

REVIEWED BY _____ DATE _____

APPROVED BY _____ DATE _____

Report discussed with and copy given to employee

BY _____ DATE _____

This report has been discussed with me
Employee's signature _____ DATE _____

Received in Personnel Office for Review
BY_____ DIRECTOR DATE _____

7

Measuring Clinical Decision Making Using a Clinical Simulation Film

Donna Ketchum Story

PURPOSE

This chapter discusses a clinical decision making measure to be used with a simulation film. The nursing performance simulation instrument, using magnitude scaling, was designed to determine the magnitude of the degree of complexity of decision making (Story, 1988). While the simulation presented here employs film, the instrument can be readily adapted for use with other types of simulations including computer-assisted and videodisc.

INSTRUMENT DESCRIPTION

The challenges of clinical teaching in the last decade coupled with the rapid advances in technology have been the impetus for increased emphasis on the use of simulations delivered via film, computer-assisted instruction, and interactive videodisc to assess students' clinical decision making (Weiner, Gordon, & Gilman, 1993). Further, the use of simulations in nursing in combination with clinical experience has been determined to result in more positive attitudes toward learning (Schare, Dunn, Clark, Gilman, & Soled, 1991), as well as greater clinical confidence (Weiner, Gordon, & Gilman, 1993). The conceptual basis for the nursing performance simulation instrument was drawn from decision making and measurement frameworks. Decision making is a phase of the nursing process (Yura & Walsh, 1978), a process that is comprised of a designated series of actions intended to fulfill the purposes of nursing. Nursing process is based on many theories from a variety of disciplines including general systems theory, information theory, communication theory, decision and problem solving theories, and theories of perception and human need (Banathy,

1968; Lee, 1971; Maslow, 1970; Yura & Walsh, 1978). Through the nursing process the nurse has the means to collect, designate meaning to, and make inferences about information. Lancaster and Beare (1982) described the search process for locating information about possible alternatives, including factors that affected the search. Viewing the selections of a nursing action as a decision-making process focuses attention on the application of concepts of decision theory to nursing.

Classical test theory identified by Lord and Novick (1968), Stanley (1971), and Nunnally (1978) served as the basis for the model used for assessing random measurement error. Classical test theory is a logical foundation for the method used here for the derivation of psychometric data and for estimating the reliability of empirical measurements. The measurement technique of magnitude estimation allows for the measurement of complexity of decisions.

A scale to measure the magnitude of the degree of complexity of decisions was developed from a paper-and-pencil achievement test developed by Schneider (1979), that was based on a depicted obstetrical clinical situation presented through a 16mm film designed to simulate the clinical setting. Assumptions underlying the development of the measure included:

1. The situation depicted parallels likely to have been encountered by most baccalaureate nursing students in the course of their education.
2. Nurses have been seen performing the kinds of activities customarily expected in that situation.
3. The dialogues between the nurse and patient and the physician were extensive enough to permit judgments to be made.
4. Content from a variety of disciplines (sociology, psychology, and physiology) related to the situation.
5. The quality of the film's sound and photography was such that the extraneous noise and subject matter did not interfere with an examinee's performance on the test.
6. Lack of knowledge of obstetric nursing did not affect the performance on the test.

A nursing action that involves a nursing decision was provided to the subjects through the use of a 16mm movie film depicting the real situation of a woman in labor and the birth of her baby. Subjects were then asked to make a decision based on their own rationale for the choice. The magnitude-judgment method was employed to construct a scale reflecting the complexity of each task relative to the set of tasks based on judgments made by experts. A complexity of decision score could then be obtained for each test item. A sample of a clinical decision-making measure developed for use with a specific film description of a sample film can be found at the end of the chapter.

RELIABILITY AND VALIDITY ASSESSMENT

Interrater reliability was determined between the assigned scores of the judges, and the resulting Pearson correlation coefficient was .72. Stability of the judges' scores was estimated using test-retest, and the result was .84. A group of RN completion students volunteered to view the film and respond to the 29-item tool. Internal consistency reliability for the tool was determined using student's scores; the resulting Kuder-Richardson reliability coefficient was .4899, and the alpha coefficient was .61. Logarithmic transformations of the data allowed the use of statistics requiring linear additive assumptions. The pattern of the complexity of the decision was of primary interest. Therefore, the geometric mean was obtained from the logarithmic transformations, resulting in a mean complexity score of 7.04 with a standard deviation of .2 and a score range of 6.586 to 7.372. The coefficient of determination between the correct answers and the logarithmic transformation was $r^2 = .934$. The coefficient of correlation was estimated to be .966, with a standard error of the estimate of .051.

This work demonstrates the use of magnitude-estimation techniques to produce ratio scales of the complexity of clinical decisions variable. By applying logarithmic transformations, it was possible to examine the averaged data as well as to work with individual scores and to increase the precision of the measurement by producing a ratio-level scale.

REFERENCES

Banathy, B. (1968). *Instructional systems.* Palo Alto, CA: Fearon.

Lancaster, W., & Beare, P. (1982). Decision making in nursing practice. In J. Lancaster & W. Lancaster (Eds.), *Concepts for advanced nursing practice: The nurse as a change agent* (pp. 147–170). St. Louis: C. V. Mosby.

Lee, W. (1971). *Decision theory and human behavior.* New York: John Wiley.

Lord, F. M., & Novick, M. R. (1968). *Statistical theories of mental test scores.* Reading, MA: Addison-Wesley.

Maslow, A. (1970). *Motivation and personality.* New York: Harper & Row.

Nunnally, J. C. (1978). *Psychometric theory* (2nd ed.). New York: McGraw-Hill.

Schare, B., Dunn, S., Clark, H., Gilman, B., & Soled, S. (1991). The effects of interactive video on cognitive achievement and attitude toward learning. *Journal of Nursing Education, 30*(3), 109–13.

Stanley, J. C. (1971). *Reliability.* In R. L. Thorndike (Ed.), *Educational measurement* (pp. 356–442). Washington, DC: American Council on Education.

Story, D. K. (1988). Developing a measure of clinical decision making through the use of a clinical simulation film. In O. L. Strickland & C. F. Waltz (Eds.) *Measurement of nursing outcomes: Vol. 2. Measuring nurs-*

ing performance: Practice, education, and research (pp. 202–217). New York: Springer Publishing Company.

Weiner, E. E., Gordon, J. S., & Gilman, B. R. (1993). Evaluation of a labor and delivery videodisc simulation, *Computers in Nursing, 11*(4), 191–196.

Yura, H., & Walsh, M. (1978). *The nursing process: Assessing, planning implementing, evaluating* (3rd ed.). New York: Appleton-Century Crofts.

SAMPLE OF A CLINICAL DECISION-MAKING MEASURE DEVELOPED FOR USE WITH A SPECIFIC FILM DESCRIPTION OF SAMPLE FILM

The film "Birth through the Eyes of the Mother" follows the labor process and birth of an infant as it would be seen by the mother, in this case a woman named Maureen. The camera angle is as if it were in the position of the mother's eyes. In other words, it is about $4^1/2$ to 5 feet above the ground. All of the script is in the form of people talking to the mother and her responses. There is no narration of the film, and there are no pictures of the mother. The film begins with the mother walking down the hall to the labor admission area. The nurse is giving her directions, and asking her questions about the beginning of her contractions. When the patient is on the admission table and positioned for an examination, her knees appear on either side of the screen, and the nurse's face approaches the camera. The film advances the time by looking at the clock at intervals. There are only three or four characters in the film: the mother, the nurse or nurses, and the unseen patient. The patient does not have a support person for the labor and birth process. The actions of the characters are natural and appear to be unrehearsed. The actions of the nurse are those that would be seen by many mothers. The doctor also appears in a natural role. His information and directions to the mother are the same as that given many times in an actual labor and delivery situation.

Questions used with the film "Birthday through the Eyes of the Mother."

1. The nurse asked Maureen a question that was based on the assumption that Maureen
    1. had attended an antepartal clinic.
    2. was anxious about the outcome of the pregnancy.
    3. had been timing her contractions.
    4. was knowledgeable about what to expect in subsequent stages of labor.
2. The nurse asked Maureen all of the following questions shortly after her admission. While all of the questions would be useful in establishing a nursing care plan, which one could justifiably have been postponed?
    1. "Have you been exposed recently to a communicable disease?"
    2. "Are you leaking any fluid?"
    3. "How much weight did you gain during your pregnancy?"
    4. "Do you expect to breast or bottle feed your baby?"

3. Which of these occurrences soon after Maureen was admitted would probably have diminished her confidence in the personnel?
   1. The nurse did not immediately notify the doctor of Maureen's arrival on the unit.
   2. Neither a doctor nor a nurse stayed with Maureen continuously.
   3. No one provided Maureen with information about the infant's condition.
   4. Maureen was asked the same questions by both the nurse and the doctor.

4. The doctor seemed to make several assumptions in relation to Maureen's labor and delivery. Which of them was most apparent?
   1. That Maureen was going to have a larger-than-average baby.
   2. That Maureen was going to have anesthesia.
   3. That Maureen's intrapartum course was going to be prolonged.
   4. That Maureen was going to require medication only at the end of the first stage of labor.

5. While Maureen was being shaved, it would have been desirable for the nurse to say,
   1. "Although you will experience some discomfort when the hair grows back, shaving is a necessary procedure."
   2. "Women usually complain of a tickling sensation as the hair regrows, but it shouldn't pose any great problems for you."
   3. "It's common to be embarrassed because the shaving involves a private area, but it will help to promote the safety of the birth process."
   4. "We're pretty lucky not having to shave every day, aren't we?"

6. Maureen made several comments in relation to the enema she was about to have. Which comment, if Maureen had made it, would indicate that the nurse did not prepare her adequately for the enema?
   1. "I thought I was going to drop the baby."
   2. "I had an enema as a child, but I've had none since then."
   3. "I won't be able to hold the fluid if I have a contraction."
   4. "I don't understand why an enema is so important."

7. The nurse's approach to Maureen while she was in labor appeared to be based on Maureen's
   1. socioeconomic status.
   2. prior experience with nurses and doctors.
   3. acceptance of the nurse as a helping person.
   4. preparation for childbirth.

8. All of the following are desirable nursing measures for mothers in early labor. Which one did the nurse caring for Maureen carry out?
   1. Telling the mother to relax between contractions.
   2. Encouraging the mother to relax between contractions.

3. Waiting for the mother's contraction to be over before continuing with a procedure.
4. Reassuring the mother about the baby's condition.

9. A judgment that is warranted about the doctor's sitting on Maureen's bed is that it was
   1. unsafe because patients may view such behavior as being unprofessional.
   2. unwise because patients may view such behavior as being unprofessional.
   3. acceptable as a means of establishing a closer relationship with a patient.
   4. permissible on a maternity unit, though it would not be on other hospital units.

10. After the doctor noticed that Maureen's legs were shaking, he told her that the "shaking and shivering would get worse afterwards." Which judgment of the doctor's comment is accurate? (Assume that this is Maureen's first baby.)
    1. Since chills occur less frequently after delivery today than was once true, it was an inappropriate response.
    2. Since multiparas are more susceptible to chills that are primiparas, it was an inappropriate response.
    3. Since emotionally stable patients develop chills more frequently than do emotionally labile ones, it was a premature response.
    4. Since excessive body fluid precipitates chills following delivery, it was a premature response.

11. Which of these observations about Maureen's care is most justifiable in relation to the giving of medications to her?
    1. Personnel failed to give her information about the intended effects of the medications.
    2. Measures were not taken by the nurse to allay discomfort between medications.
    3. There was a hesitancy on the part of staff to administer any medication.
    4. She was made to feel that she would be violating the principles of prepared childbirth if she were to be medicated.

12. While the doctor was examining Maureen's rectum, which of these actions by the nurse was especially undesirable in terms of Maureen's emotional needs?
    1. Leaving Maureen's lower abdomen and legs exposed.
    2. Standing in back of the doctor rather than next to Maureen.
    3. Failing to explain to Maureen what was being done.
    4. Neglecting to confer with the doctor promptly about the extent of Maureen's discomfort.

13. While Maureen was being examined by the doctor, the nurse failed to provide for
    1. proper positioning of Maureen for the procedure.
    2. disposal of the equipment used by the doctor.
    3. adequate draping of Maureen's legs.
    4. visibility of the area.

14. Maureen's comments during labor should lead one to conclude that she was
    1. unusually anxious.
    2. anticipating a prolonged labor.
    3. eager for the presence of another person.
    4. favorably impressed with the medical and nursing staffs.

15. While Maureen was in labor, the nurses giving her care failed to provide for
    1. a quiet environment conducive to rest and relaxation.
    2. instructions in how to work with contractions.
    3. physical comfort measures.
    4. equipment to promote safety.

16. The nurse coached Maureen in breathing techniques. Which judgment of the nurse's approach and method is accurate?
    1. The approach was appropriate, and the method was acceptable.
    2. The approach was appropriate, but the method was unacceptable.
    3. The approach was inappropriate, but the method was acceptable.
    4. The approach was inappropriate, and the method was unacceptable.

17. Which of these statements accurately assesses the reaction of personnel to Maureen when she was experiencing discomfort associated with contractions?
    1. The doctor was more responsive to her than were the nurses.
    2. The nurses were more supportive of her than was the doctor.
    3. There was essentially no difference between the behavior of the doctor and the nurses toward her.
    4. The actions of the admitting nurse were more like those of the doctor than were those of the nurse who cared for her later.

18. The clock in Maureen's room was visible at various times. On the basis of the passage of time gleaned from the film, which of these judgments of the length of Maureen's labor as a primigravida is warranted?
    1. Maureen's labor appeared to fit the normal pattern.
    2. The first stage of Maureen's labor was within normal limits, but the second stage was assumed to be prolonged.
    3. The first stage of Maureen's labor was unusually long, but the second stage was within the normal range.
    4. There were insufficient data to allow a conclusion about the duration of Maureen's labor.

19. On the basis of the information provided in the film, the probable rationale for the use of forceps with Maureen was to
    1. adhere to medical policy.
    2. shorten the second stage of labor.
    3. facilitate delivery of a large baby.
    4. prevent perineal tears.

20. A procedure usually carried out immediately after delivery of the placenta that was not seen in the film was
    1. administering an oxytocic.
    2. performing the "Crede" maneuver.
    3. discontinuing the intravenous infusion.
    4. evaluating the amount of blood loss.

21. The one aspect of the baby's management in the delivery room that could most justifiably be criticized was that he was
    1. not given to his mother soon enough.
    2. held by the doctor with only one hand.
    3. placed on his mother's abdomen prior to delivery of the placenta.
    4. examined rather superficially for congenital anomalies.

22. At the end of the film, when Maureen commented, "The baby was inside me for nine months and now here he is," the doctor answered, "You did a good job." Which of these assessments of his comment is justifiable?
    1. It was made before the patient's remark was clarified.
    2. It immediately reinforced positive behavior in the patient.
    3. It was a complimentary acknowledgment of the patient's reaction.
    4. It reinforced the reality of the baby's arrival for the patient.

23. Which of these interpretations is most justifiable about the nurse-doctor relationship in the film?
    1. There appeared to be an interaction commonly called "professional" between them.
    2. There seemed to be a feeling of mutual respect between them.
    3. There was little or no communication between them.
    4. There did not seem to be any independent action on the part of doctors or nurses in relation to the patient's management.

24. Which of these generalizations should a nurse have about the effect of doctor-nurse relationships on patients like Maureen in a situation such as the one depicted in the film?
    1. If any disagreement between doctors and nurses is perceived by the patient, it might be interpreted by the patient as a potential threat to her.
    2. Patients in labor are so self-centered that they are unaware of doctors' and nurses' behavior.

3. An attitude of joviality and lightheartedness on the part of doctors and nurses contributes to an anxiety-free experience for the patient.
4. The behavior of doctors and nurses as individuals is more important than the relationships between and among them.

25. From both verbal and nonverbal interactions between Maureen and the nurses, it is reasonable to infer that
    1. there was a lack of affective feelings evident in their relationships with Maureen.
    2. the nurses' behavior toward Maureen is typical of the way most nurses treat maternity patients regardless of their marital status.
    3. the calmness exhibited by the nurses is synonymous with acceptance of Maureen as a person.
    4. there was an absence of judgment on the part of Maureen and the nurses.

26. The film does not tell whether Maureen has had a baby previously or whether she has ever seen a delivery. If personnel had had such information, it would have been most useful as the
    1. basis for teaching, since knowing where the patient "is" allows the nurse to be more helpful.
    2. means by which the nurse could review and reiterate pertinent information.
    3. frame of reference for establishing a nursing care plan.
    4. mechanism by which a meaningful nurse-patient relationship could be established.

27. An assumption seemed to be made by personnel about Maureen and her baby. This assumption was that Maureen
    1. was disappointed in the baby's sex.
    2. needed help in coming to a decision about the baby's future.
    3. was uncertain about her ability to take care of the baby.
    4. planned to keep the baby.

28. The most obvious omission in the film was any reference to Maureen's
    1. feelings about giving birth.
    2. relationship with the baby's father.
    3. decision about the feeding of her baby.
    4. general health status.

29. If a group of primigravidas were to view the film, what general effect might be expected?
    1. Anxiety, because many points about labor and delivery were not covered.
    2. Satisfaction of curiosity, because some aspects of having a baby were made evident.
    3. Disappointment, because only the mother's role was shown.
    4. Disillusionment, because the joy of childbearing was not made explicit and the pain was.

8

Clinical Performance Examination for Critical Care Nurses

Barbara Clark Mims

PURPOSE

This chapter describes the **Clinical Performance Examination for Critical Care Nurses**, a criterion-referenced instrument used to measure clinical performance of nurses employed in critical care settings. It can be utilized to evaluate the impact that educational programs have on nurses' clinical performance.

INSTRUMENT DESCRIPTION

In this era of increased accountability, employers of graduates hold nursing educators accountable for producing students who achieve standards of performance that are clearly defined by professional and regulatory bodies (Redman, Lenburg, & Hinton Walker, 1999). Competency-based education has heightened interest in performance testing using a criterion-referenced approach. The evaluation of competent performance is outcome oriented and the goal is to assess the effectiveness of knowledge and skill in the practice setting (Survis & Grey, 1995). This type of performance evaluation focuses on how well an examinee is able to meet specified performance standards. The examinee's competence level is then judged on how well standards are met.

Competency-based education has gained increasing popularity among nurse educators in practice settings. Spady (as cited in Scott, 1982, p. 119) has defined competency-based education as "a data-based, adaptive, performance-oriented set of integrated processes that facilitate, measure, record, and certify within the context of flexible time parameters the demonstration of known, explicitly stated, and agreed upon learning outcomes that reflect successful functioning in life roles." These definitions support the idea that professional education should assist the learner in acquiring the ability to function successfully in the designated role. One of the most difficult tasks in implementing a competency-based learning program is the evaluation of competence. This is due to the existing measurement tools, which Spady has described as "inadequate, weak in validity, and questionable in reliability" (as cited in Scott, 1982, p. 122). Therefore, Houston and Warner (as cited in Scott, 1982, p. 123) have stated, "The future of competency-based training may well be linked to its development in three areas—new bases for specifying competencies, linking training procedures with outcome specifications and competency assessment." The notion of competence as the goal of staff development programs is attractive, as it indicates that learners will be able to function as a result of their participation.

The concept of clinical performance includes the actual observable behaviors expected of a practicing clinical nurse; that is, the way in which a nurse carries out the tasks or duties expected of her reflects her clinical performance. For the purpose of this study, clinical performance was operationalized into five categories: assessment, clinical/technical skill, communication, documentation, and general employment policies.

These categories were derived through interviews with practicing critical care nurses, including both staff nurses and nurse managers. Discussions with critical care nurse educators and a review of widely accepted critical care nursing texts confirmed that the five categories encompass the major aspects of job performance required of nurses functioning in a critical care setting. When linked together, these five categories provide a complete description of the clinical duties and responsibilities of a critical care nurse.

The five categories were divided into subcategories, each of which had one test objective. The categories and objectives were refined during reliability and validity testing. The resulting tool (Mims, 1988) has the following 24 test objectives.

> *Category I (assessment).* When caring for a critically ill adult, the nurse performs a head-to-toe assessment within 1 hr of arriving at the bedside.
>
> > Performs complete neurological system assessment.
> > Performs complete cardiovascular system assessment.
> > Performs complete pulmonary system assessment.
> > Performs complete gastrointestinal system assessment.
> > Performs complete renal/metabolic system assessment.
> > Performs complete musculoskeletal system assessment.

Category II (clinical/technical skills). When caring for a critically ill adult patient, the nurse performs the clinical/technical skills that are common in critical care nursing practice.

Adheres to safety procedures.
Performs general physical care.
Administers medications.
Administers intravenous therapy.
Performs hemodynamic monitoring.
Manages the patient-ventilator system.
Administers tube feedings.
Administers hyperalimentation.
Changes peripheral IV/arterial line dressings.
Changes central line dressings.
Changes dressings of open wounds every shift or as ordered by physician.

Category III (communication). The nurse interacts and communicates with others in a courteous and professional manner.

Participates in unit activities and interacts effectively with co-workers.
Communicates effectively with patients.
Communicates with and provides support for family members.

Category IV (documentation). The nurse completes all aspects of documentation.

Documents all nursing interventions, including patient's response when appropriate.
Maintains complete and current care plan for each patient.

Category V (general employment policies). The nurse follows hospital policy regarding dress and punctuality.

Adheres to uniform regulations.
Adheres to policies regarding punctuality.

Competency statements were developed for each of the test objectives. Since initial utilization of the tool was to be within the critical care and trauma nurse internship at Parkland Memorial Hospital, the internship faculty participated in formulating the competency statements. Documents utilized in constructing the tool included the internship evaluation tool, the quality assurance audit tools, the staff nurse job description developed at Parkland Memorial Hospital, and the American Association of Critical Care Nurses' *Standards for Nursing Care of the Critically Ill* (1981).

The final tool actually consists of 24 individual tests. Since each test is scored separately, each can be administered separately. Ideally, the tests will be treated as an aggregate, and the entire exam will be administered at one time.

Testing must take place in a critical care unit. Subjects should be given a copy of the test ahead of time and given ample notice of when the testing will take place. If all 24 tests are to be administered, the patient must have the following equipment in use: ventilator, Swan-Ganz catheter, ECG monitor, IV, and Foley catheter.

The person administering the test will observe the nurse for a minimum of 4 hrs during an 8-hr shift. Periods of observation may vary from 5 min to 1 hr. The observer will not participate in the patient's care unless an emergency arises or the patient's safety is jeopardized.

Each individual test (capital letters) within each major category (Roman numerals) is scored separately. There are four possible ratings for each item on this criterion-referenced tool. If the item was performed as stated, it is rated Done. If the nurse does not perform the item as stated or if the item is omitted, it is rated Not Done. If the item does not apply during this particular patient care situation, it is rated Not Applicable. If the item is appropriate to the patient care situation but the opportunity to observe the behavior does not arise, it is rated Not Observed.

The raw score for each test is calculated by summing the number of items rated Done. The maximum possible raw score is calculated by subtracting the number of items rated Not Applicable and Not Observed from the total number of items on the test.

In order to establish the criteria for categorizing subjects as masters or nonmasters, it was necessary to establish a cut score for each test. The panel of experts was asked to rate each test item on a scale from 1 to 10 as to its importance relative to the test objective. Each expert's ratings across all items on the test were then averaged. Finally, the mean of averages from all four experts was calculated, then converted into a proportion that became the cut score (Waltz, Strickland, & Lenz, 1991; Isaac & Michael, 1995). The cut scores and maximum obtainable raw scores are shown in Table 8.1.

Before comparing the subject's raw score to the cut score, the number of items rated Not Observed and Not Applicable is subtracted from the expert's cut score. In order for the subject to be labeled as master on the test, the raw score must equal or exceed the cut score obtained in this manner.

A percentage score is then calculated for each test (capital letters), using the following formula:

$$\text{Percentage Score} = \frac{\textit{Subject's Raw Score}}{\text{Maximum Possible Raw Score} \times 100}$$

TABLE 8.1 Cut Scores for Classifying Subjects as Master/Nonmaster

Objective (test)	Maximum possible raw score	Cut score
Category I		
A	5	5
B	10	10
C	4	4
D	5	5
E	4	4
F	3	3
Category II		
A	15	13
B	6	5
C	5	5
D	7	6
E	9	9
F	5	5
G	5	4
H	6	5
I	8	3
J	7	7
K	9	9
Category III		
A	4	3
B	7	7
C	2	2
Category IV		
A	12	9
B	3	3
Category V		
A	3	3
B	4	4

If the 24 tests are administered as an aggregate, the percentage scores for all tests (capital letters) are averaged to arrive at a score for the category (Roman numerals). Although the percentage score is not used to classify subjects as master/nonmaster, it provides useful information and enables the subject to follow his/her progress when taking the same test multiple times.

The tool was field tested in the critical care units at Parkland Memorial Hospital. Interrater reliability was established by having two trained observers simultaneously rate subjects in performing the behaviors identified in the test items. The number of subjects observed for each test ranged from 16 to 24. The subjects were critical care nurses with 1 to 5 years of experience. Most of the subjects were employed in the surgical intensive care unit. The majority were female, and most were graduates of baccalaureate nursing programs.

The statistics utilized were P_o and K. P_o represented the proportion of subjects classified the same (master/nonmaster) by both observers. K represented the proportion of persons classified the same beyond that expected by chance. The minimum acceptable K value was .50. If K was less than .50, the test items were revised or deleted. The results of interrater reliability testing are shown in Table 8.2. Out of 24 tests that were assessed for interrater reliability, six had K values less than .5. Substantial revisions were made, and the final tool appears at the end of the chapter.

RELIABILITY AND VALIDITY ASSESSMENTS

Item analysis was performed to ensure that the items on the tool represent the specified content domain. The most commonly employed criterion-referenced item analysis procedures involve either pretest/posttest measurements with one group or two independent measurements with two different groups. Neither of these approaches was appropriate for the tool under study. The tool is used to measure actual clinical practice, and it is not feasible to test a group of nurses on clinical practice before they have been taught to function in a critical care unit. Therefore, only the adjunct item discrimination index was used (Waltz, et al. 1991; Isaac & Michael, 1995).

The discrimination index was computed to measure the effectiveness of an item in relation to the total test in classifying subjects as masters/nonmasters. This was done by checking the proportion of subjects who were classified as masters and nonmasters on the overall test against the proportion of masters and nonmasters on the item (Waltz et al., 1991).

P_o, K, K_{max}, and K/K_{max} ratio are the statistics that were utilized. K_{max} indicates an upper limit value for K with a particular distribution of test results. The K/K_{max} ratio provides a value that can be interpreted on a standard scale. The upper limit of this ratio is 1.00 (Waltz et al., 1991). During this study, the minimum acceptable value for the K/K_{max} ratio was .50. If an item had an index of less than .50, the item was discarded or revised. Although there were a few items that required revision based on the adjunct item discrimination index, the mean of K/K_{max} for the 24 tests ranged from .542 to 1.00.

Content validity was considered at the item and test levels. A panel of experts was utilized to assess the relevance of items and the extent to which they measure the content domain. Since there are 24 objectives

TABLE 8.2 Results of Interrater Reliability Testing

Objective	P_o	K
Category I		
A	0.894	0.777
B	0.895	−0.006
C	0.895	0.441
D	0.875	0.733
E	0.941	0.821
F	0.944	0.770
Category II		
A	1.000	1.000
B	0.931	0.848
C	0.952	0.904
D	0.895	0.784
E	0.875	0.449
F	0.875	−0.059
G	1.000	1.000
H	1.000	1.000
I	0.944	0.870
J	0.850	0.659
K	1.000	1.000
Category III		
A	0.000	0.000
B	0.739	0.405
C	1.000	1.000
Category IV		
A	0.958	0.000
B	1.000	1.000
Category V		
A	1.000	1.000
B	1.000	1.000

on this tool, the items that are measures of each objective were treated as separate tests. The panel of experts was composed of four nurses. One was an assistant nurse coordinator for the medical intensive care unit/coronary care unit. She had a BSN and 4 years of critical care experience. She was a certified critical care registered nurse and a clinical nurse I. The second expert was a master's-prepared nurse who has worked as a clinical specialist and nurse educator in critical care. She was also a critical care registered nurse and at the time of this study, worked part-time in the surgical intensive care unit and the burn intensive care unit. The third expert had a BSN and 4 years of critical care experience and was a critical care registered nurse. She was the staff development coordinator for the medical intensive care unit. The fourth expert had a BSN and 4 years of critical care experience and was a certified critical care registered nurse. She was the staff development coordinator for the surgical intensive care unit.

Item-objective congruence was determined using the method described by Rovinelli and Hambleton (as cited in Waltz et al., 1991). Content specialists assigned a value of +1, 0, or –1 for each item, depending upon the item's congruence with the test objective. A value of +1 indicated that the item was a definite measure of the objective; a value of 0 meant that the judge was undecided; and a rating of –1 indicated that the item was not a measure of the objective. These data were then used to compute the index of item-objective congruence. The limits of this index range from –1.00 to +1.00, with +1.00 indicating perfect positive item-objective congruence. After the index was computed for each item, only those items with an index of +.80 or higher were retained.

Of a total 149 items, there were 13 with an index of item-objective congruence less than .80. Such items were refined, moved to a different section on the test, or deleted.

The content specialists were asked to rate the relevance of each item to the content domain. Interrater agreement was then determined. The P_o was calculated and reflects the items given a rating of Not/Somewhat Relevant and Quite/Very Relevant by two content specialists. Therefore, the P_o represents the "consistency of judges' ratings of the relevance of the group of items within the test to the specified content domain" (Waltz et al., 1991, p. 198). K represents P_o corrected for chance agreements. P_o was calculated to be .97, and *K*, .40.

The average congruency percentage was calculated as a further estimation of content validity. This involved calculating the proportion of items rated congruent by each judge and converting this to a percentage (Waltz et al., 1991). The average congruency percentage was then calculated by determining the mean percentage for all four judges.

Only three objectives had average congruencies of less than 90%. Items for each of these objectives were carefully scrutinized, and possible reasons for the low ratings were considered. Some of the items were then changed, some moved to a different section on the test, and some were discarded. The tool appearing at the end of this chapter includes the revisions made on the basis of the reliability and validity testing.

This study resulted in the development of a criterion-referenced tool for the objective evaluation of clinical performance of critical care nurses. The tool may be used by nurse managers, educators in practice settings, or nursing school faculty to document competence in critical care nursing. Since it provides a mechanism for competency assessment, the tool may prove useful in documenting the impact of staff development programs on clinical performance of critical care nurses.

The results of reliability testing showed that 18 of the 24 tests had evidence of interrater reliability. Substantial revisions were made in the remaining six tests.

Validity exercises indicated that the tool is valuable for assessing clinical performance of critical care nurses. When the index of item-objective congruence was computed for each of the 149 items, only 13 were found to have values less than .80. Appropriate revisions were made in these items. Interrater agreement was assessed to evaluate the relevance of items to the content domain of the test. Strong evidence of relevance was demonstrated by a *Po* of .97 and a *K* of .40. Further evidence of content validity was demonstrated when the average congruency percentage was calculated. Of 24 objectives, only three were found to have values less than 90%. Appropriate revisions were made.

Information obtained during item analysis further supported the relevance of test items to the content domain of the test. The adjunct item discrimination index was computed, and .50 for the K/K_{max} was used as a cutoff for retaining items. Although this value is fairly lenient, it was appropriate for this initial validity testing.

The Clinical Performance Examination for Critical Care Nurses was originally constructed in 1988. The focus of the examination is an evaluation of basic competency in critical care clinical practice. Although the objectives included on the tool maintain relevance today, certain competency statements are not reflective of today's standards of practice. Examples would include items referring to management of restraints (I.F.1., II.A.4.), care of Pavulonized patients (II.A.9., II.F.5.), use of single-use disposable suction catheters (II.F.2.), performance of routine IV site care (II.J.4.), and use of Betadine ointment for central line dressings (II.J.4.). Changes in Joint Commission on American Health Care Organizations (JCAHO) standards, development of new drugs and equipment, and changes in Centers for Disease Control and Prevention (CDC) guidelines mandate changes in these and possibly other areas. The tool is retained in its original form for this publication, however, as the extensive reliability and validity testing was done on the original tool. Ideally, modification in the tool and further testing will be implemented in the future. Additional work should include development of a guide to be used by examiners, specifying precisely the behaviors that must be demonstrated in order for an item to be rated Done.

Priority setting is the one aspect of clinical performance that is not addressed in this tool. A mechanism for evaluating priority setting in clinical practice needs to be incorporated as evolution of the tool continues.

REFERENCES

American Association of Critical Care Nurses. (1981). *Standards for nursing care of the critically ill.* Reston, VA: Reston Publishing.

Isaac, S., & Michael, W. B. (1995). *Handbook in research and evaluation* (3rd ed.). San Diego, CA: EdITS.

Mims, B. C. (1988). Development of a clinical performance examination for critical care nurses. In O. L. Strickland & C. F. Waltz (Eds.), *Measurement of nursing outcomes: Vol. 2. Measuring nursing performance: Practice, education, and research* (pp. 96–122). New York: Springer Publishing Company.

Redman, R. W., Lenburg, C. B., & Hinton Walker, P. (1999, September 30). Competency assessment methods for development and implementation in nursing education. *Online Journal of Issues in Nursing* [On-line serial]. Available: http://www.nursingworld.org/ojin/topic/tpc10_3.htm.

Scott, B. (1982). Competency-based learning: A literature review. *International Journal of Nursing Studies, 19*(3), 119–124.

Survis, J. P. & Grey, M. T. (1995). The anatomy of a competency. *Journal of Nursing Staff Development 11*(5), 247–252.

Waltz, C. F., Strickland, O. L., & Lenz, E. R. (1991). *Measurement in nursing research* (2nd ed.). Philadelphia: F. A. Davis.

CLINICAL PERFORMANCE EXAMINATION
FOR CRITICAL CARE NURSES

Name   Employee number

Examination date   Unit

I. Assessment

Score ____   When caring for a critically ill adult patient, the nurse per-
                 forms a head-to-toe assessment within one hour of arriving
                 at the bedside

		Done	Not done	Not observed	Not applicable
Raw Score ____ Maximum Possible Raw Score ____ Percentage Score ____ Cut Score <u>5+</u> Master ____ Nonmaster ____	A. Performs complete neurological system assessment				
	1. Assesses level of consciousness	____	____	____	____
	2. Assesses orientation	____	____	____	____
	a. person	____	____	____	____
	b. place	____	____	____	____
	c. time	____	____	____	____
	3. Check pupils				
	a. size	____	____	____	____
	b. reaction to light	____	____	____	____
	4. Evaluates ability to move extremities, purposeful or not	____	____	____	____
	5. Checks grasps				
	a. strength	____	____	____	____
	b. equality	____	____	____	____
Raw Score ____ Maximum Possible Raw Score ____ Percentage Score ____ Cut Score <u>10–</u> Master ____ Nonmaster ____	B. Performs complete cardiovascular system assessment				
	1. Obtains cardiac monitor strip	____	____	____	____
	2. Interprets cardiac monitor strip	____	____	____	____

3. Checks blood
    pressure

4. Checks heart
    rate   ____ ____   ____   ____

5. Assesses skin   ____ ____   ____   ____
    a. warm or cool   ____ ____   ____   ____
    b. moist or dry   ____ ____   ____   ____

6. Auscultates heart
    sounds   ____ ____   ____   ____

7. Palpates
    peripheral pulses   ____ ____   ____   ____

8. Checks IV   ____ ____   ____   ____
    a. patency   ____ ____   ____   ____
    b. type of fluid
       as ordered   ____ ____   ____   ____
    c. rate   ____ ____   ____   ____

9. Checks Swan-
    Ganz catheter   ____ ____   ____   ____
    a. system intact   ____ ____   ____   ____
    b. PA waveform
       visible   ____ ____   ____   ____
    c. line free of
       air bubbles   ____ ____   ____   ____

10. Checks arterial
    line   ____ ____   ____   ____
    a. evaluates
       circulation in
       extremity
       distal to
       insertion site   ____ ____   ____   ____

Raw Score ____   C. Performs complete
Maximum   pulmonary system
 Raw Score ____   assessment
Percentage
 Score ____   1. Checks oxygen
Cut Score <u>4–</u>   administration
Master ____   device   ____ ____   ____   ____
Nonmaster ____   2. Evaluates
                      respirations   ____ ____   ____   ____

3. Auscultates
    breath sounds   ____ ____   ____   ____

4. Checks chest
    tubes   ____ ____   ____   ____
    a. system intact   ____ ____   ____   ____
    b. underwater
       seal intact   ____ ____   ____   ____

c. suction set
    as ordered   ____   ____   ____   ____
d. fluctuating?   ____   ____   ____   ____
e. bubbling?   ____   ____   ____   ____
f. subcutaneous
    crepitus   ____   ____   ____   ____

Raw Score ____   D. Performs complete
Maximum   gastro-intestinal
 Possible   system assessment
 Raw Score ____   1. Checks for
Percentage   abdominal
 Score ____   distention (girth
Cut Score 5–   if applicable)   ____   ____   ____   ____
Master ____   2. Checks for
Nonmaster ____   tenderness on
                         palpation   ____   ____   ____   ____

                   3. Auscultates
                       bowel sounds   ____   ____   ____   ____

                   4. Checks NG
                       tube   ____   ____   ____   ____
                       a. color of
                           aspirate   ____   ____   ____   ____
                       b. PH if
                           appropriate   ____   ____   ____   ____
                       c. suction
                           (if ordered)   ____   ____   ____   ____

                   5. Checks
                       abdominal drains ____   ____   ____   ____
                       a. checks
                           functioning
                           of drain   ____   ____   ____   ____
                       b. describes
                           drainage   ____   ____   ____   ____

Raw Score ____   E. Performs complete
Maximum   renal/metabolic
 Possible   system assessment
 Raw Score ____   1. Checks urinary
Percentage   drainage system   ____   ____   ____   ____
 Score ____   2. Checks results
Cut Score 4–   of last SAD
Master ____   (within 1 hour
Nonmaster ____   of arrival at
                         bedside)   ____   ____   ____   ____

                   3. Takes
                       temperature   ____   ____   ____   ____

4. Checks
   hypothermia unit
   (when present) ____ ____ ____ ____

Raw Score ____   F. Performs complete
Maximum   musculoskeletal
  Possible   system assessment
  Raw Score ____
Percentage   1. Checks restraints ____ ____ ____ ____
  Score ____   a. safely applied
Cut Score 3–   b. explanation
Master ____   given to
Nonmaster ____   patient ____ ____ ____ ____

2. Checks integrity
   of skin ____ ____ ____ ____

3. Notes measures
   utilized to
   prevent decubiti ____ ____ ____ ____
   a. pillo pump ____ ____ ____ ____
   b. heel protectors ____ ____ ____ ____

II. Clinical/Technical Skills

Score ____   When caring for a critically ill adult patient, the nurse intern
performs the clinical/technical skills that are common in
critical care nursing practice

Raw Score ____   A. Adheres to safety
Maximum   procedures
  Possible
  Raw Score ____   1. Checks
Percentage   emergency
  Score ____   equipment within
Cut Score 13–   30 minutes of
Master ____   arriving at
Nonmaster ____   bedside ____ ____ ____ ____
                  a. Ambu bag ____ ____ ____ ____
                  b. flow meter ____ ____ ____ ____
                  c. O_2 tubing ____ ____ ____ ____
                  d. nipple ____ ____ ____ ____
                  e. suction ____ ____ ____ ____

2. Replaces missing
   items of
   emergency
   equipment ____ ____ ____ ____

3. Keeps side rails
   up when not at
   bedside ____ ____ ____ ____

4. Restrains wrists
of intubated
patients when
not at bedside   ____ ____   ____   ____

5. Checks cardiac
monitor alarms
for proper
functioning within
30 minutes of
arriving at bedside ____ ____   ____   ____

6. Sets cardiac
monitor limits at
25% +/− heart
rate   ____ ____   ____   ____

7. Checks to be sure
disconnect alarm
(low pressure or
low volume) on
ventilator is on
and functioning
within 30 minutes
of arriving at
bedside   ____ ____   ____   ____

8. Maintains secure
position of
endotracheal/
tracheostomy tube ____ ____   ____   ____

9. Tapes eyelids
closed if patient is
Pavulonized   ____ ____   ____   ____

10. Verifies NG tube
placement prior
to instilling fluids/
medications   ____ ____   ____   ____

11. Covers stopcock
ports with
injection caps   ____ ____   ____   ____

12. Ensures that
patient is wearing
a legible arm band ____ ____   ____   ____

13. Washes hands
prior to
performing
"clean"
procedures   ____ ____   ____   ____

14. Washes hands after performing "dirty" procedures ____ ____ ____ ____

15. Ensures that special electrical equipment has current certification label ____ ____ ____ ____

Raw Score ____
Maximum
 Possible
 Raw Score ____
Percentage
 Score ____
Cut Score 5–
Master ____
Nonmaster ____

B. Performs general physical care

1. Turns immobilized patients at least every 2 hours (unless contra-indicated by patient's condition) ____ ____ ____ ____

2. Provides for privacy when giving bath, bed-pan, etc. ____ ____ ____ ____

3. Applies heel protectors if indicated ____ ____ ____ ____

4. Gives passive ROM to immobilized patients 1 × per shift (unless contraindicated) ____ ____ ____ ____

5. Performs Foley care 1 × per shift ____ ____ ____ ____

6. Correctly measures and records I & O: ____ ____ ____ ____
   a. Measures and records urine output +/– 10 minutes of the hour ____ ____ ____ ____
   b. Records all IV fluids infused during shift ____ ____ ____ ____

c. Measures
amounts in all
drainage bags/
bottles and
records at end
of shift (or as
indicated)
(NG, CT,
axioms, etc.) ____ ____ ____ ____
d. Totals I's and
O's correctly ____ ____ ____ ____
e. Leaves IV
credits for
next shift ____ ____ ____ ____

Raw Score ____   C. Administers medications
Maximum
 Possible
 Raw Score ____
Percentage
 Score ____
Cut Score <u>5–</u>
Master ____
Nonmaster ____

     1. Looks up
medications prior
to administering
if unfamiliar with
normal dose,
action, side
effects, and route ____ ____ ____ ____

2. Checks
appropriate
parameters prior
to giving medica-
tions (blood
pressure with
antihypertensives,
SAD/dextrostik
with insulin,
PCWP, UOP, K+
with Lasix, HR
and K+ with dig,
BP with MS,
Valium, etc.) ____ ____ ____ ____

3. Administers all
medications
within 30 minutes
before or after
time due ____ ____ ____ ____

4. Clamps NG tube
for 30 minutes
after instilling
medications
(not including
antacids) ____ ____ ____ ____

5. Signs out controlled substances and follows correct wastage procedure ___ ___ ___ ___

Raw Score ___
Maximum
 Raw Score ___
Percentage
 Score ___
Cut Score <u>6–</u>
Master ___
Nonmaster ___

D. Administers intra-venous therapy

1. Maintains flow rate within 10% +/– ordered rate ___ ___ ___ ___

2. Time tapes IV bag (unless KO rate) ___ ___ ___ ___

3. Changes IV tubing according to unit routine ___ ___ ___ ___

4. Calculates mcg/kg/min of cardiovascular infusions within 15 minutes of changing infusion rate ___ ___ ___ ___

5. Calculates mcg/kg/min of cardiovascular infusion within 1 hour of arrival at bedside ___ ___ ___ ___

6. Identifies line for emergency drug infusion within 1 hour of arrival at bedside ___ ___ ___ ___

7. Checks reference source to determine amount of fluid and infusion rate of PB medications ___ ___ ___ ___

Raw Score ___

Maximum
 Possible
 Raw Score ___

Percentage
 Score ___

Cut Score _9–_

Master ___

Nonmaster ___

E. Performs
hemodynamic
monitoring

1. Levels air fluid
interface with
right atrium
(4th ICS,
midaxillary line)   ___   ___   ___   ___

2. Calibrates
monitor prior
to obtaining
first readings
each shift   ___   ___   ___   ___

3. Assures that
pressure gauge
on blood pump
is set at
300 mmHg   ___   ___   ___   ___

4. Changes flush
bag and tubing
according to
unit policy   ___   ___   ___   ___

5. Obtains PA
systolic, diastolic,
mean, and PCWP
correctly and
records every
2 hours
(or as ordered)   ___   ___   ___   ___

6. Displays Swan-
Ganz wave form
on oscilloscope to
monitor for
wedging of Swan   ___   ___   ___   ___

7. Checks cuff BP
and compares to
arterial line BP
within 1 hour of
arrival at bedside   ___   ___   ___   ___

8. Draws blood
specimens
correctly from
arterial line   ___   ___   ___   ___

9. Obtains cardiac
output values
correctly   ___   ___   ___   ___

Raw Score ____
Maximum
  Possible
  Raw Score ____
Percentage
  Score ____
Cut Score <u>5–</u>
Master ____
Nonmaster ____

F. Manages patient-
   ventilator system

1. Keeps ventilator
   tubing free of
   water (empties
   into receptacle,
   not into cascade) ____ ____ ____ ____

2. Suctions patient
   PRN ____ ____ ____ ____

   a. Recognizes
      when patient
      needs to be
      suctioned ____ ____ ____ ____

   b. Sets suction
      regulator at
      –80 to –120
      mmHg ____ ____ ____ ____

   c. Maintains
      sterile
      technique
      during entire
      suctioning
      process;
      discards
      catheter if
      contaminated
      and begins
      again if task is
      not completed ____ ____ ____ ____

   d. Places finger
      over hole and
      withdraws
      catheter using
      a rotating
      motion ____ ____ ____ ____

   e. Uses
      continuous
      suction and
      limits suction
      time to a
      maximum of
      10 seconds ____ ____ ____ ____

   f. Observes the
      cardiac
      monitor for
      dysrhythmias
      and patient
      for signs
      of distress ____ ____ ____ ____

g. Disposes of
   contaminated
   catheter   ____   ____   ____   ____

3. Calculates SEC
   (per unit routine
   or if asked
   to do so)   ____   ____   ____   ____

4. Takes appropriate
   action when
   alarms sound
   or can describe
   these actions
   when asked   ____   ____   ____   ____

5. Administers
   sedatives PRN
   for patients
   receiving
   Pavulon   ____   ____   ____   ____

Raw Score ____   G. Administers tube
Maximum   feedings   ____   ____   ____   ____
 Possible
 Raw Score ____   1. Rinses
Percentage   administration
 Score ____   bag and tubing
Cut Score <u>4–</u>   with tap water
Master ____   when adding
Nonmaster ____   new formula   ____   ____   ____   ____

2. Delivers correct
   formula   ____   ____   ____   ____

3. Maintains correct
   flow rate   ____   ____   ____   ____

4. Hangs new
   formula every
   8 hours   ____   ____   ____   ____

5. Irrigates feeding
   tube every 4 hours
   with 10 cc saline   ____   ____   ____   ____

Raw Score ____   H. Administers
Maximum   hyperalimentation
 Possible
 Raw Score ____   1. Check label on
Percentage   bottle with
 Score ____   physician's
Cut Score <u>5–</u>   order sheet   ____   ____   ____   ____
Master ____
Nonmaster ____

2. Checks patient's latest SMA results (K+, glucose) and notifies physician of abnormalities ____ ____ ____ ____

3. Hangs bottle using aseptic technique ____ ____ ____ ____

4. Checks fluid level with time tape every 2 hours ____ ____ ____ ____

5. Checks SADs every 6 hours ____ ____ ____ ____

6. Changes IV dressing and tubing to hub according to unit policy ____ ____ ____ ____

Raw Score ____
Maximum
 Possible
 Raw Score ____
Percentage
 Score ____
Cut Score <u>8–</u>
Master ____
Nonmaster ____

I. Changes peripheral IV/arterial line dressings

1. If needed, changes IV tubing to catheter hub prior to cleansing IV site ____ ____ ____ ____

2. Dons sterile gloves ____ ____ ____ ____

3. Cleanses IV site with Betadine solution ____ ____ ____ ____

4. Applies Betadine ointment ____ ____ ____ ____

5. Covers IV site with sterile dressing ____ ____ ____ ____

6. Documents appearance of IV site ____ ____ ____ ____

7. Writes date, time, and initials on new dressing ____ ____ ____ ____

8. Maintains sterile
technique
throughout
dressing change ____ ____ ____ ____

Raw Score ____
Maximum
 Possible
 Raw Score ____
Percentage
 Score ____
Cut Score <u>7–</u>
Master ____
Nonmaster ____

J. Changes central
line dressing

1. Dons sterile
gloves ____ ____ ____ ____

2. Cleanses
insertion site
with acetone
if soiled ____ ____ ____ ____

3. Cleanses with
Betadine solution ____ ____ ____ ____

4. Applies Betadine
ointment and
Benzoin
(if needed) ____ ____ ____ ____

5. Applies tape ____ ____ ____ ____

6. Writes date, time,
and initials on
new dressing ____ ____ ____ ____

7. Maintains sterile
technique
throughout
dressing change ____ ____ ____ ____

Raw Score ____
Maximum
 Possible
 Raw Score ____
Percentage
 Score ____
Cut Score <u>9–</u>
Master ____
Nonmaster ____

K. Changes dressing of
open wound every
shift or as ordered
by physician

1. Dons mask, cap,
and nonsterile
gloves ____ ____ ____ ____

2. Removes and
deposits old
dressing in plastic
bag. If unable to
remove entire
dressing, dons
sterile gloves to
remove inner
layers ____ ____ ____ ____

3. Changes sterile
   gloves   ____ ____   ____   ____

4. Cleanses wound
   with 4 × 4 soaked
   with solution
   ordered   ____ ____   ____   ____

5. Dresses wound
   according to
   physician's order   ____ ____   ____   ____

6. Secures dressing
   correctly   ____ ____   ____   ____

7. Notifies MD of
   any deteriorating
   change in wound
   appearance (dusky
   appearance,
   necrotic areas)   ____ ____   ____   ____

8. Closes bag
   containing old
   dressing and
   deposits in trash   ____ ____   ____   ____

9. Maintains sterile
   technique
   throughout
   dressing change   ____ ____   ____   ____

III. Communication

Score ____

The nurse intern interacts and communicates with others in a courteous and professional manner

Raw Score ____
Maximum
 Possible
 Raw Score ____
Percentage
 Score ____
Cut Score _3–_
Master ____
Nonmaster ____

A. Participates in unit
   activities and interacts
   effectively with
   co-workers

   1. Readily assists
      other nurses
      when indicated   ____ ____   ____   ____

   2. Gives thorough,
      concise, verbal
      reports using
      systems approach ____ ____   ____   ____

3. States name of
    unit and own
    name when
    answering
    telephone   ____ ____ ____   ____

4. Refrains from
    inappropriate
    conversation at
    the bedside   ____ ____ ____   ____

Raw Score ____   B. Communicates
Maximum   effectively with
 Possible   patients
 Raw Score ____   1. Introduces self
Percentage   to patient at
 Score ____   beginning of
Cut Score 7–   shift   ____ ____ ____   ____
Master ____
Nonmaster ____   2. Orients patient
                         to time and place
                         if necessary   ____ ____ ____   ____

                     3. Provides means
                         of communica-
                         tion for patients
                         who are
                         intubated   ____ ____ ____   ____

                     4. Informs patient
                         prior to drawing
                         blood, giving
                         injections, etc.   ____ ____ ____   ____

                     5. Provides verbal
                         support and
                         comfort during
                         painful procedures
                         (Swan-Ganz, CVP,
                         arterial line, CT
                         insertion)   ____ ____ ____   ____

                     6. Refrains from
                         discussing patient
                         at the bedside   ____ ____ ____   ____

                     7. Ensures that call
                         light is within
                         reach when not
                         present at the
                         bedside   ____ ____ ____   ____

Raw Score ____
Maximum
 Possible
 Raw Score ____
Percentage
 Score ____
Cut Score <u>2–</u>
Master ____
Nonmaster ____

C. Communicates with
    and provides support
    for family members

1. If family is
    available, makes
    contact with
    them at least
    once per shift   ____ ____   ____   ____

2. Stays with family
    during visits at
    bedside to
    provide support
    and answer
    questions   ____ ____   ____   ____

IV. Documentation

Score ____

The nurse intern completes all aspects of documentation

Raw Score ____
Maximum
 Possible
 Raw Score ____
Percentage
 Score ____
Cut Score <u>9–</u>
Master ____
Nonmaster ____

A. Documents all nursing
    interventions, including
    patient's response when
    appropriate

1. Charts complete
    physical assess-
    ment within 3
    hours of arriving
    at bedside   ____ ____   ____   ____

2. Records within
    10 minutes of
    taking vital signs   ____ ____   ____   ____

3. Documents all
    medications
    within 10 minutes
    of administering   ____ ____   ____   ____

4. Documents
    effects of PRN
    medication   ____ ____   ____   ____

5. Documents lab
    results within 30
    minutes of
    receiving   ____ ____   ____   ____

6. Documents support of family or significant others   ____   ____   ____   ____

7. Documents explanations/ patient teaching performed   ____   ____   ____   ____

8. Documents patient's anxiety and appropriate nursing interventions   ____   ____   ____   ____

9. Completes patient classification units each shift   ____   ____   ____   ____

10. Uses no unauthorized abbreviations   ____   ____   ____   ____

11. Signs name using first name, last name, R.N.   ____   ____   ____   ____

12. Documents verbal orders on physician's order sheet   ____   ____   ____   ____

Raw Score ____
Maximum
 Possible
 Raw Score ____
Percentage
 Score ____
Cut Score <u>3–</u>
Master ____
Nonmaster ____

B. Maintains complete and current care plan for each patient

1. Ensures that care plan includes one problem in each of the following areas:
   a. physical   ____   ____   ____   ____
   b. psychosocial   ____   ____   ____   ____
   c. teaching   ____   ____   ____   ____

2. Includes long-term or discharge goals on care plan   ____   ____   ____   ____

3. Updates Kardex on a daily basis   ____   ____   ____   ____

V. General Employment Policies

Score ____   Follows hospital policy regarding dress and punctuality

Raw Score ____   A.   Adheres to uniform
Maximum   regulations
 Possible
 Raw Score ____   1.   Wears white
Percentage   uniform, light-
 Score ____   colored top over
Cut Score <u>3–</u>   white uniform
Master ____   pants, or scrub
Nonmaster ____   clothes   ____   ____   ____   ____

                       2.   Wears I.D. card
                            or name badge   ____   ____   ____   ____

                       3.   If hair is longer
                            than shoulder
                            length, wears
                            it pulled back
                            or pinned off
                            the neck   ____   ____   ____   ____

9

Clinical Performance Measure*

Kathryn S. Hegedus, Eloise M. Balasco, and Anne S. Black

PURPOSE

This tool was developed to measure the clinical performance of advanced-level nurses at Children's Hospital in Boston (Hegedus, Balasco, & Black, 1990). It was part of a larger effort to define three levels of practice and develop measures for each. The measurement tool flows from a body of work of the following Professional Advancement and Evaluation Committee members: Pat Kraepelian-Bartels, RNC, MS, head nurse; Jill Stanely-Brown, RN, BSN, BA, staff nurse; Ann Colangelo, RN, BSN, staff nurse; Ruth Fisk, RNC, MS, clinical specialist; Roberta Harding, RN, MSN, head nurse; Ann Jenks, RN, BSN, head nurse; and Susan Shaw, RN, head nurse.

INSTRUMENT DESCRIPTION

Professional nursing practice incorporates the elements of competency, accountability, scientific inquiry, leadership, and humanistic orientation to individuals and the community. Attempts to measure these variables have been elusive, and the elements in existing tools most frequently address processes nurses use to provide care. While it is important to know what the nurse does, the behaviors that identify the qualitative dimensions inherent in progressive practice and to identify them in ways that can be reasonably measured have not been adequately described.

Delineating behaviors that describe the complex knowledge and competencies that nurses are expected to exhibit is central to principles of autonomy and accountability.

---

*This tool may be obtained from Kathryn S. Hegedus, RN, DNSc, University of Connecticut, School of Nursing, Storrs, CT 06269.

The purpose of the Professional Advancement Program at the Children's Hospital is to define nursing practice behaviors descriptive of movement toward expert practice and to recognize and reward that practice (A. Black, Memorandum, The Children's Hospital, 1984). The program now recognizes three levels of practice, which are described in performance criteria. A formal process for advancement is in place.

The system is built on the premise that the staff nurse I role is the first level of nursing practice that is a fully acceptable level of practice. Certain nurses, within varying time frames, will choose to seek advancement beyond the staff nurse I role. Progression beyond this first designation requires high levels of competency in professional practice, combined with distinctive integration of leadership, educational, and research competencies and activities. The characteristics ascribed to a staff nurse III are the ability to reason intuitively, reduce artifacts, and quickly grasp the whole. They rely less on deliberative analysis of the clinical situation; thus, their performance is more holistic. This is in contrast to staff nurses I and II, who perform in a more incremental manner and rely to a higher degree on procedure and process.

Responsibilities for seeking promotion to advanced practice levels reside primarily with each individual nurse. A board of review of the Professional Advancement Program has been established to provide a strong component of peer review for all candidates seeking promotion to staff nurse III. The board affirms attainment of staff nurse III role requirements, recommends for or against appointment, assures standardization of expectations and processes, monitors system equity, and compiles system data relevant to staff nurse III profiles.

A criterion refers to a set standard of behavior. Criterion-referenced measurement is used to determine an individual's performance against specific behavioral criteria. The measurement tool devised to examine the clinical performance of the staff nurse III utilizes a criterion-referenced approach to measurement.

Within the framework of the Professional Advancement Program, the following four practice domains have been identified for the staff nurse III level: (a) clinical practice, (b) clinical leadership, (c) professional growth/continuing education, and (d) nursing research. Stem statements that operationalize the domain in a qualitative way were generated. In addition, for each stem, critical elements were developed that describe specific behaviors for each domain. The final tool has a total of seven stems and 27 critical elements. Table 9.1 provides an example of a stem and the critical elements.

This tool is a rating scale that allows the supervisor or head nurse to rate the nurse's performance, or the nurse may do a self-rating.

The instrument has two columns or possible choices for determining performance as being present either "consistently" or "intermittently." Data that follow provide findings using this model, but it is recognized that this portion of the tool requires further evaluation. Acceptable performance levels specifying the percentage of items or specific items in each practice domain that must receive a rating of "consistently" have not yet been determined by the tool's developers.

RELIABILITY AND VALIDITY ASSESSMENTS

Members of the Professional Advancement and Evaluation Committee were responsible for devising the tool utilizing content from a long progression of developmental work and incorporating the work of Benner (1984). The committee membership includes directors of nursing, clinical specialists, head nurses, and staff nurses, all of whom serve as content specialists in the establishment of the criteria.

A pilot test of the instrument was conducted to assess the congruence between the self-ratings of nurses in the staff nurse III role and that of their supervisors. Each nurse in the staff nurse III role utilized the tool independently to evaluate the performance of the nurse or nurses reporting to her. It is important to note that for purposes of the piloting phase, persons were asked to utilize the tool at the time of entry into the role, although the tool is designed to be used both as a pre-entry guide and as an assessment tool for the nurse designated as a staff nurse.

TABLE 9.1 Sample Items: Stem and Critical Elements Showing Domain of Nursing Research

Demonstrates competency in nursing research	*Consistently*	*Intermittently*
1. Critically analyzes research studies to justify the inclusion/exclusion of findings in the rationale for nursing decisions		
2. Collaborates in the research activities of colleagues as appropriate		
3. Identifies researchable problems and communicates these in a spirit of inquiry		
4. Designs and implements research studies and reports these findings at professional meetings or in professional publications		

The pilot sample of staff nurses consisted of five women, four of whom held a bachelor's degree and one of whom held a master's degree. They ranged in age from 30 to 32, having practiced in nursing between 6 and 10 years, with 5 to 7 of those years at the Children's Hospital.

Because of the small sample size and limited variability in scores, a measure of internal consistency was not obtained. As sample size increases, the Kuder-Richardson 20 statistic will be used to obtain a reliability measure.

Content validity (Waltz, Strickland, & Lenz, 1991) was established by using a panel of qualified experts (three staff nurses and three head nurses who were not members of the committee). They determined, independently of one another, the adequacy of each critical element for representing the domain of practice. The range for percentage of agreement was from 74% to 100% (Table 9.2) This tool was determined to be valid and was used for the pilot test.

Each staff nurse III and her respective manager received a package containing the tool and directions for completion of the tool. The directions for completion of the instrument required placing a check mark for each of the 27 items in the column (either consistently or intermittently) that best described their current practice in relation to each of the items, and in working independently of others.

The staff nurses rated their performance by marking the critical elements "consistent" 80% of the time, in comparison to the head nurses, who marked the items as "consistent" 89% of the time. The staff nurses

TABLE 9.2 Percentage of Agreement for the Stems and Critical Elements

Stem	No. of items	% Agreement
Clinical practice		
I	5	100
II	4	74
Clinical leadership		
III	3	100
IV	3	96
Professional growth/ continuing education		
V	4	88
VI	4	96
Nursing research		
VII	4	96

chose "intermittent" 20% of the time in contrast to the head nurses, who made this choice 11% of the time. The 9% discrepancy between staff nurses and head nurses occurred predominantly in the areas of professional growth/continuing education and nursing research. The domains of clinical practice and clinical leadership were congruent.

When the scores for the staff nurse III self-ratings and ratings by the head nurses were correlated for the five subjects, the Pearson product-moment correlation coefficient was $r = .85$. This provides a validity index that reflects a fairly high level of congruence between the self-ratings and the head nurse rating.

Clearly, the issues of scoring need further assessment and continuing development. One possible new approach is the assignment of a combined score from the subject's assessment of his/her own performance and that of a peer evaluator. Another strategy that might be applied to the tool is factor analysis by subscale. This second strategy would result in a measure of internal consistency, thereby providing an additional reliability estimate (i.e., theta coefficient) (Armor, 1974).

Additional work is needed for establishing pass or cut scores. It is recognized that the final tool will allow for differences in proficiency level and that some domains will have higher standards than others. For example, clinical practice and clinical leadership would require high levels of competency, whereas professional growth/continuing education and research could have lower passing points.

This study demonstrates the value of research directed toward measurement of behaviors associated with advancing clinical practice. The valuable involvement of staff nurses in the research process has also been described.

Members of he Professional Advancement and Evaluation Committee of the Children's Hospital have utilized the four domains described in the staff nurse III criteria and devised critical elements to examine the performance of staff nurses I and II. A panel of experts has established content validity, and these tools are now ready for further testing. All of these tools allow for assessment of nursing competencies and move in the direction of examining behaviors, not processes. The comparison of the three instruments now indicates the need to revise the tool for staff nurse III.

Implications for nursing are seen from the perspective of both the individual and the discipline. The interface between the two is based on the assumption that nursing is a practice discipline; thus, its theory base can best be described and tested in the arena of care.

The ability to establish measures that would identify practice behaviors along a continuum from novice to expert allows for the portrayal of nursing with all of its complex scientific and artistic dimensions. The tool permits examination of individual performance, and from this description, patterns of practice emerge that signify a body of knowledge inductively built. In turn, hypotheses are formulated and tested with implications for strengthening and building a science of practice. The tool has been used in a study by Hegedus (1994).

REFERENCES

Armor, D. F. (1974). Theta reliability and factor scaling. In H. L. Costner (Ed.), *Sociological methodology* (pp. 17–50). San Francisco: Jossey-Bass.

Benner, P. (1984). *From novice to expert: Excellence and power in clinical nursing practice.* Menlo Park, CA: Addison-Wesley.

Hegedus, K. S., Balasco, E. M., & Black, A. S. (1988). Measuring clinical performance. In O. L. Strickland & C. F. Waltz (Eds.), *Measurement of nursing outcomes: Vol. 2. Measuring nursing performance: practice, education, and research* (123–132). New York: Springer Publishing Company.

Hegedus, K. S. (1994). Caring and learning: A mosaic. In D. A. Du Gaut, A. Boykin (Eds.). *Caring as healing: Renewal through hope* (pp. 265–273). New York: National League for Nursing.

Waltz, C. F., Strickland, O. L., & Lenz, E. R. (1991). *Measurement in nursing research* (2nd ed.). Philadelphia: F. A. Davis.

10

Measuring Quality of Nursing Care for DRGs Using the HEW-Medicus Nursing Process Methodology*

Elizabeth A. Barrett

PURPOSE

This chapter discuses the **HEW-Medicus Nursing Process Methodology** (H-MNPM), a measure of nursing care in relation to Diagnosis Related Groups (DRGs). This measurement protocol was undertaken (Barrett, 1988) to develop and test a methodology to score quality monitoring data, using specific DRGs as the level of analysis (Jelinek, Haussmann, Hegyvary, 1977; Haussmann, Hegyvary, & Newman, 1976).

INSTRUMENT DESCRIPTION

Health care records can be an effective, comprehensive source of data for determining the quality of health care outcomes (Richardson, Selby-Harrington, Krowchuk, Cross, & Williams, 1994). Advantages of using health care records for this purpose include access to large representative data samples at relatively low cost and accuracy (Krowchuk, Moore, & Richardson, 1995). The outcome variable was the quality of nursing care scores for specific case-mix categories. Quality of nursing care was measured by an assessment of the nursing process (H-MNPM). A methodology was developed to utilize case-mix categories—specifically, the New York state system of DRGs—as the level of analysis rather than the nursing unit. The outcome was the quality of care indicator(s) for patients

---

* Available from U.S. Government Printing Office, Washington, DC, DHEW Publication No. HRA 76-25.

with particular DRGs. This project had as its specific goal to develop and test a methodology for converting raw data from the H-MNPM into quality scores for patients with particular DRGs rather than into quality scores for particular nursing units. In future research, quality of nursing care scores for patients can be related to revenue aspects of patient care.

Available tools for measuring quality of nursing care in a hospital setting were evaluated to determine their usefulness for the current project. As a result of this analysis, the H-MNPM was selected because of the rigor with which it was developed and tested and because of the evidence for reliability and validity resulting from several revisions and retesting (Hegyvary, Gortner, & Haussmann, 1976). A description of the development and testing of this measure follows.

The H-MNPM was developed through a contract from the Division of Nursing Health Resources Administration, U.S. Department of Health, Education and Welfare with the Rush-Presbyterian-St. Luke's Medical Center and through them to the Medicus Corporation (Jelinek et al., 1974).

The H-MNPM (Ward & Lindeman, 1979) measures the quality of nursing care by an assessment of the nursing process defined as the assessing, planning, implementing, and evaluating components of care. From a master set of 357 evaluative criteria, a computer-generated set of criteria were produced for 32 subobjectives that fall within a framework of six major objectives: the plan of care is formulated; the physical needs of the patient are attended; the nonphysical (psychological, emotional, mental, and social) needs of the patient are attended; achievement of nursing care objectives is evaluated; unit procedures are followed for the protection of all patients; and the delivery of nursing care is facilitated by administrative and managerial services. Subobjectives were selected according to patient classification: self-care, partial care, complete care, and intensive care.

Ten percent of a nursing unit's one-month patient census—usually about 20 patients—is reviewed. Observations are randomly distributed across days, patients, and day and evening shifts. Interrater reliability of a minimum of .85 needs to be established by raters prior to each period of data collection. A computer program was developed to produce quality indices for each of the 32 subobjectives and the 6 objectives for each of the monitored units.

An initial set of 900 items was developed by reviewing existing methodologies. The items were examined for measurability and redundancy, and a revised list of approximately 220 items was used in a pilot study in two hospitals. The criteria were then revised, expanded, and field tested in 19 hospitals to establish reliability and validity. Item analyses were included in the reliability studies. The claims for construct validity were based on (a) analysis of scores from 19 hospitals, which indicated that the scores were predictable based on current nursing practices; (b) current trends in nursing education and practice, which led to the hypothesis that components of the nursing process were highly correlated in terms of quality.

The hypothesis was supported by analysis of quality scores from the 19 hospitals ($p = .001$). There was little evidence for concurrent or predictive validity. This methodology represents one of the most widely tested means for measuring quality of nursing care, and features careful attention to conceptual framework, detail, planning, testing, and evaluation. Ward and Lindeman (1979) noted that although the instrument was expensive in terms of resources, it has potential for making a significant contribution to the nursing profession.

The H-MNPM was operational in what was then the current investigator's employing institution, which is a 1,171-bed hospital within a major metropolitan medical center. In addition to being conceptually sound and methodologically sophisticated, advantages to its use in the current project included the consideration of patient classification in generation of items and the availability of alternate forms that were developed according to patient classification and clinical area from the master list of criteria. In addition, the tool had been widely used to assess quality of nursing care for medical, surgical, obstetric, pediatric, and psychiatric patients.

Since the H-MNPM had been developed using the nursing process model as its conceptual basis, this model was also employed as the basis underlying the methodology to provide quality scores for patients with particular DRGs. For this project, the nursing process model was conceptually defined as the assessment of the patient and family, the planning of care based on needs or problems, the implementation of physical and nonphysical aspects of the care plan, and the evaluation of response to care. The nursing process model was operationally defined by selected criteria that fall within the rubric of 32 subobjectives and 6 major objectives. The model contained aspects of clerical and support services since they impact on the nursing process, especially if nurses engage in those activities (Hegyvary, Gortner, & Haussmann, 1976). The operationalization of the framework is presented in Table 10.1.

As stated, the major objective of the current study was to use existing reliable raw data collected for monitoring quality of nursing care on a nursing unit to obtain scores indicative of quality of nursing care for specific case-mix categories of patients. The data collection procedures used in the investigator's institution remained the same. Before each data collection period, a 7.5-hr orientation for data collection was given, and inter-rater reliability established. During data collection, master's-prepared nursing staff educators randomly selected patients for monitoring. Use of these data for the current project provided for a cost-effective and reliable means of data collection. Data concerning DRG classification were available for only a one-year period in which approximately 1,550 patients were monitored and represented numerous DRGs. Small sample size per DRG limited the procedures that could be undertaken for reliability and validity testing within the context of the current study.

TABLE 10.1 Nursing Process Framework

1.0 The plan of nursing care is formulated.
    1.1 The condition of the patient is assessed on admission.
    1.2 Data relevant to hospital care are ascertained on admission.
    1.3 The current condition of the patient is assessed.
    1.4 The written plan of nursing care is formulated.
    1.5 The plan of nursing care is coordinated with the medical plan of care.

2.0 The physical needs of the patient are attended.
    2.1 The patient is protected from accident and injury.
    2.2 The need for physical comfort and rest is attended.
    2.3 The need for physical hygiene is attended.
    2.4 The need for supply of oxygen is attended.
    2.5 The need for activity is attended.
    2.6 The need for nutrition and fluid balance is attended.
    2.7 The need for elimination is attended.
    2.8 The need for skin care is attended.
    2.9 The patient is protected from infection.

3.0 The nonphysical (psychological, emotional, mental, and social) needs of the patient are attended.
    3.1 The patient is oriented to hospital facilities on admission.
    3.2 The patient is extended social courtesy by the nursing staff.
    3.3 The patient's privacy and civil rights are honored.
    3.4 The need for psychological-emotional well-being is attended.
    3.5 The patient is taught measures of health maintenance and illness prevention.
    3.6 The patient's family is included in the nursing care process.

4.0 Achievement of nursing care objectives is evaluated.
    4.1 Records document the care provided for the patient.
    4.2 The patient's response to therapy is evaluated.

5.0 Unit procedures are followed for the protection of all patients.
    5.1 Isolation and decontamination procedures are followed.
    5.2 The unit is prepared for emergency situations.
    5.3 Medical-legal procedures are followed.
    5.4 Unit safety and protective procedures are followed.
6.0 The delivery of nursing care is facilitated by administrative and managerial services.
    6.1 Nursing reporting follows prescribed standards.
    6.2 Nursing management is provided.
    6.3 Clerical services are provided.
    6.4 Environmental and support services are provided.
    6.5 Professional and administrative services are provided.

In cooperation with the medical records department, patient names and identification of specific versions of the tool used for data collection were obtained from a control sheet. The purpose of the control sheet was to avoid monitoring the same patient twice on successive days. The control sheet was essential to link data to a particular patient because neither names nor identification numbers appeared on the data collection instrument in order to protect confidentiality.

Patient names, monitoring data, and nursing units were used to access, via microfiche, patient identification numbers from medical records. The patient ID numbers were used to retrieve the patient's DRG from computerized reports that provide this information. When the number of cases per DRG was determined, two DRGs having the highest number of cases ($n = 43$) were selected for investigation in this study. Quality data were retrieved from the original data collection answer sheets for those patients with the DRGs that were being considered in the study. Information recorded included patient identification number, DRG, and raw data scores for each item monitored during data collection. Patient names were not used in order to ensure confidentiality.

Scoring occurred as described for the H-MNPM, using as the unit of analysis the particular case-mix category. In this study, however, scores were produced only for the first four objectives and subobjectives. The first four objective scores were combined to provide an index of quality of nursing care. This score could be compared with the total index score, which would consider the six subobjectives. Variability by case-mix category could also be explicated for the two total scores: (a) assessing, planning, implementing, and evaluating quality of nursing care; (b) assessing, planning, implementing, and evaluating quality of nursing care, unit procedures, and administrative and managerial services. Although this is a criterion-referenced test, wide variability in scores, in addition to lack of a cutoff score to substantiate achievement of quality, suggested a norm-referenced interpretation. For purposes of this project, percentage scores were used.

RELIABILITY AND VALIDITY ASSESSMENTS

The two highest volume DRGs were selected for reliability and validity testing: normal mature newborn ($n = 43$), and schizoaffective psychosis, manic-depressive psychosis (a single DRG category, $n = 20$).

Interrater reliability for the current project was .94. In addition, item-to-total correlations were computed to test for homogeneity of the criteria in each dimension of the nursing process (objectives 1 to 4). The range for normal mature newborn was .32 to .89, and the range for schizoaffective psychosis, manic-depressive psychosis was .00 to .94. Only subobjectives 1.1, 1.3, 2.3, 3.3, and 3.7 for schizoaffective psychosis, manic-depressive psychosis had item-to-total correlations below .30. Alpha coefficients for the normal mature newborn were .49, .14, .72, and .20 for objectives 1 through 4, respectively. Alpha coefficients for schizoaffective psychosis, manic-depressive psychosis were .32, .13, .47, and .31 for objectives 1 through 4, respectively. Due to small sample size, interpretation should be made cautiously.

Since the instrument was not altered, basic validity remained intact and thus, no attempt was made to assess item content validity as a measure of the extent to which the item was a measure of the content domain. To determine validity of the scoring methodology, whereby quality monitoring data were linked to the patient's DRG rather than to the nursing unit, scores were compared for the normal newborn nurseries (units) with scores for normal newborn patients (DRG). Because not all subobjective items are included in the various versions of the H-MNPM instrument, objective scores are based on an average of subobjective scores, each of which was weighted by the number of items used to measure that subobjective. The scores are not expected to be identical since the DRG sample ($n = 43$) is a subset of data within the larger sample ($n = 64$) representing the nursing units. Differences in sample size are primarily due to inability to retrieve DRG data for all patients and the finding that some patients in the normal newborn nurseries had DRG classifications other than normal newborn. However, scores were similar and supported the validity of the DRG scoring methodology.

Because the psychiatric units had considerable variability regarding DRG classification, a similar comparison was not appropriate.

In summary, results indicate that the proposed methodology is workable. However, procedures should be replicated with a larger sample size allowing more thorough investigation of reliability and validity issues, including factor analysis and/or cluster analysis to assess construct validity.

REFERENCES

Barrett, E. A. (1988). Measuring quality of nursing care for DRGs using the HEW-Medicus nursing process methodology. In O. L. Strickland & C. F. Waltz (Eds.), *Measurement of nursing outcomes: Vol. 2. Measuring nursing performance: practice, education, and research* (154–177). New York: Springer Publishing Company.

Haussmann, R. K. D., & Hegyvary, S. T. (1977). *Monitoring quality of nursing care: Part III* (DHEW Publication No. HRA 77–70). Washington, DC: U.S. Government Printing Office.

Haussmann, R. K. D., Hegyvary, S. T., & Newman, J. F. (1976). *Monitoring quality of nursing care: Part IV* (DHEW Publication No. HRA 76–7). Washington, DC: U.S. Government Printing Office.

Hegyvary, S. T., Gortner, S. R., & Haussmann, R. K. D. (1976). Development of criterion measures for quality of care: The Rush-Medicus experience. In *Issues in Evaluation Research* (pp. 106–114). Kansas City, MO: American Nurses' Association.

Jelinek, R. C., Haussmann, R. K. D., Hegyvary, S. T., & Newman, J. F. (1974). *A methodology for monitoring quality of nursing care* (DHEW Publication No. HRA 76–25). Washington, DC: U.S. Government Printing Office.

Krowchuk, H. V., Moore, M. L. & Richardson, L. (1995). Using health care records as sources of data for research. *Journal of Nursing Measurement, 3*(1), 3–12.

Richardson, L. A., Selby-Harrington, M. L., Krowchuk, H. V., Cross, A. W., & Williams, D. (1994). Comprehensiveness of well-child checkups for children on Medicaid: A pilot study. *Journal of Pediatric Health Care, 8,* 212–220.

Ward, M. J., & Lindeman, C. A. (Eds.). (1979). *Instruments for measuring practice and other health care variables* (Vols. 1–2). Hyattsville, MD: U.S. Department of Health, Education & Welfare (DHEW Publication Nos. 78–53, 78–54).

11

Clinical Evaluation Tool

Carol L. Rossel, Barbara A. Kakta,
Gail A. Vitale, Peggy R. Rice,
Katherine N. McDannel, and Pamela A. Martyn

PURPOSE

The purpose of the **Clinical Evaluation Tool** is to evaluate sophomore, junior, and senior baccalaureate nursing students clinically throughout and at the completion of each clinical course. The intent was to develop an instrument with sufficient flexibility to accommodate various learning experiences, courses, and settings while demonstrating reliability and validity in measuring students' performance. While terminal characteristics may vary by program, the format of the instrument and the evaluation process are considered applicable to other settings.

INSTRUMENT DESCRIPTION

Clinical practice is the essence of nursing for practitioners, educators, researchers, and students. Evaluation of that clinical practice is critical for assurance of patient safety, development and refinement of nursing practice, progression of students, promotion of staff, and justification of funding. Cognitive, psychomotor, and affective learning are accomplished in a myriad of classroom and laboratory settings where control of the learning and concomitant evaluation can be readily achieved. Evaluation of nursing students' clinical experience, however, presents a challenge in that these experiences often vary. Moreover, contemporary student practice occurs in more settings and/or in different kinds of settings than in the past. Thus, for clinical nurse educators evaluation of student learning is most challenging.

Evaluation of student clinical performance has undergone substantial change since the pre-1960's era when the teacher's subjective general impressions of the student's performance were communicated to the student at the end of the clinical rotation (Abrahason, 1985). Today judgments of student performance are based on established standards and include both formative and summative components (Billings & Halstead, 1998).

Schools of nursing are expected to identify terminal characteristics for their graduates and demonstrate how the curriculum provides for their achievement. Characteristics expected of students at the completion of each program level demonstrate student's development of increasingly complex competence toward the mastery of terminal characteristics. Terminal characteristics define the graduate from that educational program. Nursing programs should strive to prepare new nurses for entry level into current nursing practice, as well as motivate graduates for continued growth and development in their professional practice (Acord, 1998).

The conceptual framework selected to guide the development of the instrument incorporates competency-based measurement to evaluate students' progress in clinical practice toward the terminal characteristics. Specifically, criterion-referenced measurement (CRM) was utilized in the development of the instrument.

The instrument reported here is a revision of one developed by Rossel and Kakta (1990). Modifications made to the original tool reflect recommendations in the Pew Health Professions Commission's final report (Bellack & O'Neil, 1998) that challenge educators to incorporate more interdisciplinary, ambulatory practice, and public service experiences in the curriculum, and to produce nurses with group management skills, clinical management skills, technological capabilities, critical thinking, and professional judgment who are ready to practice in community-based settings. Thus, the modified Clinical Practice Evaluation tool provides for changes in the practice arena of nursing and incorporation of new objectives that could be used in nontraditional, as well as traditional settings.

The eight steps of the process undertaken in developing this tool included: (a) development of terminal objectives; (b) development of level outcome characteristics; (c) identification of conceptual areas of content; (d) identification and labeling of tracks; (e) identification and labeling within tracks; (f) placement of concepts within courses; (g) development of syllabi for each course; and (h) development of the clinical evaluation tool based upon the terminal objectives.

Initially, terminal characteristics were revised and refined by the faculty at large. Then level characteristics and conceptual areas of content were developed using a "brainstorming" and voting process.

Eight terminal outcome characteristics and 63 subcharacteristics of graduates at the completion of the sophomore, junior, and senior years were identified. Subcharacteristics for each level derived from the terminal characteristics guided the development of the instrument. While the eight terminal characteristics addressed by the tool are specific to the developers school of nursing, the format of the instrument and the evaluation process are considered applicable to other settings. The terminal characteristics and examples of level subcharacteristics appear in Table 11.1.

Conceptual areas were identified by faculty and matched with the appropriate outcome characteristic. Conceptual areas were then leveled for implementation. Examples of conceptual areas appear in Table 11.2.

Five "tracks" that cut across the five semesters of nursing courses were identified and labeled as sophomore, professional development, wellness/health promotion, health maintenance/ restoration, and child/family. Courses were identified and labeled with each track and appear in Table 11.3.

Concepts were then placed within the appropriate course(s). Clinical objectives were developed for each course, and then clinical outcomes based upon terminal objectives. Course outcomes were placed in the tool format as professional behavior, implementation of the nursing process, leadership, personal/professional growth, and clinical objectives. An example of the first pages of the tool and select professional behaviors are found at the end of the chapter for foundations of clinical nursing; health maintenance and restoration: adulthood; and health promotion.

Administration and scoring procedures for the tool take into account that evaluation and learning must be separate events. Thus, it is essential that the Clinical Evaluation Tool be shared with the student during the first week of the clinical grading period, with expectations and outcomes defined. The student should then receive ongoing formative evaluation until the last part of the grading period. The faculty teaching the clinical courses should schedule evaluation observation periods with each student. Behaviors are evaluated and scored as "P" for pass and "F" for fail. "Critical" behaviors designated by an asterisk on the tool must be achieved. The lead teacher for each course determines the number of behaviors students must achieve to pass the clinical.

RELIABILITY AND VALIDITY ASSESSMENTS

The original, Clinical Evaluation Tool was pilot tested for reliability and validity (Rossel & Kakta, 1990) in a college of nursing located in a medium-sized, midwestern Catholic university. The clinical settings consisted of one medium-sized, long-term care facility for the elderly and one rehabilitation unit in a large VA hospital. A total of 9 of the 10 generic students in a junior-level clinical aged section and 4 of the 9 students in a senior-level clinical rehabilitation section volunteered to participate in the pilot study. A sample instrument format for the original tool is included at the end of the chapter.

TABLE 11.1 Terminal Characteristics and Examples of Level Subcharacteristics

Terminal Characteristics	Sophomore Subcharacteristics	Junior Subcharacteristics	Senior Subcharacteristics
Develop a personalized professional identity	Develop beginning concept of self in a professional nurse role	Demonstrate self-confidence and self-respect in an evolving professional identity	Demonstrate independence in a newly acquired professional nurse identity
Apply in interactions with clients the concept of holistic person in interaction with the total environment	Recognize the client's self-determination rights in decision making that affects their perception of well-being	Begin to collaborate with clients in mutual goal setting and ongoing evaluation that affects their perception of well-being	Collaborate with clients in mutual goal setting and ongoing evaluation that affects their perception of well-being
Utilize critical inquiry in professional roles	Explain and begin to organize data	Organize, interpret and validate data	Bring multiple perspectives into the differentiation and interpretation of data
Demonstrate effective communication in a variety of professional nursing roles	Describe effective communication techniques directed toward client care	Incorporate effective communication patterns in the provision of direct nursing care	Incorporate effective communication patterns as a member of the health care team
Demonstrate competence in the role of care giver (G), educator (E), and counselor (C)	Begin to develop technical skills related to nursing practice	Utilize technical skills related to nursing practice	Integrate technical skills into nursing practice

TABLE 11.1 (*continued*)

Terminal Characteristics	Sophomore Subcharacteristics	Junior Subcharacteristics	Senior Subcharacteristics
Assume professional responsibility for addressing social issues and concerns which affect the health of all members of society	Identify independent functions of the nurse in a variety of settings	Participate in independent nursing practice in a variety of settings	Adapt independent nursing practice to a variety of settings
Assume leadership and management roles to assure quality nursing practice in the delivery of health services	Define various leadership concepts	Utilize principles of leadership while functioning as a member of the health care team	Utilize leadership skills in coordinating delivery of health care services
Value and assume responsibility for self-directed interactive learning as a lifelong process	Participate in the learning process	Begin to initiate self-directed learning activities	Incorporate self-directed learning activities in the learning process

TABLE 11.2 Examples of Conceptual Areas by Terminal Characteristic

Terminal characteristics	Examples of conceptual areas
1.	Ethical dimensions of professional nursing
2.	Family wellness
3.	Nursing theories, nursing process
4.	Individual, group, and therapeutic communication
5.	Growth and development
6.	Vulnerable populations
7.	Health care resources
8.	Self-directed learning

The pilot study was conducted in two clinical settings to establish reliability of the instrument. The instrument was pilot tested during a 1-month period of a spring semester. Data were collected by the two researchers on 2 clinical days in each setting. The first day was used for practice with observations of client care, and the second day's observations were used for calculating the reliability coefficients. Care plans were evaluated once on either the first or second day. Postconference observations occurred on the first day only for the aged clinical section and on both days for the rehabilitation section. Observations of students' client care, 10 minutes in length, were scheduled with the student to occur during a period of planned activity. No attempt was made to observe all students performing the same behaviors.

An oral explanation of the research was given to the clinical faculty and students. Permission was obtained from the dean of the college of nursing, the clinical agency, and the students. The researchers briefly introduced themselves to the client upon entering the room and before beginning the observations.

To determine interrater reliability, coefficients for P_o, P_c, K, K_{max}, and K/K_{max} were calculated between the observations of the two researchers (Waltz, Strickland, & Lenz, 1991). For the aged section, the K/K_{max} values ranged from .83 to 1.00, with the components of skills and leadership exceeding the .90 level. For the rehabilitation section, the K/K_{max} values were 1.00 for care plan and skills. The percentage of clinical behaviors observed for the aged section were as follows: care plan, 46%; skills, 28%; postconference, 35%; and leadership, 12%. For the rehabilitation section, the percentage of observed behaviors was 56%, 29%, 0%, and 0%, respectively.

TABLE 11.3 Courses By Track

Sophomore	Professional development	Wellness health promotion	Health maintenance restoration	Child/ family
Foundations of Nursing	Nursing Research	Health Promotion Across the Life Span I	HMR: Adulthood I	HMR: Children
Foundations of Clinical Nursing	Professional Development I	Health Promotion Across the Life Span II	HMR: Adulthood II	HMR: Childbearing Families
Health Assessment	Professional Development II	Promoting Healthy Communities	HMR: Adulthood III	
	Professional Development III		HMR: Crisis	
	Role Transition Practicum			

Validity was assessed using the average congruency percentage test. This test was used to determine if the general behaviors were representative of the terminal characteristics. For the first assessment, percentages ranged from 86.6% to 100%, with two characteristics below the 90% average congruency level established as a minimal acceptable level. The revised general behaviors were reassessed by the two raters with the following results: values, 100%; cognitive learning, 100%; nursing process, 93.04%; adaptation/professional roles, 100%; leadership and management, 100%; research, 91.67%; and continued growth, 100%.

The content validity index (CVI) was calculated for the course content behaviors for the aged and rehabilitation sections using two faculty members for each course. The coefficients for the seven terminal characteristics for the aged clinical course were as follows: values, .88; cognitive learning, .86; nursing process, .84; adaptative/professional roles, .67; leadership and management, .55; research, .67; and continued growth, .80. The coefficients for the seven terminal characteristics for the rehabilitation clinical course were .93, .64, .86, .67, .70, 1.00, and .25, respectively. Only course behaviors rated as quite relevant or very relevant by both raters were retained for instrument development to achieve the .90 cutoff. For the aged section, 22.5% of the course behaviors were omitted, and for the rehabilitation section, 20% were omitted.

Interrater reliability coefficients for content-specific behaviors were calculated for proportion observed, proportion chance agreements, and adjusted values for each of the four components. Values for proportion observed (P_o) reached or approached the .90 acceptable level. Values adjusted for chance agreement (K) were somewhat lower as expected. Subsequent analysis utilizing K/K_{max} was completed. While these values reached or approached acceptable levels, they should be interpreted with caution. To avoid overestimating the interrater reliability coefficients, calculations were based only on behaviors observed on at least one occasion by either observer. The proportion of behaviors observed was low, ranging from 0% to 56% of the total behaviors for individual components of the instrument. For two areas, postconference and leadership on the rehabilitation instrument, no behaviors were observed. Interrater reliability coefficients were not computed for these two components.

Following the observation sessions, the researchers discussed behaviors that were not observed by either person. Behaviors were labeled either "clear, no opportunity to observe" or "unclear."

For items identified as "clear, no opportunity to observe," situations in which these behaviors can be observed need to be delineated. One possible explanation for the lack of opportunity to observe select behaviors may have been the time intervals utilized in the pilot study. Ten-minute observation periods may have been insufficient to observe all behaviors. In addition, the observation sessions were not conducted in all clinical settings used by students in the aged and rehabilitation courses. For example, the aged section instrument was piloted in the long-term care facility, while the rehabilitation section instrument was piloted on one of three units. An alternative reason for the relatively high number of behaviors unobserved is that no opportunities were provided for students to demonstrate these behaviors.

For items identified as "unclear," clarification statements in the form of written guidelines were indicated. The researchers reviewed, clarified, and/or revised these problematic items with content expert faculty. Following these alterations, interrater reliability for the modified instrument was established.

Acceptable average congruency levels were achieved for general behaviors of terminal characteristics. Therefore, there are no plans to modify the identified general behaviors.

CVI values for course-specific behaviors or general behaviors were lower than expected. For the aged section, none of the seven characteristics met the .90 level, and only four approached this level. For the rehabilitation section, two of the seven characteristics reached the .90 level, and another approached this level.

Future plans for development of the instrument include a review and revision of those items for which there was disagreement between the experts. A follow-up rating by different content experts and subsequent recalculation of an index of content validity was indicated.

Reliability for the modified tool was addressed a priori in that the tool is designed so that same/similar behaviors are evaluated from course to course and semester to semester as well as behaviors unique to a particular course/clinical. The format for the health promotion I course found at the end of the chapter illustrates comparative evaluation of level sub-characteristics for the sophomore, junior, and senior program levels. There are 15 professional behaviors and five steps of the nursing process common to all course tools. The four leadership behaviors for the junior year are the same for both health promotion courses. Likewise, the four personal/professional growth behaviors are the same for the junior year in all courses. All clinical courses use a similar format. The narrative remarks of faculty on a leadership behavior of "Displays appropriate decision-making skills" can be tracked for each student throughout the five-semester nursing program. For some of the clinical courses, such as health promotion, the student receives clinical evaluation from three faculty members, providing an opportunity for determination of interrater reliability.

Validity was also addressed in the development of the tool by deriving clinical course behaviors from terminal characteristics identified and agreed upon by faculty experts and based on the current literature.

Reliability and validity for the revised Clinical Evaluation Tool, when employed, should be tested empirically as well. A sample of the revised Clinical Evaluation Tool format is included at the end of the chapter.

In summary, for the original tool, utilizing the average congruency percentage procedure, acceptable validity levels were achieved for general behaviors. Content-specific behaviors were developed. Content validity indices for specific behaviors were somewhat lower than anticipated. Preliminary interrater reliability coefficients for content-specific behaviors reached acceptable levels. Reliability and validity testing using similar procedures should be undertaken for the revised Clinical Evaluation Tool.

REFERENCES

Abrahason, S. (1985). Assessment of student clinical performance: The state-of-the-art. *Evaluation and the Health Professions, 8*(4), 413–427.

Acord, L. G. (ed.). (1998). *The essentials of baccalaureate education for professional nursing practice.* Washington, DC: American Association of Colleges of Nursing.

Billings, D. M., & Halstead, J. A. (1998). *Teaching in nursing: A guide for faculty.* Philadelphia: W. B. Saunders Co.

Bellack, J. P., & O'Neil, E. H. (2000). Recreating nursing practice for a new century: Recommendations and implications of the Pew Health Programs Commissions final report. *Nursing Health Care Perspectives, 21*(1), 14–21.

Rossel, C. L., & Kakta, B. A. (1990). Clinical evaluation of nursing students: A criterion-referenced approach to clinical evaluation based on terminal characteristics. In O. L. Strickland & C. F. Waltz (Eds.), *Measurement of nursing outcomes: Vol. 3. Measuring clinical skills and professional development in education and practice* (pp. 17–30). New York: Springer Publishing Company.

Waltz, C. F., Strickland, O. L., & Lenz, E. R. (1991). *Measurement in nursing research.* (2nd ed.). Philadelphia: F. A. Davis.

CLINICAL EVALUATION TOOL
SAMPLE INSTRUMENT FORMAT
(ORIGINAL TOOL)

	With Assistance		Without Assistance		Comments
	Sem	S/U	Sem	S/U	
1. CARE PLAN					
a. assessment					
Behavior #1	1				
Behavior #2		2			
b. plan					
Behavior(s)	1				
c. nursing orders					
Behavior(s)			1		
d. rationale					
Behavior(s)			1		
e. evaluation					
Behavior(s)			2		
2. OBSERVATION OF PATIENT CARE					
a. communication					
Behavior(s)			1		
b. organization					
Behavior(s)	1				
c. skills					
Behavior(s)	1				
3. POSTCONFERENCE					
Behavior(s)	1				
4. LEADERSHIP					
Behavior(s)	1				

Key: S = Satisfactory; U = Unsatisfactory.

Front Page of Foundations of Clinical Nursing

Lewis University/College of Nursing

CLINICAL EVALUATION (Revised)
N230 Foundations of Clinical Nursing

STUDENT _____

FACULTY _____

CLINICAL SITE _____

DATES _____ TO _____

In order to receive a pass clinical grade, the student must
pass *all* critical behaviors
Clinical Grade: PASS _____   FAIL _____

	Service Hours ___	Service Activity ___
	Service Hours ___	Service Activity ___
	Service Hours ___	Service Activity ___

P = PASS   F = FAIL   W = WITH ASSISTANCE   WO = WITHOUT ASSISTANCE

IF ANY OBJECTIVE IS FAILED, DETAILED ANECDOTALS MUST BE ATTACHED.

I. PROFESSIONAL BEHAVIOR	P	F	COMMENTS
A. General			
*1. Arrives on time (wo)			
*2. Is attired in accord with college/faculty/agency requirements (wo)			
*3. Demonstrates a professional approach in appearance, care of clients, and in interactions with members of the health care team (wo)			
*4. Notifies faculty of absence prior to expected time of arrival (see individual faculty for policy in assigned agency) (wo)			
*5. Brings equipment and/or resource material(s) to clinical setting as needed (wo)			
*6. Provides for client safety in the following ways: a) Obtains a report on the client before initiating care (wo).			

_____

* Critical behaviors.

154

Personal/Professional Growth Behaviors From the HMR: Adulthood I Tool, Front Page

Lewis University/College of Nursing

CLINICAL EVALUATION

N331 Health Maintenance and Restoration: Adulthood I

STUDENT _____

FACULTY _____

CLINICAL SITE _____

DATES _____ TO _____

In order to receive a pass clinical grade, the student must pass *all* critical behaviors

Clinical Grade: PASS _____   FAIL _____

P = PASS   F = FAIL   W = WITH ASSISTANCE   WO = WITHOUT ASSISTANCE

Service Hours   Service Activity _____
Service Hours   Service Activity _____
Service Hours   Service Activity _____

IF ANY OBJECTIVE IS FAILED, DETAILED ANECDOTALS MUST BE ATTACHED.

I. PROFESSIONAL BEHAVIOR	P	F	COMMENTS
A. General			
*1. Arrives on time (wo)			
*2. Is attired in accord with college/faculty/agency requirements (wo)			
*3. Demonstrates a professional approach and appearance the care of clients and in interactions with members of the health care team (wo)			
*4. Notifies faculty of absence prior to expected time of arrival (see individual faculty for policy in assigned agency) (wo)			
*5. Brings equipment and/or resource material(s) to clinical setting as needed (wo)			

* Critical behaviors.

155

Health Promotion I, Front Page

Lewis University/College of Nursing

CLINICAL EVALUATION
N330 Health Promotion I

STUDENT _____

			Service Hours _____	Service Activity _____
Faculty (Peds)	_____	Clinical Site	Service Hours _____	Service Activity _____
			Service Hours _____	Service Activity _____
Faculty (Peds)	Clinical Site	Dates	Days Absent _____	Tardy _____
Faculty (Adult)	Clinical Site	Dates	Days Absent _____	Tardy _____
Faculty (Aged)	Clinical Site	Dates	Days Absent _____	Tardy _____

In order to receive a pass clinical grade, the student must pass *all* critical behaviors.

Clinical Grade: Pass _____ Fail _____

P = PASS   F = FAIL   W = WITH ASSISTANCE   WO = WITHOUT ASSISTANCE

IF ANY OBJECTIVE IS FAILED, DETAILED ANECDOTALS MUST BE ATTACHED.

COMMENTS

I. Professional Behavior	P	F	Faculty: Peds	Faculty: Adult	Faculty: Aged
A. General *1. Arrives on time (wo) *2. Is attired in accord with college/faculty/agency requirements (wo)					

* Critical Behaviors.

156

12

Clinical Competence Rating Scale

Linda J. Scheetz

PURPOSE

The **Clinical Competence Rating Scale** (CCRS) measures the dimensions of clinical competence of baccalaureate nursing students including problem solving, application of theory to practice, and psychomotor skill performance. The instrument was designed to be generic in nature, flexible enough to be utilized in a variety of clinical settings, easily administered, and easily scored (Scheetz, 2000).

INSTRUMENT DESCRIPTION

Clinical competence is conceptually defined as the demonstration of skills that reflect learning at the higher levels of the cognitive, affective, and psychomotor domains (Field, Gallman, Nicholson, & Dreher, 1984; Reilly, 1975). It is demonstrated by the ability of the student to utilize the skills of problem solving, to apply theory to practice, and to perform psychomotor skills. Bloom's (1956) taxonomy of the cognitive domain offers a relatively concise model for the analysis of intellectual skills in the areas of problem solving and application of theory to practice. Krathwohl, Bloom, and Masia's (1964) taxonomy of the affective domain describes the emotive basis for learning. Harrow (1972) developed a taxonomy of behaviors in the psychomotor domain that provides a theoretical model for the development of clinical competence in the area of nursing practice. While problem solving is considered to be a cognitive process, the judgments and decision making that are part of this process reflect the student's level of affective development.

Harrow's (1972) taxonomy of the psychomotor domain assumes learning in the cognitive and affective domains as a requisite to the correct implementation of a technical skill. The hierarchical structure of the domain reflects progress in the acquisition of a psychomotor skill. To perform a psychomotor skill efficiently and effectively, the individual must demonstrate learning at the higher levels of Harrow's taxonomy. If such is the case, the individual is able to perform the skill in a variety of situations with ease. The performance of the skill merely becomes a means to an end, not an end in itself.

The original Clinical Competence Rating Scale (Scheetz, 1990) consists of 53 measurable nursing behaviors utilizing a 6-point Likert-type scale. The nursing behaviors are organized into three subscales: problem solving (29 items); application of theory to practice (14 items); and psychomotor skill performance (10 items). The student's level of competence for each behavior is rated as follows: independent, supervised, assisted, marginal, dependent, or not observed. Statements of behaviors were derived from standards and characteristics of baccalaureate graduates, the Midwest Alliance in Nursing's competency statements for baccalaureate graduates (Primm, 1986), and a review of the literature to identify specific behaviors for expected competencies. Panels of experts critiqued the tool and revisions were made accordingly. The criterion-referenced descriptive rating scale labels were developed and field tested by Bondy (1984). Each of the five descriptive rating scale labels reflects behavior according to standards of practice, quality of performance, and the amount of assistance needed. A sixth label, "not observed," was added for this instrument. A sample of items from the original Clinical Competence Rating Scale is included at the end of the chapter.

The rater should be a registered nurse with a minimum of a baccalaureate degree and at least 1 year of clinical practice experience. The rater should be trained in the use of the instrument. The rater observes the student's performance over a three-day period. Information regarding the student's performance can be gathered through direct observation of the student and discussion with the student. At the completion of the observation period, the rater completes the rating scale.

The assigned level of performance for any item on the rating scale should indicate performance according to all criteria with that performance level. Point values are assigned as follows: independent (5 points), supervised (4 points), assisted (3 points), marginal (2 points), and dependent (1 point). Summative scoring is employed to derive subscale scores and a total scale score. Raw scores ranges for subscales and total scores are 29–145 for problem solving; 14–70 for application of theory to practice; 10–50 for psychomotor skill performance; and 53–265 for total scale score. The range of mean scores is 1–5. The higher the score, the more competent the student. To use the CCRS for student evaluation purposes, faculty must determine, prior to utilizing the instrument, acceptable scores for the assignment of pass/fail or letter grades. Included at the end of the chapter is a copy of the CCRS adapted in 1992 by faculty in the Division of Nursing at Mount Saint Mary College, New York, for use in adult health nursing clinical courses in the baccalaureate curriculum.

Initially, there was some resistance to the use of the instrument by faculty teaching courses other than medical-surgical nursing. After careful examination of the items on the original CCRS, faculty determined that the items were applicable to a variety of settings. To clarify applicability, faculty listed specific examples of student behaviors under each item that were applicable to their clinical setting. Because behaviors on the psychomotor skill subscale are often not observed for students practicing in a psychiatric-mental health setting, faculty indicate this on the instrument.

Faculty use the adapted CCRS to complete midterm and final clinical evaluations for all students in each clinical area. Since the instrument is so comprehensive and specific, there is sufficient documentation of clinical strengths and weaknesses to allow students time to focus attention on areas needing improvement. A final page was added to the instrument for narrative comments by faculty and students at midterm and the end of the semester.

The faculty's adaptation of the CCRS consisted of the following:

1. Reorganizing the scale items to "fit under" course objectives. The CCRS subscale headings were deleted, and scale items were moved under the most appropriate course objective.
2. Addition of behavioral examples for each item on the instrument. Faculty believed such an addition was necessary to provide clarification of items and to assist them in using the instrument in settings other than medical-surgical nursing. Behavioral examples are identified for most rating scale behaviors. For example, one CCRS item states, "Utilizes therapeutic communication skills with client." One behavioral example for this item is, "Introduces self to client at beginning of clinical day." Additional behaviors are added by faculty to provide clarification of the rating scale item and applicability to various clinical settings. Faculty teaching in labor and delivery have added site-specific behavioral examples to the item, "Assesses client's physical status."
3. The rating scale label "marginal" was changed to "provisional" since faculty believed that marginal had a negative connotation.
4. Eleven items were selected as critical elements. To earn a passing grade, students must meet all critical elements at the stipulated level (which is one level higher than noncritical elements). Failure to meet any of the critical elements results in clinical failure, regardless of the ratings of other behaviors on the scale.
5. Level standards for determination of pass/fail were developed. The curriculum has three levels: Level I in the first half of the junior year, Level II in the second half of the junior year, and Level III in the senior year. The passing standard is raised as students move through the levels.

- Students at Level I (the first medical-surgical nursing course) must achieve a score of *assisted* on all critical elements and *marginal* on all noncritical elements.
- Students at Level II (second medical-surgical nursing course, care of the childbearing family, and psychiatric-mental health nursing course) must achieve a score of *supervised* on all critical elements and *assisted* on all noncritical elements.
- Students at Level III (community health, pediatric, and critical care nursing courses) must achieve a score of *independent* on all critical elements and *supervised* on all noncritical elements.

Because the curriculum is based on the concepts of simple to complex client care/health system variables and dependent to independent student performance, identifying different levels of expected behavior for students as they move through the curriculum is rational.

Using one evaluation instrument for all clinical courses, for which levels of expected clinical performance correspond with curriculum levels, enables faculty to track student progress throughout the curriculum. Moreover, it is an educational and legally defensible system of clinical evaluation in that there is consistency in the method of evaluation. Students perceive the instrument as being fair.

The adapted CCRS has been in use in the baccalaureate nursing program at Mount Saint Mary College for 9 years. Although the curriculum has undergone modifications, the instrument remains applicable, since the items were derived from expected competencies of baccalaureate graduates. The instrument is evaluated periodically for its applicability; each time faculty have determined that it remains applicable.

RELIABILITY AND VALIDITY ASSESSMENTS

The tool has been used by nurse educators, researchers, and staff development professionals worldwide to measure clinical competence in baccalaureate nursing students and novice nurses. Reliability and validity evidence obtained by the developer and others who have used the tool is presented in Table 12.1.

REFERENCES

Bloom, B. (1956). *Taxonomy of educational objectives. Handbook I: Cognitive domain.* New York: David McKay.

Bondy, K. (1984). Clinical evaluation of student performance: The effects of criteria on accuracy and reliability. *Research in Nursing and Health, 7*(1), 25–33.

Field, W., Gallman, L., Nicholson, R., & Dreher, M. (1984). Clinical competencies of baccalaureate nursing students. *Journal of Nursing Education, 23*(7), 284–293.

Harrow, A. (1972). *A taxonomy of the psychomotor domain.* New York: David McKay.

Krathwohl, D., Bloom, B., & Masia, B. (1964). *Taxonomy of educational objectives: The classification of educational goals. Handbook II: Affective domain.* New York: David McKay.

Oermann, M. H., & Navin, M. A. (1991). Effect of extern experiences on clinical competence of graduate nurses. *Nursing Connections, 4*(4), 31–38.

Primm, P. (1986). Entry into practice: Competency statements for BSNs and ADNs. *Nursing Outlook, 334*, 135–137.

Reilly, D. (1975). *Behavioral objectives in nursing: Evaluation of learner attainment.* New York: Appleton-Century-Crofts.

Ryan, F. (1998). *Preceptorship and clinical competence.* Unpublished master's thesis, University of Phoenix, Phoenix, Arizona.

Scheetz, L. (1989). Baccalaureate nursing student preceptorship programs and the development of clinical competence. *Journal of Nursing Education, 28*(1), 29–35.

Scheetz, L. (1990). Measuring clinical competence in baccalaureate nursing students. In O. L. Strickland & C. F. Waltz (Eds.), *Measurement of Nursing Outcomes: Vol. 3. Measuring clinical skills and professional development in education and practice* (pp. 3–16). New York: Springer Publishing Company.

Scheetz, L. (In press). Use of the Clinical Competence Rating Scale to measure baccalaureate nursing students' performance in varied clinical settings. In Scheetz, L. (Ed.), *Nursing faculty secrets* (pp.). Philadelphia: Hanley & Belfus Medical Publishers.

TABLE 12.1 CCRS Reliability and Validity Testing

Study citation	*Sample and characteristics*	*Reliability evidence*	*Validity evidence*
Scheetz, L. (1989)	Two samples of junior and senior generic baccalaureate nursing students, females aged 18–25 enrolled in accredited nursing programs in Eastern U.S.	**Interrater reliability** Sample 1 = 10 Sample 2 = 12 Rates 2 RNs observing over 2-day period; clinical instructors paired with RN with primary responsibility for patient. **Sample 1** Spearman rank order coefficients: problem solving .83, application theory to practice .84, psychomotor skill .66, total CCSR .80 **Sample 2** 3-day observation period by paired raters, students' preceptor and unit head nurse. Spearman rank order coefficients: problem solving .91, application theory to practice .93,	**A priori content validity** Review of standards, essential literature **Content validity** Panel of 10 masters and PhDs prepared content; experts rated each item to domain of competence using scale of 1, not relevant, to 4, very relevant. Content validity index (CVI) .90 **Concurrent validity** 22 senior students' performance rated after 3 days observation during week 7 of semester. Criterion measures: NLN Comprehensive Achievement Test (1986 edition). Spearman coefficient: problem solving .66, application theory .68

TABLE 12.1 *(continued)*

Study citation	Sample and characteristics	Reliability evidence	Validity evidence
		psychomotor skill .80, total CCSR .86 **Internal consistency** Sample 1 = 67 seniors and junior Sample 2 = 72 seniors **1st sample** alpha coefficient: problem solving .93, application theory to practice .91, psychomotor skill .92, total CCSR .96 **2nd sample** alphas: problem solving .98, application theory to practice .96, psychomotor skill .98, total CCSR .97	**Construct validity** Contrasted groups' approach Low group, 28 junior students High group, 36 senior students. One-way analysis of variance to assess differences on each subscale and total score. Problem solving: $F = 4.20$, $df = 1.62$, $P = .0419$. Application theory: $F = 7.96$, $P = .006$, $df = 1.62$. Psychomotor: $F = 6.94$, $P = .010$, $df = 1.62$. Total CCSR: $F = 6.15$, $df = 1.62$, $P = .0151$. **Sensitivity to changes in clinical competence** $N = 40$ seniors $N = 27$ juniors Rated 5 weeks before end of semester and at end of semester

TABLE 12.1 *(continued)*

Study citation	Sample and characteristics	Reliability evidence	Validity evidence
			One way ANOVA Juniors Problem solving: $F = 16.18$, $P = .000$, $df = 1.51$ Application theory: $F = 10.97$, $df = 1.51$, $P = .002$ Psychomotor skill: $F = 15.91$, $P = .000$, $df = 1.51$ Total CCSR: $F = 15.20$, $df = 1.51$, $P = .0005$. **Seniors** Problem solving: $F = 6.91$, $P = .010$, $df = 1.59$. Application theory: $F = 14.09$, $df = 1.59$, $P = .0006$. Psychomotor skill: $F = 12.51$, $df = 1.57$, $P = .0011$. Total CCSR: $F = 9.96$, $df = 1.59$, $P = .0028$.
Ryan (1998)	New Navy nurses who participated in preceptorship programs during their BSN education and during	**Internal consistency reliability** Alpha: Problem solving, 0.997; Application theory, 0.959;	**Construct validity, hypothesis:** "precepted new nurse would indicate a higher level of clinical competency

TABLE 12.1 *(continued)*

Study citation	Sample and characteristics	Reliability evidence	Validity evidence
	orientation to first nursing position	Psychomotor skill, 0.949; Total CCSR, 0.989.	than unprecepted new nurses." Results unclear.
Oermann and Navin (1991)	24 pairs of graduate nurses and their preceptors on CCRS		**Construct validity** Examined effect of nursing student externships on development of clinical competence of new graduate nurses. Findings: 1. Significant differences between new graduates' preceptors and their own clinical competence and new graduates' clinical competence as rated by their preceptors. 2. New graduates who partici-pated in externships as students rated themselves higher on each of CCRS

TABLE 12.1 *(continued)*

Study citation	Sample and characteristics	Reliability evidence	Validity evidence
			subscales than did new grads who did not participate in student externships. 3. Preceptors noted no difference in clinical competence between new grads who did and did not participate in student externship experiences.
M. Miller (personal communication, August, 1991) Aurora Heath Care Milwaukee, Wisconsin	New staff nurses after completing an internship program	**Internal consistency reliability** Subscales and overall greater than .91.	**Construct validity** Pretest/posttest design using CCRS to measure clinical competence in new staff nurses after completing an internship program. Findings: No changes in groups

CLINICAL COMPETENCE RATING SCALE, SAMPLE ITEMS
(ORIGINAL TOOL)

	I	S	A	M	D	NO
Problem Solving						
Collects relevant health data from client and other sources	—	—	—	—	—	—
Assesses client's ability to communicate verbally	—	—	—	—	—	—
Assesses client's physical status	—	—	—	—	—	—
Interprets client's nonverbal behavior	—	—	—	—	—	—
Formulates nursing diagnoses and/or problem list	—	—	—	—	—	—
Seeks client input to develop a plan of care	—	—	—	—	—	—
Organizes activities to promote efficiency	—	—	—	—	—	—
Application of Theory to Practice						
Develops a plan of care for client based on assessment data	—	—	—	—	—	—
Plans nursing activities that will facilitate the achievement of client outcomes	—	—	—	—	—	—
Implements nursing activities to meet client's needs	—	—	—	—	—	—
Incorporates theoretical knowledge and scientific principles into nursing care	—	—	—	—	—	—
Reacts to signs and symptoms of physical distress in client	—	—	—	—	—	—
Psychomotor Skill Performance						
Demonstrates manual dexterity with equipment	—	—	—	—	—	—
Adapts psychomotor skill performance to client situation	—	—	—	—	—	—
Maintains client safety	—	—	—	—	—	—
Documents nursing interventions on client's chart	—	—	—	—	—	—

CLINICAL COMPETENCE RATING SCALE
FOR USE IN AN ADULT HEALTH NURSING CLINICAL COURSE

Directions: Observe the clinical performance of the nursing student for at least three days before rating his/her performance. Place a check mark in the column that most accurately describes the performance. Definitions of the rating scale labels are provided below. Please note that each descriptive phrase within each definition *may not* apply to each item on the scale.

I (Independent) *Safe, accurate performance* according to accepted standards; the desired outcome is obtained each time; affect is *appropriate;* the student is *proficient, coordinated, confident; occasional expenditure* of excess energy is noted; task is completed within a *reasonable* time period; *no supporting cues* are needed.

S (Supervised) *Safe, accurate performance* according to accepted standards; the desired outcome is obtained *each time;* affect is *appropriate;* the student is *efficient, coordinated, confident; some expenditure* of excess energy is noted; task is completed within a *reasonable* time period; *occasional supporting* cues are needed.

A (Assisted) *Safe, accurate performance* according to accepted standards; the desired outcome is obtained *most of the time;* affect is *appropriate most of the time;* skillful *in parts* of the behavior; the student is *inefficient and uncoordinated;* student *expends excess* energy to accomplish the task; task is completed within a *delayed time period; frequent* verbal and occasional physical directive cues are needed in addition to supportive cues.

M (Marginal) *Safe, but not alone;* student *performs at risk;* student is *not always* accurate; the desired *outcome is obtained only occasionally;* student's *affect is appropriate only occasionally; unskilled, inefficient* performance; *considerable expenditure* of energy noted; task completed within a *prolonged time period; continuous* verbal and frequent physical directive cues are needed.

D (Dependent) *Unsafe, unable* to demonstrate behavior; student lacks *confidence, coordination, efficiency; continuous* verbal and physical cues are needed.

NO/NA Not observed or not applicable.

Scoring. To assign a numerical grade for clinical performance, the following values may be used:

Independent (I)	5
Supervised (S)	4
Assisted (A)	3
Marginal (M)	2
Dependent (D)	1

Determine a cutoff value for each subscale or for the total instrument to use as a passing standard. The user might also wish to identify critical elements which must be met. Alternatively, faculty may wish to specify level of performance (I, A, S, M, D) to be met as a passing standard for each course or level of the curriculum.

NUR 301, Clinical Evaluation

	Midterm Eval						Final Eval					
	I	S	A	M	D	NO NA	I	S	A	M	D	NO NA
Course objective 1: Provides comprehensive professional nursing care to diverse adult populations in an acute care setting.												
1. Utilizes therapeutic communication skills with client												
1.1 introduces self to client at beginning of clinical day												
1.2 orients client to time and place if necessary												
1.3 provides alternate means of communication as needed												
1.4 uses facilitators of communication												
1.5 avoids the use of communication barriers												
1.6 informs client prior to any interventions												
1.7 provides verbal support during painful procedures												
1.8 refrains from discussing client within hearing distance												
1.9 ensures call light is within reach when not in room												
1.10 refrains from inappropriate conversation within hearing distance of client												
2. Anticipates client's responses to therapeutic interventions												
3. Implements nursing activities to meet client's needs												

NUR 301, Clinical Evaluation (*continued*)

	Midterm Eval						Final Eval					
	I	S	A	M	D	NO NA	I	S	A	M	D	NO NA
4. **Reacts to signs and symptoms of physical distress in client***												
4.1 reports abnormal laboratory finding to appropriate individual												
4.2 reports abnormal vital signs to appropriate individual												
5. Conveys attitude of acceptance and empathy toward client												
6. Acts in a nonjudgmental manner toward client												
6.1 refrains from the use of any judgmental remarks or nonverbal behavior												
7. Demonstrates manual dexterity with equipment												
8. ***Performs psychomotor skills with minimal discomfort to client**												
9. Gathers necessary equipment and supplies prior to performance a psychomotor skill												
10. **Maintains medical asepsis**												

* Critical element that must be met.

NUR 301, Clinical Evaluation (continued)

	Midterm Eval						Final Eval					
	I	S	A	M	D	NO NA	I	S	A	M	D	NO NA
Course objective 2: Analyzes knowledge from nursing theories, the humanities, and sciences in the provision of nursing care.												
1. Assesses client's ability to communicate verbally												
2. Assesses client's physical status												
2.1 completes physical assessment within 1 hour of arriving												
2.2 is aware of all physician's orders pertaining to client												
2.3 conducts appropriate assessment												
3. Assesses client's psychosocial status												
4. Assesses client's developmental level												
4.1 identifies developmental level so that interactions and expectations are appropriate												
5. Assesses client's environmental safety needs												
5.1 checks emergency equipment within 30 minutes of arrival at bedside												
5.2 ensures client is wearing a legible ID band												

NUR 301, Clinical Evaluation (*continued*)

	Midterm Eval						Final Eval					
	I	S	A	M	D	NO NA	I	S	A	M	D	NO NA
5.3 checks all alarm systems on equipment												
5.4 checks appropriate position of all tubes												
6. Assesses impact of illness on client and significant others												
7. Assesses learning needs of client and significant others												
7.1 assesses level of knowledge												
7.2 states client-family's willingness/interest/availability for learning												
7.3 states client-family's psychological and physical readiness to learn												
7.4 describes client-family's proficiency in performing psychomotor skills												
7.5 describes client-family's behaviors indicating learning needs in affective domain												
7.6 evaluates cultural patterns influencing teaching-learning												
8. Differentiates subjective and objective client data												

NUR 301, Clinical Evaluation (*continued*)

	Midterm Eval						Final Eval					
	I	S	A	M	D	NO NA	I	S	A	M	D	NO NA
9. Interprets client's nonverbal behavior												
10. Considers client's cultural background when planning care												
11. *Recognizes signs and symptoms of distress in client												
12. *Evaluates client's response to therapeutic interventions												
13. *Adapts psychomotor skill performance to client situation												
14. *Recognizes hazards to client												
14.1 states "potential" nursing diagnoses based on individual assessment												
14.2 maintains bed in low position												
14.3 checks client's immediate environment for electrical hazards												
14.4 places client's articles within reach												
14.5 uses side rails for all confused, elderly, seizure, and post-op clients												
15. *Maintains surgical asepsis when appropriate												

NUR 301, Clinical Evaluation (*continued*)

	Midterm Eval					Final Eval				
	I	S	A	M	D	NO NA	I	S	A	M	D	NO NA
Course objective 3: Uses the nursing process in a dependent/ interdependent manner to provide nursing care to individuals and families.											
1. Collects relevant health data from client and all available sources											
2. Formulates nursing diagnoses and/or problem list											
2.1 nursing diagnoses flow directly from assessment											
2.2 prioritizes the nursing diagnoses											
3. Develops a plan of care for client based on assessment data											
3.1 able to state planned interventions for assigned client											
4. Formulates a plan of care consistent with client's values											
5. Documents nursing interventions and client responses											
5.1 charts complete nursing assessment											
5.2 records all medications within 10 minutes of administration											
5.3 documents effects of PRN medications											

NUR 301, Clinical Evaluation (*continued*)

	Midterm Eval						Final Eval					
	I	S	A	M	D	NO NA	I	S	A	M	D	NO NA
5.4 documents client's response to specific nursing interventions												
5.5 records client-family teaching performed												
6. Evaluates client's progress toward desired outcomes												
6.1 notes whether client met stated outcomes during clinical time												
6.2 utilizes measurable client outcomes												
7. Revises plan of care when indicated												
8. Detects salient aspects of client's behavior												
8.1 assesses adverse reactions to interventions												
8.2 assesses reaction to hospitalization												
Course objective 4: Accepts responsibility and accountability for one's own actions.												
1. *Seeks assistance when needed												

NUR 301, Clinical Evaluation (continued)

	Midterm Eval						Final Eval					
	I	S	A	M	D	NO NA	I	S	A	M	D	NO NA
1.1 utilizes clinical instructor appropriately												
1.2 utilizes hospital staff appropriately for assistance and information												
1.3 utilizes peers appropriately for assistance and information												
1.4 verbally accepts responsibility for inappropriately seeking assistance												
2. *Maintains client safety												
Course objective 5: Applies beginning leadership skills and a knowledge of the political system to enhance the delivery of professional nursing care to individuals.												
1. Demonstrates ability to effectively manage time in the clinical setting												
2. Demonstrates ability to prioritize planned nursing interventions												
3. Schedules nursing activities to promote client comfort												
4. Organizes activities to promote efficiency												

NUR 301, Clinical Evaluation (*continued*)

	Midterm Eval						Final Eval					
	I	S	A	M	D	NO/NA	I	S	A	M	D	NO/NA
Course objective 6: Applies selected research findings to professional nursing practice.												
1. Plans nursing activities that will facilitate the achievement of client outcomes												
1.1 states current research findings that support nursing interventions for planned interventions and outcomes												
2. Incorporates theoretical knowledge and scientific principles into nursing care												
2.1 states scientific rationale for nursing interventions												
Course objective 7: Consults with colleagues and the general public to promote the health and well-being of individuals and families.												
1. Seeks client input to develop a plan of care												
2. Consults with other members of the health care team												
2.1 communicates with dietary re: dietary questions												
3. Develops rapport with client and health team members												

NUR 301, Clinical Evaluation (*continued*)

	Midterm Eval						Final Eval					
	I	S	A	M	D	NO NA	I	S	A	M	D	NO NA
3.1 utilizes appropriate interpersonal skills												
4. Reports pertinent client information to appropriate health team members												
5. Incorporates client's significant others into plan of care when appropriate												
6. Plans nursing activities that are congruent with the prescribed medical plan												
Course objective 8: Articulates conflicts in medical, legal, and ethical aspects of nursing practice.												
1. Supports client's right to a personal philosophy, lifestyle												
2. Allows client to choose freely among alternative actions												
3. *Maintains client-family confidentiality*												

NUR 301, Clinical Evaluation (*continued*)

	Midterm Eval					Final Eval				
	I	S	A	M	D	NO NA	I	S	A	M	D	NO NA

	I	S	A	M	D	NO/NA	I	S	A	M	D	NO/NA
Course objective 9: Analyzes emerging nursing roles needed to meet the health needs of the general public in a changing society.												
1. Acts as an advocate for the client												
2. Anticipates client's needs after discharge												
2.1 identifies community resources needed by client post-discharge												
2.2 reviews discharge information with client												
2.3 makes appropriate referrals for discharge												
3. Carries out client teaching												
3.1 provides client with necessary and appropriate information for following prescribed treatment plan												
3.2 provides necessary information for safe administration of prescribed medication												

NUR 301, Clinical Evaluation (*continued*)

	Midterm Eval						Final Eval					
	I	S	A	M	D	NO NA	I	S	A	M	D	NO NA
Course objective 10: Demonstrates an evolving growth of professionalism.												
1. Presents self in clinical area in a professionally dressed and groomed manner												
2. Demonstrates consistent punctuality												
3. Accepts responsibility for clinical assignment without excuses												
4. Demonstrates qualities consistent with leadership characteristics												
4.1 develops increasingly complex time management skills												
4.2 develops prioritization skills appropriately to meet client needs												
4.3 cares for more than one client												
4.4 appropriately delegates to other team members												
4.5 identifies areas of needed change in the clinical setting												
5. Participates in activities that contribute to individual professional development												

NUR 301, Clinical Evaluation (*continued*)

	Midterm Eval						Final Eval					
	I	S	A	M	D	NO NA	I	S	A	M	D	NO NA
5.1 participates in professional organization												
5.2 contributes to disseminating health care information to the community/public and political officials												
5.3 demonstrates autonomous continuous learning outside of the classroom												
5.4 attends a professional conference or in-house education program												
5.5 demonstrates initiative in seeking new learning experiences												

Note. Rating scale adapted from "Clinical evaluation of student performance: The effects of criteria on accuracy and reliability," by K. Bondy, 1984, *Research in Nursing and Health, 7*(1), 25–33. Adapted with permission.
* Copyright 1988, Dr. Linda Scheetz.

Midterm Comments

Faculty:

Student:

End of Semester Comments

Faculty:

_____ _____
Signature   Date

_____ _____
Signature   Date

_____ _____
Signature   Date

13

Clinical Evaluation Tool

Elizabeth P. Howard

PURPOSE

This chapter describes the **Clinical Evaluation Tool**, which enables nursing faculty to measure student achievement of clinical objectives. A baccalaureate nursing program in a private liberal arts college located in the northeast region of the country served as the setting for the study.

The evaluation tool was developed specifically for the nursing program in which it was tested, and thus was organized according to the program's clinical objectives. Although this instrument is designed for one program, the Tylerian model of development and testing described here, which involves comparing measured performance with behavioral standards, has broad applicability (Issac & Michael, 1995). Nursing faculty may replicate the steps to develop an evaluation tool as well as replicate the reliability and validity assessments. The resulting clinical evaluation tool would be specific to the nursing program, having the clinical objectives serve as the organizing framework for the instrument.

INSTRUMENT DESCRIPTION

The conceptual basis for the development of this tool was the behavioral objective or goal-based evaluation model that is designed to provide explicit information to decision makers who try to arrive at a single judgment. Utilization of this model as a framework for clinical evaluations provides specific data to faculty who must decide whether a student has satisfactorily achieved the clinical objectives.

Under the behavioral objectives evaluation approach (Tyler, 1950, 1991), faculty use educational objectives as guidelines for selecting relevant clinical experiences and facilitating the learning process. The model assumes faculty development of appropriate and measurable objectives. Specific nursing behaviors serve to define the objectives and provide the structure to collect data, enabling faculty to assess whether the clinical objectives have been achieved.

Through a review of various instruments currently used as clinical evaluation tools, a list of 70 nursing behaviors was extracted. Initially, four content experts were asked to sort the 70 nursing behavioral items according to the clinical objectives. All content experts were directed to match each behavioral item with the most relevant clinical objective. A "not applicable" category was added to the list of clinical objectives for nursing behaviors that were not related to any of the clinical objectives. The nursing behaviors sorted by the clinical objectives with 75% agreement were included on the initial measure. From the initial sorting of the 70 nursing behaviors with the most relevant clinical objectives, there were 46 nursing behaviors matched with the nine clinical objectives, with a minimum of 75% agreement among the content experts for the 46 nursing behaviors. The initial measure became a tool with nine subscales, one subscale for each clinical objective. The numbers of nursing behaviors in each subscale ranged between 3 and 12.

Eight of the subscales of nursing behaviors had a content validity index of 75% or greater. One subscale of nursing behaviors associated with Clinical Objective I had a content validity index of 67% (see Table 13.1).

The subscale for Clinical Objective I consisted of three nursing behaviors. Faculty rated two of the three behaviors as "very relevant." The remaining behavior received a rating of "somewhat relevant" by one evaluator and "very relevant" by the other. This discrepancy resulted in a content validity index of 67% for the subscale. Because only two faculty members

TABLE 13.1 Content Validity Index for Subscales of Nursing Behaviors

Clinical Objective *(Subscale)*	*Content Validity Index* % Agreement
I	67
II	90
III	100
IV	100
V	100
VI	75
VII	100
VIII	92
IX	83

assessed the content validity of the behavior and there were only three behaviors for this subscale, no changes were made. However, faculty were expected to further evaluate the nursing behaviors associated with Clinical Objective I following initial implementation of the instrument.

The tool is designed to be utilized by faculty to evaluate student achievement of each clinical objective at the completion of the first semester in the nursing program. They evaluate student performance of the nursing behaviors using a 4-point rating scale. This scale is defined by the following terms: *consistently performs* (performs 90%–100% of the time), *usually performs* (performs 80%–89% of the time), *occasionally performs* (performs 60%–79% of the time), and *fails to perform* (performs less than 60% of the time). The rating scale has assigned values of 4, 3, 2, and 1, respectively.

The average rating for each subscale is calculated by summing the rating for each nursing behavior and dividing the sum by the total number of behaviors for the particular subscale. For example, if a subscale consisted of six nursing behaviors, the rating for each behavior would be added together, and this sum would be divided by 6. The resulting value represents an average rating for the subscale or clinical objective. The overall average rating of the student's clinical performance is calculated by summing the average rating for each subscale and dividing this sum by 9, the total number of subscales.

Implementation of this scoring procedure provides faculty and students with data regarding achievement of individual clinical objectives as well as an overall assessment of clinical performance.

RELIABILITY AND VALIDITY ASSESSMENTS

The reliability of the clinical evaluation tool was estimated by implementing interrater agreement procedures for criterion-referenced measures (Howard, 1990). These procedures assess the consistency of classifications by two raters evaluating one group of individuals, using the same measurement tool on the same occasion. In a pilot study, two faculty members evaluated a group of eight nursing students at the same time, using the clinical evaluation tool.

The average rating for each student was calculated and rounded to the nearest whole number, which represented one of four classifications. All students were classified into one of two groups: "usually performs the nursing behaviors" (80%–89% of the time) and "occasionally performs the nursing behaviors" (60%–79% of the time). The resulting P, the proportion of observed agreements in classification of both raters for eight students on the measure of clinical performance was .50. K, the proportion of nonchance agreements was .50. These results indicate the need to further evaluate the reliability of the instrument following each administration. A detailed discussion of the application and interpretation of the rating scale among faculty members who use the tool may serve to increase the consistency in measuring student clinical performance.

Four additional content experts were given the list of clinical objectives and the corresponding nursing behaviors that resulted from the initial sorting. The content experts assigned a value of +1, 0, or –1 for each item depending on the item's congruence with the clinical objective. The scale was defined by the following terms: +1, item is a definite measure of the objective; 0, uncertain about whether the item is a measure of the objective; and –1, item is not a measure of the objective.

Following this rating, the index of item-objective congruence was calculated for each nursing behavior. The desired index cutoff score was .75. Of the 46 items on the initial measure, 38 nursing behaviors had an index score of .75 or greater. The initial measure was revised to include the 38 nursing behaviors and the corresponding clinical objectives.

The next phase of the project involved an evaluation of the relevancy of each behavior to the clinical objective. Two nursing faculty members, who would eventually use the clinical evaluation tool that resulted from this project, were asked to participate in this phase. The faculty members were asked to independently evaluate the relevancy of each nursing behavior to the clinical objective using the following rating scale: 1, not relevant; 2, somewhat relevant; 3, quite relevant; and 4, very relevant. The proportion of nursing behaviors given a rating of quite relevant or very relevant by both raters was calculated. The resulting percentage was the content validity index (CVI) for each subscale of nursing behaviors used to measure achievement of the clinical objectives. Table 13.1 lists the content validity index for each subscale of nursing behaviors. The nine subscales of nursing behaviors represent the nine clinical objectives and their associated nursing behaviors.

The protocol specified here may be adapted for use in other nursing programs. Using a generic set of nursing behaviors, faculty may correlate these behaviors with the clinical objectives. The procedures for establishing the reliability and validity of the instrument then may be replicated.

The goal-based, or behavioral objectives evaluation, approach (Tyler, 1950) provides a suitable avenue for the development and implementation of a clinical evaluation tool. Clarity regarding faculty expectations of student performance is enhanced when the standards and criteria are stated explicitly. This model also allows for a logical consistent approach to evaluating achievement of educational outcomes.

The evaluation of student clinical performance is a continuing challenge. The measure described here is one attempt to meet the challenge and create a method for objectively assessing achievement of clinical objectives. In addition to evaluating student performance, the tool provides a vehicle for feedback to students and may be regarded as a method for measuring program implementation.

REFERENCES

Howard, E. P. (1990). *Measurement of student clinical performance.* In C. F. Waltz & O. L. Strickland (Eds.), *Measurement of nursing outcomes: Vol. 3. Measuring clinical skills and professional development in education and practice* (31–43). New York: Springer Publishing Company.

Issac, S., & Michael, W. B. (1995). *Handbook in research and evaluation* (3rd ed.). San Diego, CA: EdITS.

Tyler, R. W. (1950). *Basic principles of curriculum and instruction.* Chicago: University of Chicago Press.

Tyler, R. W. (1991). General statement on program evaluation. In M. W. McLaughlen & D. C. Phillips (Eds.). *Nineteenth yearbook of the National Society for the Study of Education: Pt. II. Evaluation and education at quarter century.* Chicago, IL: National Society for the Study of Education.

CLINICAL EVALUATION TOOL

Instructions

1. This evaluation tool should be used by students and faculty for evaluating the student's clinical learning.
2. Determine the performance level of the student for each behavior listed under the clinical objectives by using the rating scale specified.
3. Each objective must be achieved at a "satisfactory" level in order to achieve an overall satisfactory evaluation.
4. Satisfactory level is defined by an average rating of 2.5 or greater.
5. Please comment with specific examples on each objective.
6. A student must pass the clinical practice component of the course with a satisfactory evaluation.

Rating Scale

4—consistently performs (performs behaviors 90%–100% of the time)
3—usually performs (performs behaviors 80%–89% of the time)
2—occasionally performs (performs behaviors 60%–79% of the time)
1—fails to perform (performs behaviors less than 60% of the time)
0—not applicable

I. Relate knowledge from nursing, the natural, behavioral and social sciences, and the humanities to the nursing care of client systems.

1. Use theoretical and empirical knowledge in the nursing process.	4	3	2	1	0
2. Utilize knowledge of group dynamics in nursing practice.	4	3	2	1	0
3. Evaluate behavior based on knowledge of human responses and stages of growth and development.	4	3	2	1	0

Comments:

II. Utilize leadership and management skills to organize nursing care for client systems requiring primary and tertiary prevention.

    1. Encourage the client to participate in own care.   4   3   2   1   0

    2. Distinguish between nursing role and other health professionals' roles in the health care delivery system.   4   3   2   1   0

    3. Recognize the importance of their future role as leaders.   4   3   2   1   0

    4. Value the contributions of all persons involved in providing health care.   4   3   2   1   0

    5. Utilize the principles of change to achieve goals with individuals and groups.   4   3   2   1   0

Comments:

III. Utilize results of nursing and related research in the delivery of nursing care to the client systems.

    1. Use research findings to improve nursing practice.   4   3   2   1   0

Comments:

IV. Identify own learning needs in collaboration with faculty.

    1. Seek resources to improve own level of practice based on evaluation by self and others.   4   3   2   1   0

Comments:

V. Identify the client's rights and advocacy needs related to health care.

    1. Encourage the client to select own goals.   4   3   2   1   0

    2. Encourage the client to participate in own care.   4   3   2   1   0

    3. Involve the client/family in assessing, planning, implementing and evaluating nursing care.   4   3   2   1   0

Comments:

VI. Demonstrate professional accountability to client systems for the provision of quality nursing care within the bounds of the beginning student experiences.

1. Apply theoretical concepts   4   3   2   1   0
   of nursing and management to
   own practice.
2. Participate in formal   4   3   2   1   0
   activities designed to evaluate
   the quality of nursing care.
3. Evaluate interpersonal relationships   4   3   2   1   0
   with other health professionals.
4. Appreciate the importance of   4   3   2   1   0
   participating in professional
   organizations and community activities.

Comments:

VII. Communicate with client systems and members of the nursing team to promote system stability.

1. Assess communication of and   4   3   2   1   0
   families based on knowledge and
   techniques of interpersonal
   communications.
2. Use appropriate communication   4   3   2   1   0
   techniques in nursing practice.
3. Communicate effectively through   4   3   2   1   0
   utilization of oral and written
   methods.

Comments:

VIII. Utilize the nursing process in the provision of nursing care to client systems experiencing potential stressors impacting the flexible line of defense.

1. Involve the client/family in   4   3   2   1   0
   assessing, planning, implementing,
   and evaluating nursing care.
2. Implement a plan of nursing   4   3   2   1   0
   intervention that is consistent with
   ANA Standards of Practice.
3. Determine the need for nursing   4   3   2   1   0
   intervention based on data analysis.
4. Develop nursing diagnosis.   4   3   2   1   0
5. Collect data about the   4   3   2   1   0
   health status of clients.

6.	Develop objectives based on identified nursing diagnosis.	4	3	2	1	0
7.	Evaluate the effectiveness of a plan based on an understanding of the dependent functions of the nurse.	4	3	2	1	0
8.	Implement the teaching plan designed to improve or maintain health.	4	3	2	1	0
9.	Recognize the independent function of the teaching role.	4	3	2	1	0
10.	Evaluate the effectiveness of the teaching plan based on an understanding of the interdependent functions of the nurse.	4	3	2	1	0
11.	Evaluate the effectiveness of the teaching plan based on an understanding of the independent functions of the nurse.	4	3	2	1	0
12.	Revise the nursing care plan based on the evaluation of outcomes.	4	3	2	1	0

Comments:

IX. Utilize systems theory to identify social, political, and economic stressors on the client system.

1.	Seek current knowledge of the political, social, and economic factors that affect nursing practice.	4	3	2	1	0
2.	Demonstrate an appreciation for cultural and societal factors that affect health promotion/ maintenance, restoration, and rehabilitation.	4	3	2	1	0
3.	Analyze how personal, social, and cultural values influence decision making in providing care to individuals or groups.	4	3	2	1	0

4. Collaborate with the individual   4   3   2   1   0
    or group in identifying alternative
    actions available to promote,
    maintain, or restore health
    consistent with their cultural values.

5. Discern the influence of ethical   4   3   2   1   0
    legal issues on the provision of
    nursing care.

6. Determine community resources   4   3   2   1   0
    for promotion of optimal level
    of wellness for client/family.

Comments:

14

Measuring RN Students' Clinical Skills via Computer

Linda Finke, Patricia Messmer, Marie Spruck,
Barbara Gilman, Elizabeth Weiner,
and Lou Ann Emerson

PURPOSE

The clinical simulation exam tests the nurse's ability to gather pertinent information about clients and to make appropriate decisions based on that data. Successful completion of the clinical simulation exam by the RN serves as validation of the required competency level to enter an RN completion program. The purpose was to design and implement a prototype for testing the reliability and validity of an existing computer simulation that can be readily adapted for use across varied computer simulations.

INSTRUMENT DESCRIPTION

The use of computers is becoming increasingly important in nursing education as a means to facilitate students development of clinical and diagnostic reasoning skills using patient simulations (Stamler, Thomas, & McMahon, 1999; Lange et al., 1997). Predicted benefits of such computer applications include better preparation for critical thinking and reasoning (Poirrier, Wills, Broussard, & Payne, 1996) and opportunities to experience practical applications that cannot be provided in the classroom alone (Stamler, Thomas, & McMahon, 1999). In this tool (or instrument), four clinical situations were referenced to measure the desired competencies of RNs entering a BSN-MSN educational mobility program. The question driving the study was: Does the technology of the computer provide a medium for an efficient, confidential, and consistent evaluation of the student?

Available simulations were reviewed by a core of faculty and the decision made to utilize the software, Clinical Simulations in Nursing: Medical-Surgical Nursing Simulations I & II (1986), to determine the clinical competencies of the RN seeking clinical credit assessment. Clinical Simulations in Nursing (CSN) is a software package developed by the Medical Examination Publishing Company to be used on Apple or IBM equipment. At the time of this study, reliability and validity had not been determined for the CSN. The minimal competencies to be validated were based on those established by a Midwest Alliance in Nursing (MAIN) project funded by the W. K. Kellogg Foundation (Primm, 1986).

The MAIN practice model has three major and three minor components. Major components include provision of direct care, communication, and management of care. Minor components are patient teaching, coordination with other disciplines, and delegation of care. Competencies for the MAIN for the ADN and BSN were differentiated by MAIN according to each component of the nursing practice model. The competencies were examined by a core group of faculty, who reached consensus that the following competencies were minimal expectations for the RN before beginning nursing courses in the program:

1. Direct care competencies
   a. Expanding the collection of data to identify complex health care needs.
   b. Organizing and analyzing health pattern data in order to select nursing diagnoses from an established list.
   c. Establishing goals with the focal client to develop a comprehensive nursing plan of care from admission to postdischarge.
   d. Developing and implementing an individualized nursing plan of care using established nursing diagnoses and protocols to promote, maintain, and restore health.
   e. Interpreting the medical plan of care into nursing activities to formulate approaches to nursing care.
   f. Evaluating focal client responses to nursing interventions and altering the plan of care as necessary to meet client needs.
2. Communication competencies
   a. Developing and maintaining goal-directed interactions to promote effective coping behaviors and facilitate change in behavior.
   b. Modifying and implementing a standard teaching plan in order to restore, maintain, and promote health.
   c. Documenting and communicating data for clients with common, well-defined nursing diagnoses to provide continuity of care.

      d.   Using established channels of communication to implement an effective health care plan.

3.   Management competencies

      a.   Prioritizing, planning, and organizing the delivery of comprehensive nursing care in order to use time and resources effectively and efficiently.

      b.   Recognizing the need for referral and conferring with appropriate nursing personnel for assistance to promote continuity of care.

      c.   Working with other health care personnel within the organizational structure to manage client care.

The four simulations available in CSN I—"A Surgical Patient," "A Patient with Abdominal Pain," "A Patient"—with Cardiopulmonary Distress, and An Unconscious Patient, were given to students in random order. Students were required to pass the simulations with an average score of 65% in order to be considered successful. Two attempts to pass the simulations were given. The second attempt was made on the same four simulations in CSN II.

The scoring process is inherent in the simulation program. Both a raw score and percentage for information gathering and decision making are presented at the end of a simulation. The student is scored on each option selected as the student proceeds through the simulation on a scale of +3 to −3. The scoring rationale is as follows:

+3 Of central importance to good patient care. Omission would result in serious damage to the patient in terms of cost, time, pain, or risk of morbidity and/or mortality.

+2 Strongly contributes to good patient care.

+1 Mildly contributes to good patient care.

0   Does not contribute to patient care, but does not cause the patient any harms in terms of increased cost, time, pain, or risk.

−1 Mildly detrimental to good patient care.

−2 Seriously detrimental to patient care.

−3 Gravely damaging to patient care and very costly to patient welfare in terms of cost, time, pain, or risk (Medical Examination Publishing Company & Elsevier Science [Instructor's Manual], 1986, pp. 11–12).

Prior to taking the exam, students were given study guides with references for review purposes and were also provided with the opportunity to practice using the computer by completing a clinical simulation not included in the challenge exam (i.e., maternity, psychiatric simulation).

RELIABILITY AND VALIDITY ASSESSMENT

Fifty-four RNs seeking admission into the BSN-MSN program were included in the reliability analysis (Finke et al., 1988). Student ages ranged from 22 to 57 years; 21 were nurses with a diploma in nursing and 23 held an associate degree in nursing. The parallel measures model used to assess the reliability of the simulations. The consistency of paired simulations was analyzed to determine Cohen's kappa. The "A Surgical Patient" and "A Patient with Cardiopulmonary Distress" simulations were paired against the "A Patient with Abdominal Pain" and "An Unconscious Patient." The proportion of students consistently classified as pass or fail on both pairs of simulations (P_o) was .87. Four percent ($n = 2$) of the students failed the surgical/cardiopulmonary paired simulation. None of the students failed the abdominal pain/unconscious patient paired simulation. Cohen's kappa was .24; the adjusted kappa (proportion of nonchance agreements over the highest possible agreements) was 1.0. Caution should be exercised in interpreting this result in that the adjusted reliability may not be consistent due to the fact that the test had a cutoff point and a very homogeneous group was measured (Waltz, Strickland, & Lenz, 1991).

Validity was examined using three methods (content, construct, and decision-making validity) appropriate for criterion-referenced tests to determine the extent that the simulations measured the clinical competency of the RNs (Finke et al., 1988).

Content validity was determined using a panel of four expert judges who scored the extent to which each competency was measured in each simulation. A content validity index (CVI) was determined for each simulation and two simulations were paired as stated above. The CVI for the surgical patient/cardiopulmonary distress pair was .88, and for the abdominal pain/unconscious patient pair, .81.

Construct validity was investigated using contrasted groups. Sophomore students, a group not expected to possess the clinical competencies, were compared with the RNs. The mean score of 22 sophomores was compared with the mean for the RNs using a t test for each simulation. Significant differences were found between the scores on all simulations except "A Patient with Abdominal Pain" [$t(58) = 1.13$, $p > .05$]. When scoring for both groups on this simulation was examined in more detail, it was determined that the mean scores on information gathering were significantly different [$t(58) = 1.96$, $p < .05$], as well as the mean scores on decision making [$t(5) = 4.52$, $p < .05$]. It was only after averaging the information gathering scores and the decision-making scores that there was not a significant difference at the .05 level.

Decision-making validity was calculated by computing the correlation between the mean scores on the clinical simulations and the clinical course grades of the RNs from the first clinical course taken by them after entering the program using the Pearson product-moment correlation coefficient. Mean ranges for the four simulations were 67% to 81%, and the mean ranges from the clinical grades were 80% to 100%. The correlation was $r = .37$, $p < .05$. Each simulation was also correlated with the clinical grades. The unconscious patient simulation yielded the highest correlation ($r = .52$, $p = < .002$).

In summary, the computer simulations were shown to be a reliable and valid tool to test the clinical competencies of RN students seeking admission to the BSN-MSN educational mobility program for RNs. Evidence was found for content, construct, and decision-making validity. In addition, students in this study could be tested simultaneously in less than four hours, suggesting that computer simulations are a cost-effective alternative in terms of faculty and student time for making observations in the clinical setting.

REFERENCES

Finke, L., Messmer, P., Spruck, M., Gilman, B., Weiner, E., & Emerson, L. (1990). Measuring clinical skills via computer for RNs in a BSN-MSN educational mobility program. In O. L. Struckland & C. F. Waltz (Eds.), *Measurement of nursing outcomes: Vol. 3. Measuring clinical skills and professional development in education and practice* (pp. 44–53). New York: Springer Publishing Company.

Medical Examination Publishing Company, & Elsevier Science. (1986). *Clinical simulations in nursing: Medical-surgical nursing simulations I & II.* [Computer Software]. New York: Authors.

Lange, L. L., Haak, S. W., Lincoln, M. J., Thompson, C. B., Turner, C. W., Weir, C., Foerster, V., Nelasina, D., & Reeves, R. (1997). Use of Iliad to improve diagnostic performance of nurse practitioner students. *Journal of Nursing Education, 36,* 36–45.

Poirrier, S. P., Wills, E. M., Broussard, P. C., & Payne, R. L. (1996). Nursing information systems: Application in nursing curricula. *Nurse Educator, 21* (1), 18–22.

Primm, P. (1986). Defining and differentiating AND and BSN competencies. *Issues, 7*(1), 1–8.

Stamler, L. L., Thomas, B., & McMahon, S. (1999). Nursing students respond to a computer assignment. *Journal of Professional Nursing, 15*(1), 52–58.

Waltz, C., Strickland, O., & Lenz, E. (1991). *Measurement in nursing research* (2nd ed.). Philadelphia: F. A. Davis.

PART II
Measuring Educational Outcomes

15

Influence of Review Course Preparation on NCLEX-RN Scores

Nelda Samarel

PURPOSE

The purpose of this study was to determine how review course participation influenced NCLEX-RN scores. In this case, the NCLEX-RN exam is the measurement tool.

PROJECT DESCRIPTION

Interest in various strategies to facilitate student success on the NCLEX-RN remains high. Among the strategies reported in the literature are cooperative learning groups (Ross, 2000) and computerized practice examinations (e.g., Ross, Nice, May, & Billings, 1996). Examples of such software reviewed in the literature include Billings et al. (1996) and Riner et al. (1997).

Noting the popularity of review courses, Samarel (1990) explored the influence of participation in these courses on NCLEX-RN scores. Of particular interest were questions of whether these courses were helpful and whether their impact on NCLEX-RN scores was positive. The conceptual basis was an eclectic blend of learning theories drawing on the work such as that of McDonald (1966) and Gagne (1975). Learning was viewed as a three-part process: input, operation, and feedback. A review course involving knowledge acquisition, repetition, and practice was hypothesized to further develop knowledge retention, recall, and generalization in nursing school graduates that would in turn positively impact on NCLEX-RN scores. Three hypotheses were posed: (a) participants in a review course would perform better than nonparticipants on the NCLEX-RN; (b) participants would demonstrate greater improvement over pretest scores than nonparticipants; and (c) those scoring poorly on the pretest would demonstrate greater benefit from participating in a review course than graduate nurses who scored well on the pretest. The project design was quasi-experimental.

The outcome measure was the NCLEX-RN. The pretest was the National League for Nursing Comprehensive Nursing Achievement Test (NLNC-NAT), which has been acknowledged as a strong predictor of NCLEX-RN performance (Breyer, 1984, 1986). The NLNCNAT was administered to subjects in January of their senior year, 6 months before taking the NCLEX-RN. The NCLEX-RN was taken in July following graduation and 6 weeks after review courses were completed by participants.

Subjects were graduates ($N = 28$) of an entire class from a BSN program at a state university. The 21 who participated in review courses took either a 5-day course ($n = 2$) or an 8-day university-sponsored course ($n =19$). The remaining seven students did not participate in a review course. While review course participants scored higher on the NCLEX-RN than did nonparticipants, the difference was not statistically significant. Pretest scores of the nonparticipants in a review course were higher than those of participants, which indicated the need for using pretest scores as a covariate. This re-analysis revealed a positive effect of review course participation on NCLEX-RN scores, although the results were not statistically significant. Those who participated in the review courses had a statistically significant gain in scores between NLNCNAT and NCLEX-RN administrations. Those with lower scores on the NLNCNAT benefited more from review course participation, although this effect was not statistically significant. In summary, of the three hypotheses posed, only the second was statistically significant.

Results have generally positive implications for participation in review courses, particularly for those identified as at risk by low NLNCNAT scores. Further research with larger sample sizes of graduates from various types of educational programs was recommended (Samarel, 1990).

REFERENCES

Billings, D., Hodson-Carlton, L., Kirkpatrick, J., Aaltonen, P., Dillard, N., Richardson, V., Siktberg, L., & Vinten, S. (1996). Computerized NCLEX-RN preparation programs: A comparative review. *Computers in Nursing, 15*(5), 255–267.

Breyer, F. J. (1984). The Comprehensive Nursing Achievement Test as a predictor of performance on the NCLEX-RN. *Nursing and Health Care, 5*(4), 193–195.

Breyer, F. J. (1986). *The Comprehensive Nursing Achievement Test, 1986 edition as a predictor of performance on the NCLEX-RN: A validity update.* New York: National League for Nursing.

Gagne, R. M. (1975). *Essentials of learning for instruction*. Hinsdale, IL: Dryden Press.

McDonald, F. J. (1966). *Educational psychology*. Belmont, CA: Wadsworth.

Riner, M. E., Mueller, C., Ihrke, B., Smolen, R. A., Wilson, M., Richardson, V., Stone, C., & Zwirn, E. E. (1997). Computerized NCLEX-RN and NCLEX-PN preparation programs: Comparative review. *Computers in Nursing, 15*(5), 255–267.

Ross. B., Nice, A., May, F. E., & Billings, D. M. (1996). Assisting students at risk: Using computer NCLEX-RN review software. *Nurse Educator, 21*(2), 39–43.

Ross, C. A. (2000). Benefits of cooperative learning groups when preparing for the NCLEX-RN examination. *Nurse Educator, 25*(3), 124.

Samarel, N. (1990). Effect of review course participation on NCLEX-RN scores of graduate nurses. In C. F. Waltz & O. L. Strickland (Eds.), *Measurement of nursing outcomes: Vol. 3. Measuring clinical skills and professional development in education and practice* (pp. 361–372). New York: Springer Publishing Company.

16

Influence of English Language on Ability to Pass the NCLEX-RN

Joan Gittins Johnston

PURPOSE

The purpose of this study was to determine if the NCLEX-RN is a reliable and valid measure of minimum competence in new graduate nurses whose primary language is not English.

PROJECT DESCRIPTION

Numerous reports focus on identifying key predictors of nursing school graduate success (e.g., Barkley, Rhodes, & DuFour, 1998) and failure (e.g., Wendt, Worcester, & Loquist, 1998) on the NCLEX-RN. English as a second language is an important consideration, particularly when foreign-born graduates are included in such studies (e.g., Endres, 1997).

The author undertook this project after having noted the higher failure rate on the NCLEX-RN by respondents whose primary language is not English (see Johnston, 1990). This project was also an attempt to identify possible predictors of NCLEX-RN failure in ethnically and linguistically diverse students.

The study was conducted in a school where 95% of students were ethnically diverse; Haitian Creole or Spanish was the primary language of approximately 40% of the students. NCLEX-RN pass rates of school graduates were low, and the mean scores of those who did pass were below the state mean.

Key variables of interest were: (a) primary language (from student self-report, faculty knowledge, or both); (b) science grade-point average (from grades on two 4-credit anatomy and physiology courses and two 4-credit chemistry courses); and (c) enrollment in remedial courses (on basis of

College Skills Assessment test scores in math, English, and reading). Data on these variables were obtained via record review; NCLEX-RN scores were obtained from the state board of nursing.

In the first phase of this project, data on primary language and NCLEX-RN scores (percentage pass/fail for each language group) were obtained on 290 graduates. Of these, English was the primary spoken language for 184; 31 were bilingual; Spanish was the primary spoken language for 26; 38 spoke Creole; and 11 reported another language as their primary spoken language. In this group, NCLEX-RN pass rates varied widely. Bilingual graduates had the highest pass rate (100%), followed by those with English as their primary spoken language (79.9%), dominant Creole speakers (57.9%), dominant Spanish speakers (46.2%), and finally, a low of 36.4% among those graduates reporting "other" as their primary spoken language.

In the next phase, data for 142 graduates of the 290 in the first phase who had completed all of their education in the same program were obtained on the key variables and coded dichotomously: (a) English/non-English; (b) science grade point average (SPGA) above or below 2.2; and (c) remediation, yes/no. NCLEX-RN scores (percentage pass rates) were categorized by these variables as seen in Table 16.1.

When variables were considered in combination, students whose first language was English, regardless of their academic record, had a likelihood of passing the NCLEX-RN of between 67.7% and 95%. If English was a second language, the NCLEX-RN pass rate dropped to between 33.3% and 47% (Johnston, 1990).

In the third phase, regression analysis was conducted to explore the relative contribution of each of the three key variables to explaining variance in NCLEX-RN scores. Together the amount of variance explained was 36%, with language alone accounting for 20%.

This project points to language skills as a key factor in passing the NCLEX-RN examination. The author recommends future work on the NCLEX-RN to help ensure that tests are as free as possible of cultural and linguistic bias.

TABLE 16.1 Language and Academic Variables   NCLEX Pass Rate (%)

Key Variables and	NCLEX Pass Rate
English	84.9
Non-English	45
SGPA above 2.2	77.3
SGPA below 2.2	58.6
Remedials	60.9
No remedials	92.1

REFERENCES

Barkley, T. W. Jr., Rhodes, R. S., & DuFour, C. A. (1998). Predictors of success on the NCLEX-RN among baccalaureate nursing students. *Nursing and Health Care Perspectives, 19*(3), 132–137.

Endres, D. (1997). A comparison of predictors of success on NLCEX-RN for African American, foreign-born, and white baccalaureate graduates. *Journal of Nursing Education, 36*(8), 365–371.

Johnston, J. G. (1990). The influence of English language on the ability to pass the NCLEX-RN. In C. F. Waltz & Strickland, O. L. (Eds.), *Measurement of nursing outcomes: Vol. 3. Measuring clinical skills and professional development in education and practice* (pp. 373–383). New York: Springer Publishing Company.

Wendt, A., Worcester, P., & Loquist, R. (1998). Update on NCLEX-RN candidate diagnostic profiles: Candidates who fail the examination. *Computers in Nursing, 16*(3), 142, 144.

17

Criterion-Related Validity of the NCLEX-RN

Muriel W. Lessner

PURPOSE

This project assessed the effect of a type of integrated versus noninte-grated curriculum or curriculum characteristics on performance on the **NCLEX-RN** exam.

DESCRIPTION

The literature continues to offer numerous reports relating to the crite-rion validity of the NCLEX-RN, and the most frequently studied variables are academic. Such studies, including this one, generally focus on aca-demic achievement indicators collected at various points in student edu-cation preparation or program of study (e.g., Alexander & Brophy, 1997; Schmidt, 2000).

The conceptual basis for this project is systems theory, in which the cur-riculum is viewed as an open system. The focus was on the "output" of this system—professionally educated nurses and the extent of their educational preparation as measured on the licensing examination. Students are clearly the "input" in this conceptualization. However, the "throughput," or deliv-ery of the educational process, varies. For example, in baccalaureate nurs-ing education, this process may be described as integrated, which "is generally thought to eliminate teaching the same content in several basic courses and to allow more time to give students a greater amount of expo-sure to more knowledge" (Pardue, 1979, p. 305); or nonintegrated, which is subject centered and sometimes described as blocked (Lessner, 1990).

Conducting a study of whether differences existed in student outcomes depending on whether their nursing education had been in integrated or nonintegrated baccalaureate programs also provided an opportunity to concurrently explore criterion-related validity of the National Council Licensure Examination for Registered Nurses (NCLEX-RN). The NCLEX-RN became the national licensing examination for registered nurses in 1982. It is organized around the nursing process, which was a change from the special-area structure of the examination previously used which was the State Board Test Pool Exam (SBTPE). Both are standardized examinations meeting criteria as described in Waltz, Strickland, & Lenz (1991).

Several measures were used in this retrospective study. Scores from a pre-college entrance test [the College Aptitude Test (ACT) or the Scholastic Aptitude Test (SAT)], and the SBTPE or the NCLEX-RN were considered. The ACT addresses four areas: English usage (possible score range, 1 to 33) and mathematics (1 to 36), and reading in social studies (1 to 34) and natural science (1 to 35). A mean composite ACI score is also produced, ranging from 1 to 35. The SAT measures verbal and mathematical abilities; scores on each of these can range from 200 to 800. Both are used to predict an individual's potential for success in college. The passing score for the SBTPE on each of the sections (medical, surgical, maternity, pediatric, and psychiatric) was 350, with the possible range of scores from 200 to 800. On the NCLEX-RN, the passing score is 1600 with the possible range of scores from 800 to 3200. Each of four measures had reported evidence of reliability and validity. In addition, data on high-school rank, as well as grade point averages (GPAs) for high school, the end of the sophomore year, nursing theory courses, nursing process (clinical) courses, and cumulative for the baccalaureate degree were collected. The source of data was student records. Fifty records were randomly selected from each of the six classes from 1979 to 1984 from each of two public research universities. As noted previously, the NCLEX-RN replaced the SBTPE in 1982 (Lessner, 1990).

With ACT and SAT scores as covariates to control for potential differences in student abilities between those in integrated and nonintegrated curricula, both SBTPE ($n = 289$) or NCLEX-RN ($n = 299$) scores were statistically significantly different, with those from nonintegrated curricula having higher scores. Students from nonintegrated curricula also had higher scores on the ACT or SAT. On inspection, mean GPAs for the students from the nonintegrated program were higher at all points in time reported (high school GPA was not reported). Predictors of NCLEX-RN performance were identified using stepwise multiple regression analyses. Nursing theory GPA and nursing process GPA together accounted for 50% of the variance in NCLEX-RN scores in students from integrated programs. In students from nonintegrated programs, three predictors entered the equation. Together, nursing theory GPA, total ACT score, and high school GPA accounted for a total of 54% of the variance in NCLEX-RN scores. The only common predictor of NCLEX-RN scores identified between the two programs was nursing theory GPA (Lessner, 1990).

Given that various predictors of NCLEX-RN scores vary in importance across reported studies, the author (1990) recommended that each program may wish to identify the rank order of predictors for its graduates, as well as further study to increase the amount of variance explained in NCLEX-RN scores (Lessner, 1990).

REFERENCES

Alexander, J. E., Brophy, G. H. (1997). A five-year study of graduates' performance on NLEX-RN. *Journal of Nursing Education, 36*(9), 443–445.

Lessner, M. W. (1990). Student outcomes of integrated and nonintegrated baccalaureate nursing programs. In C. F. Waltz & O. L. Strickland (Eds.), *Measurement of nursing outcomes: Vol. 3. Measuring/clinical skills and professional development in education and practice* (pp. 349–360). New York: Springer Publishing Company.

Pardue, S. F. (1979). Blocked- and integrated-content baccalaureate nursing programs: A comparative study. *Nursing Research. 28*(5), 305–311.

Schmidt, A. E. (2000). An approximation of a hierarchical logistic model used to establish the predictive validity of scores on a nursing licensure exam. *Educational and Psychological Measurement. 60*(3), 463–478

Waltz, C. F., Strickland, O. L., and Lenz, E. R. (1991). *Measurement in nursing research* (2nd ed.). Philadelphia: F. A. Davis.

18

Self-Assessment Leadership Instrument

Bonnie Ketchum Smola

PURPOSE

The purpose of the **Self-Assessment Leadership Instrument** (SALI) is to measure leadership characteristics in baccalaureate nursing students or nurses in practice.

INSTRUMENT DESCRIPTION

Leadership in nursing is critical at multiple levels (Fagin, 1996; Fralic, 1999), from preparing students for leadership roles (DiSimone, 1996) to preparing leaders in clinical settings for institutionalizing evidence-based practice (Stetler et al., 1998). Measures of leadership characteristics such as the SALI are integral components of outcome measurement in leadership development.

The definition of leadership used in development of the SALI is drawn from the work of Copi (1961) and articulated as "the process of influencing the behavior of other persons in their efforts toward goal setting and goal achievement; this implies defining and planning for nursing in an interactional setting" (Smola, 1988, p. 314).

The SALI is based on the Leadership Behavior Tool developed by Yura (1970). Yura's work in turn drew upon sources such as the Leadership Behavior Description Questionnaire (LBDQ) by Halpin (1957) as well as literature related to leadership behavior in nursing.

Aspects of various theories are identified as components of the conceptual framework used in developing the SALI. These include: psychological attributes of the group, follower, situations, interpersonal relationships, and communication (Tannenbaum, Weschler, & Massarik,

1961); the leader's interactions with others as well as position in the structure of the organization (Argyis, 1962); behavior of the individual within a group structure (Stogdill, 1958); and decision making (Griffith, 1958). General effects of behavior of an individual in a particular situation (Cartwright & Zander, 1960) and specific leadership behaviors and their effect on group members' behavior (Wenrich & Wenrich, 1974) as well as measurement theories (Martuzza, 1977; Waltz, Strickland, & Lenz, 1991) are also included in the theoretical bases used.

As part of her dissertation research, Yura (1970) developed the 70-item Leadership Behavior Tool for use with 300 nursing faculty in various parts of the United States to explore their perceptions of behavior indicating leadership potential of baccalaureate nursing students. Items were grouped into several categories: self, critical thinking and decision making, interpersonal relationships, group relations, and job relations. Using the frequency data reported by Yura (1970), Smola (1988) conducted chi-square analyses and confirmed an association of item responses with the above categories, which supported Yura's conceptualization.

Using Yura's (1970) instrument, the author collected data from nursing students ($N = 90$) from three colleges to explore their perceptions of nursing leadership behavior. Internal consistency was estimated using the Kuder-Richardson formula; the value obtained was .93. These student scores were not statistically significantly different from those of faculty in the Yura study.

Next, item analysis was carried out using data from this administration. Item difficulty level and discrimination indices were computed. On this basis of these two steps, 46 items were retained. These 46-items were reworded into a self-report format designed for self-administration. Items asking whether the respondents considered themselves to be leaders and whether the respondents had completed a leadership course were added. The response format was a 5-point, Likert-type scale with anchors of 0 = usually not and 4 = almost always. By summing item responses, a total score was obtained, with higher scores indicating higher self-assessment of leadership characteristics. A copy of the SALI is included at the end of the chapter.

RELIABILITY AND VALIDITY ASESSMENT

Test-retest reliability was estimated from data provided by 24 students who completed a second administration of the SALI 10 days after the first. Cohen's K coefficient was used to estimate reliability; the result was 55% agreement.

Five judges, all doctorally prepared with expertise in leadership, reviewed the SALI for aspects of content validity. Clarity and relevance were rated using modified semantic differential scales, and as a result six items were eliminated. Items were also reviewed for congruence with their respective objectives. Items were not eliminated as a result of this process. However, because there was limited agreement (ranging from 0% to 47%) among the judges as to the fit of items in the categories posited by Yura, all items were considered as covering the broad domain of leadership rather than conceptualized into categories. The resulting SALI consists of 40 items.

To estimate construct validity, contrasted groups of nurses identified by peers, head nurses, or directors of nursing as leaders (n = 42) or non-leaders (n = 20) were identified and asked to complete the SALI. Mean item scores were significantly different between these two groups on two-thirds of the items. When asked if they considered themselves to be leaders, 100% of the leader group said yes, and in the nonleader group, 25% said yes. Further use of the SALI should include administration in different circumstances; factor analysis with content analysis of items loading on each factor; and establishment of a cut score/standard to distinguish leaders from nonleaders.

REFERENCES

Argyris, C. (1962). *Interpersonal competences and organizational effectiveness.* Homewood, IL: Dorsey.

Cartwright, R. & Zander, A; (1960). *Group dynamics: Research and theory* (2nd ed.). Evanston, IL: Rowe, Peterson.

Copi, I. (1961). *Introduction to logic.* New York: Macmillan.

DiSimone, B. B. (1996). Transforming curriculum for a nursing leadership course: a collaborative approach. *Journal of Professional Nursing, 12*(2), 111–118.

Fagin, C. M. (1996). Executive leadership: Improving nursing practice, education, and research. *Journal of Nursing Administration, 26*(3), 30–37.

Fralic, M. F. (1999). Nursing leadership for the new millennium: essential knowledge and skills. *Nursing and Health Care Perspectives, 20*(5), 260–265.

Griffith, D. (1958). Administration as decision-making. In A. Halpin (Ed.), *Administrative theory in education* (pp. 199–149). Chicago: University of Chicago, Midwest Administrative Center.

Halpin, A. W. (1957). *Manual for the Leader Behavior Questionnaire.* Columbus, OH: Ohio State University, Bureau of Business Research.

Martuza, V. R. (1977). *Applying norm-referenced and criterion-references measurement in education.* Boston: Allyn and Bacon.

Smola, B. K. (1988). Refinement and validation of a tool measuring leadership characteristics of baccalaureate students. In O. L. Strickland & C. F. Waltz (Eds.), *Measurement of nursing outcomes: Vol. 2. Measuring nursing performance* (pp. 314–336). New York: Springer Publishing Company.

Stetler, C. B., Brunell, M., Giuliano, K. K., Morsin, D., Prince, L., & Newell-Stokes, V. (1998). Evidence-based practice and the role of nursing leadership. *Journal of Nursing Administration, 28*(7–8), 45–53.

Stogdill, R. M. (1958). *Individual behavior and group achievement.* New York: Oxford University Press.

Tannenbaum, R., Weschler, I., & Massarik, F. (1961). *Leadership and organization.* New York: McGraw-Hill.

Waltz, C. F., Strickland, O. L, & Lenz, E. R. (1991). *Measurement in nursing research* (2nd ed.). Philadelphia: F. A. Davis.

Wenrich, R. C., & Wenrich, J. W. (1974). *Leadership in administration of vocational and technical education.* Columbus, OH: Charles E. Merrill.

Yura, H. (1970). *Faculty perceptions of behavior indicating leadership potential of baccalaureate nursing students.* Unpublished doctoral dissertation, Catholic University of America, Washington DC.

SELF-ASSESSMENT LEADERSHIP INSTRUMENT

About the Questionnaire:

Please consider the following behaviors as they relate to your leadership. You should consider your reaction to each behavior and mark the rating accordingly.

A 5-point numerical scale (4 ... 3 ... 2 ... 1 ... 0) is used to indicate the rating. The interpretation of the extreme point on the continuum ranges from:

4—Almost always behave in this manner
0—Usually not behave in this manner

Thus the ratings:

4.........	3.........	2.........	1.........	0
Almost always	More than $1/2$ time	About $1/2$ time	Less than $1/2$ time	Usually not

Directions: 1. Read each statement of behavior.
2. Indicate your judgment of how often you use this behavior.
3. Place the number that most closely indicates your estimate (i.e., 4 or 3 or 2 or 1 or 0) in the space provided at the end of the statement.
4. Respond to *every* statement.

Statement of Leadership Behavior	Rating
1. Evaluate your own needs	(____)
2. Fully grasp the ideas of the problem	(____)
3. Are aware of how you communicate with others	(____)
4. Are able to persuade groups to agree on specific issues	(____)
5. Organize your thoughts clearly and logically	(____)
6. Listen attentively for meaning and feelings	(____)
7. Get others to work together effectively	(____)
8. Predict the consequences of your decisions	(____)
9. Aware of the perceptions of other	(____)
10. Encourage the understanding of point of view of other group members	(____)
11. Plan ahead for what should be done	(____)
12. Recognize and locate resources in order to solve a problem	(____)

13. Show a willingness to make changes (_____)
14. Influence a group in goal setting (_____)
15. Make decisions on a factual basis (_____)
16. Alter your own behavior to meet a situation (_____)
17. Strive to understand other people (_____)
18. Assume responsibility for action taken based on your own decisions (_____)
19. Try to learn what impact you make on others (_____)
20. Grasp essentials of a problem, see solutions, and choose a course of action (_____)
21. Hold the attention of others while presenting pertinent ideas (_____)
22. Try new ideas on a group (_____)
23. Delegate responsibility appropriately (_____)
24. Feel good about face-to-face exchanges of ideas (_____)
25. Discriminate between relevant, irrelevant, essential, and accidental data (_____)
26. Get others to follow your advice and direction (_____)
27. Encourage group members to work as a team (_____)
28. Direct group members or instruct them on what to do (_____)
29. Originate new approaches to problems (_____)
30. Have group member share in the decision making (_____)
31. Look for ways to improve yourself (_____)
32. Initiate action for new and better procedures and policies (_____)
33. Know how to proceed to get something done (_____)
34. Are friendly and approachable (_____)
35. Stand up for a group even if it makes you unpopular (_____)
36. Can define your role in a situation (_____)
37. Explain the reason for criticism (_____)
38. Encourage group members to express their ideas and opinions (_____)
39. Encourage slow-working members to improve their effort (_____)
40. Give credit when credit is due (_____)

19

Evaluation of Learning According to Objectives Tool

Joan M. Johnson

PURPOSE

The purpose of the **Evaluation of Learning According to Objectives Tool** is to measure student perceptions of their competency at the end of a baccalaureate program.

INSTRUMENT DESCRIPTION

The assessment of clinical competence and the difficulty in evaluating nursing performance in an objective, reliable, and valid way remain salient concerns (O'Connor, Pearse, Smith, Vogeli, & Walton, 1999).

The theoretical definition of competence used in developing the Evaluation of Learning According to Objectives Tool was "the student's perceived achievement of clearly specified behavioral objectives, established to characterize competency in nursing, based on the University of Wisconsin-Oshkosh curriculum" (Johnson, 1988, p. 338).

The conceptual basis of the instrument was the University of Wisconsin-Oshkosh curriculum, which builds on the humanities, natural and social sciences, and prenursing courses. The nursing content is developed along the health-illness continuum with individual, environment, health, and nursing as key components.

The program's terminal objectives are:

1. Use the nursing process to maintain, promote, or improve health of individuals, groups, and communities.
2. Use teaching methods to improve nursing and other health care.

3. Make informed decisions concerning the delivery of comprehensive health care.
4. Establish effective interpersonal relationships based on knowledge of human behavior.
5. Collaborate in independent, dependent, and interdependent role relations to promote, restore, and maintain the health of individuals, groups, and communities.
6. Assume professional responsibility for providing quality nursing care.
7. Assume responsibility for own personal and professional growth (Johnson, 1988, p. 340).

There are 57 performance indicators for these terminal curriculum objectives. These indicators were used to develop the 67 items comprising the Evaluation of Learning According to Objectives Tool. The instrument is a paper-and-pencil measure designed to be self-administered at or near the end of the baccalaureate nursing program. Respondents are asked to indicate the extent to which they are able to perform each of the terminal behaviors listed using a 5-point, Likert-type scale response format (5 = very well to 1 = not at all). A total score is obtained from the summing of item scores. Relevant item scores can also be summed for each of the terminal objectives. A copy of the tool is included at the end of the chapter.

RELIABILITY AND VALIDITY ASSESSMENT

Internal consistency reliability was estimated from data provided by 60 senior nursing students three weeks before graduation. They were asked to rate how well they could carry out each behavior listed in items without assistance. The alpha value obtained was .96 for the total instrument. Alpha values for categories of items reflecting each of the seven objectives ranged from .79 (objective I) to .996 (objective II).

The test-retest reliability estimate was based on data from the initial administration and another carried out three weeks later on the last day of class. Coefficients were statistically significant ($p = .05$ to $.001$) for each of the categories of items by objective and ranged from $r = .255$ to $.748$.

Ratings of the relevance of each item to the curriculum and its objectives implemented by two faculty members were used to estimate content validity. Because the content validity index obtained was .91, all 67 items on the instrument were retained.

Evidence for predictive criterion validity was the statistically significant relationship between students' scores and subsequent scores on the state board examination ($r = .749$; $p < .01$). Ten faculty ratings of student competence were correlated with scores of respective students; this correlation was not statistically significant, nor were correlations between scores on the Evaluation of Learning According to Objectives Tool and National League for Nursing test scores.

The author recommends further work to accrue additional evidence for the validity of the measure, as well as further research using the tool. Use of the instrument within other curricula may require modification to tailor items to objectives of the program in which it will be employed. Items relate to objectives in the three major areas of cognitive, affective, and psychomotor functioning (Menix, 1996) of nursing practice, which may facilitate usefulness within other schools.

REFERENCE

Johnson, J. M. (1988). Assessing students in relation to curriculum objectives. In O. L. Strickland & C. F. Waltz (Eds.), *Measurement of nursing outcomes: Vol. 2. Measuring nursing performance* (pp. 337–348). New York: Springer Publishing Company.

Menix, K. D. (1996). Domains of learning: Interdependent components of achievable learning outcomes. *Journal of Continuing Education in Nursing, 27*(5), 200–208.

O'Connor, S., E., Pearse, J., Smith, R. L., Vogeli, D., & Walton, P. (1999). Monitoring the quality of pre-registration education: Development, validation and piloting of competency based performance indicators for newly qualified nurses. *Nurse Education Today 1999, 19*(4) 334–341.

EVALUATION OF LEARNING ACCORDING TO CURRICULUM OBJECTIVES

We are interested in how well your program has prepared students to implement program goals. Indicate the extent to which you are able to perform each of the following terminal behaviors.

	Very Well				Not At All
1. Use research findings to improve nursing practice.	5	4	3	2	1
2. Use theoretical and empirical knowledge in the application of the nursing process.	5	4	3	2	1
3. Collect data about the health status of clients.	5	4	3	2	1
4. Collect data about the health status of a group or community.	5	4	3	2	1
5. Determine the need for nursing intervention based on data analysis.	5	4	3	2	1
6. Develop nursing diagnoses.	5	4	3	2	1
7. Develop objectives based on identified nursing diagnoses.	5	4	3	2	1
8. Evaluate the goals of nursing care, using knowledge from physical and behavioral science and nursing theories.	5	4	3	2	1
9. Encourage the client to select own goals.	5	4	3	2	1
10. Encourage the client to participate in own care.	5	4	3	2	1
11. Determine care activities which require the specialized skills of the professional nurse.	5	4	3	2	1
12. Determine community resources for promotion of optimal level of wellness for client/family.	5	4	3	2	1
13. Implement a plan of nursing intervention which is consistent with scientific rationales.	5	4	3	2	1
14. Implement a plan which facilitates health seeking behaviors with a select population within a community.	5	4	3	2	1
15. Evaluate the effectiveness of nursing practice.	5	4	3	2	1
16. Revise the nursing care plan based on evaluation of outcomes.	5	4	3	2	1
17. Recognize the *independent* function of the teaching role.	5	4	3	2	1
18. Recognize the *interdependent* function of the teaching role.	5	4	3	2	1

19. Recognize the *dependent* function of the   5   4   3   2   1
    teaching role.
20. Assume responsibility for initiating teaching   5   4   3   2   1
    appropriate to the learner's needs.
21. Apply the principles of teaching and   5   4   3   2   1
    learning in nursing practice.
22. Design a teaching plan which integrates   5   4   3   2   1
    plans of other disciplines.
23. Analyze individual teaching plan based on   5   4   3   2   1
    an understanding of the *independent*
    functions of the nurse.
24. Analyze individual teaching plan based on   5   4   3   2   1
    an understanding of the *interdependent*
    functions of the nurse.
25. Analyze individual teaching plan based on   5   4   3   2   1
    an understanding of the *dependent*
    functions of the nurse.
26. Implement the teaching plan designed to   5   4   3   2   1
    improve or maintain health.
27. Initiate action with other health team   5   4   3   2   1
    members to meet the learning needs
    of clients.
28. Evaluate the effectiveness of the teaching   5   4   3   2   1
    plan based on the understanding of the
    independent functions of the nurse.
29. Evaluate the effectiveness of the teaching   5   4   3   2   1
    plan based on the understanding of the
    interdependent functions of the nurse.
30. Evaluate the effectiveness of the teaching   5   4   3   2   1
    plan based on the understanding of the
    dependent functions of the nurse.
31. Demonstrate an appreciation for the   5   4   3   2   1
    cultural and societal factors which affect
    health promotion/maintenance, restoration,
    and rehabilitation.
32. Analyze how personal, social, and cultural   5   4   3   2   1
    values influence decision making in providing
    care to individuals or groups.
33. Support the individual/group's need to   5   4   3   2   1
    participate in beliefs and practices
    meaningful to their lifestyle.
34. Collaborate with the individual or group   5   4   3   2   1
    in identifying alternative actions available
    to promote, maintain, or restore health
    consistent with their cultural values.

35. Utilize a systematic decision-making process   5   4   3   2   1
to achieve goals with individuals and groups.
36. Utilize the principles of change to achieve   5   4   3   2   1
goals with individuals and groups.
37. Discern the influence of ethical and legal   5   4   3   2   1
issues on the provision of nursing care.
38. Evaluate the effectiveness of decision making   5   4   3   2   1
in meeting the needs of individuals or groups.
39. Assess communication of clients and families   5   4   3   2   1
based upon knowledge and techniques of
interpersonal communication.
40. Use appropriate communication techniques   5   4   3   2   1
in nursing practice.
41. Utilize knowledge of group dynamics in   5   4   3   2   1
nursing practice.
42. Communicate effectively through utilization   5   4   3   2   1
of oral and written methods.
43. Evaluate behavior based on knowledge of   5   4   3   2   1
human responses and stages of growth and
development.
44. Evaluate interpersonal relationships   5   4   3   2   1
with clients.
45. Evaluate interpersonal relationships   5   4   3   2   1
with peers.
46. Evaluate interpersonal relationships with   5   4   3   2   1
other health professionals.
47. Involve the client/family in assessing,   5   4   3   2   1
planning, implementing, and evaluating
nursing care.
48. Cooperate with other health personnel to   5   4   3   2   1
promote congruency and continuity of care.
49. Value the contributions of all persons   5   4   3   2   1
involved in providing health care.
50. Accept responsibility to identify the role of   5   4   3   2   1
all persons involved in providing health care
to other health care professionals.
51. Distinguish between nursing role and other   5   4   3   2   1
health professionals' roles in the health care
delivery system.
52. Establish effective working relationships   5   4   3   2   1
with other health team members.
53. Identify issues that impact on the   5   4   3   2   1
professional nursing role in health care.
54. Appreciate the historical developments   5   4   3   2   1
which have had an impact on the
professional nursing role.

55. Relate the significance of the changes   5   4   3   2   1
    effected by nurses and the nursing
    profession to the present and future role
    of the professional nurse.
56. Apply theoretical concepts of nursing and   5   4   3   2   1
    management to own practice.
57. Demonstrate the ability to carry out the   5   4   3   2   1
    nursing process in a variety of settings.
58. Assume total nursing care responsibility   5   4   3   2   1
    for clients.
59. Implement a plan of nursing intervention   5   4   3   2   1
    which is consistent with American Nurses'
    Association Standards of Practice.
60. Design plans for directing care given by   5   4   3   2   1
    ancillary personnel.
61. Take necessary action when resources for   5   4   3   2   1
    care are not provided.
62. Evaluate others who give nursing care to   5   4   3   2   1
    promote quality care.
63. Participate in formal activities designed to   5   4   3   2   1
    evaluate the quality of nursing care.
64. Recognize the importance of their future   5   4   3   2   1
    role as leaders.
65. Seek resources to improve own level of   5   4   3   2   1
    practice based on evaluation by self and others.
66. Seek current knowledge of the political,   5   4   3   2   1
    social, and economic factors which affect
    nursing practice.
67. Appreciate the importance of participating   5   4   3   2   1
    in professional organizations and
    community activities.

Thank you for your assistance with this project.
               Do Not Sign This Questionnaire

Demographic Data:

Have you had experience as a nurse's aid/assistant? _____Yes _____ No
    If yes, length/amount of experience: _____ months or _____ years

Are you a Licensed Practical Nurse? _____Yes _____ No
    If yes, length/amount of experience: _____months or _____years

Have you participated in State Board Review Sessions? _____Yes _____ No

                    Thank you!

20

Student Stress and Coping Inventory

Barbara Jaffin Cohen

PURPOSE

The purpose of the **Student Stress and Coping Inventory (SSCI)** (Cohen, 1990) is to identify psychological stress factors in nursing students' environments and the ways students cope with this stress.

INSTRUMENT DESCRIPTION

Both clinical (Oermann, 1998) and academic (Kirkland, 1998) stressors have been documented along with some information on coping strategies used by students. Sawatzky (1998) points to the need for comprehensive research in this area of stress.

The transactional model of stress (Parkes, 1984; Vicino, 1987; Zweig, 1988) and the concepts of problem-focused and emotion-focused coping strategies operationalized by Lazarus and Folkman (1984) served as the conceptual basis for instrument development. Stress was defined for respondents as something in a person's environment that he/she believes or feels is upsetting, threatening, or endangering to him/her. Coping was defined for respondents as the actions or thoughts a person uses to attempt to manage, reduce or alleviate the stress associated with a situation or experience. The SSCI elicits self-reports of stress and coping in five areas specific to the nursing student's college environment: nursing classrooms, nursing clinical experiences, other (than nursing) classrooms and laboratories, the college environment, and the social/personal environment. In addition to identifying situations that a student deems stressful and related patterns of coping, the SSCI obtains respondents' biographical information.

Items were generated from the literature and from 21 tape-recorded interviews with baccalaureate nursing students enrolled in the nursing division of a large publicly funded university in the northeastern United States. Students interviewed, who were randomly selected from among the 300 students enrolled, were given definitions of stress and coping and asked to respond to 10 open-ended questions requiring them to name stressful situations or conditions associated with being a student nurse and the efforts/strategies they employed to minimize or alleviate these feelings of stress. Respondents represented sophomore, junior, and senior levels of the nursing program. Two nursing faculty members from the same university, a social worker, and an intern in social work from the office of student affairs were also interviewed. These four individuals were chosen because of their experience in counseling students and/or previous research in the area of student stress. Their remarks validated student responses to interview questions.

The resulting instrument consists of five stress subscales containing a total of 89 items: nursing classrooms (20 items); nursing clinical experiences (24 items); other classrooms and laboratories (20 items); college environment (14 items), and social/personal environment in relation to attending school (11 items). Items are rated on a 4-point Likert scale, with 1 indicating "not at all stressful" to 4 indicating "extremely stressful." A 22-item coping scale was generated from three existing scales (Jalowiec, Murphy, & Powers, 1984; Jalowiec, 1988; Lazarus & Folkman, 1984; Murphy, 1984) by asking five reviewers with nursing and psychology backgrounds to identify items from the three scales that had corresponding content. Each item considered by at least four of the five raters to be represented in all three scales were considered for inclusion on the SSCI. Items were then constructed that incorporated the key words from the corresponding items in the three scales. Phrases from student interviews were also included, in which they clarified the meaning of items. For the 22 coping items, respondents were asked to indicate on a 4-point Likert scale the extent to which a response or reaction was used, with 1 "not used" to 4 "used a great deal." For each item the five stress areas were also listed for students to indicate the use or nonuse of each strategy for each area. All items were reviewed for clarity by two nursing faculty members and five senior level nursing students who had not participated in the interviews.

The SCCI is designed to be administered no earlier than 4 weeks into a semester to allow students to have sufficient clinical experience on which to base their responses. Administration during highly stressful periods such as during examinations should be avoided. Approximately 20 minutes are required to complete the instrument. Scores are summed for each of the five stress subscales and for the coping scale and then divided by the number of valid responses. If respondents do not answer more than 10% of the items in any one of the scales, the questionnaire should be excluded. A total stress score is obtained by summing the scores for the five areas, with a possible range of 5 to 20. A coping usage score for each of the five areas is obtained by counting the number of strategies used for the respective area, with a possible range of 0 to 22 for each area. Total coping is determined by counting across the five areas, with a possible range of 0 to 110. Higher scores indicate higher degrees of stress or usage of coping strategy. A copy of the SCCI is included at the end of the chapter.

RELIABILITY AND VALIDITY ASSESSMENT

During instrument development content validity indices (CVI) were computed for the five stress subscales and the coping scale. Judges who rated the scale items were nursing faculty members experienced in conducting stress workshops for nursing students and other members of the college community. Resulting CVIs were: .625, nursing classroom; .79, clinical situations; .675, other classrooms and laboratories; .50, college environment; 1.00, social/personal environment; and 1.00, coping.

Internal consistency reliability and concurrent validity were examined with a volunteer sample of 298 baccalaureate nursing students enrolled in three different baccalaureate nursing programs, two public and one private, located in the New York metropolitan area. The sample included students representative of each level of the nursing program. A total of 89% were enrolled in nine or more credits; 13% were RNs; and 77% were minorities. Subjects ranged in age from 18 to 43 years, with 69% 27 or younger; 25% were married; 34% had children living with them; and 81% were employed. Annual family income was less than $25,000 for 56% of the students. Internal consistency reliability was assessed using Cronbach's alpha coefficients. Resulting alphas for each of the subscales were: .85, nursing classroom; .91, nursing clinical situations; .91, other classes and laboratories; .84, college environment; .85, social/personal environment; .81, total stress; and .76, coping.

Concurrent validity for the five stress subscales was examined by correlating these scores with three variables: state anxiety, trait anxiety (Speilberger, Gorsuch, Lushene, Vagg, & Jacobs, 1977), and college life experiences as measured by the College Schedule of Recent Experience (Anderson, 1972). Resulting alpha coefficients for each of the criterion tools used in this study were .93, .91, and .83, respectively. Pearson product-moment correlation coefficients for the stress subscales and total scores with the three stress-related measures were positive and ranged from .11 (college environment stress with state anxiety) to .44 (nursing clinical stress with trait anxiety). Concurrent validity of the coping scale was examined by correlating the coping score with the stress scores resulting in correlation coefficients that ranged from .20 (nursing clinical) to .30 (social/personal environment). The correlations were all positive and statistically significant.

Further testing of the instrument will explore the unidimensionality of the SCCI scales. A preliminary factor analysis of the 89 items that constitute the five stress subscales suggests that certain factors may overlap some of these areas. A factor analysis of the 22 coping items suggests that coping may be unidimensional. Effects of the demographic characteristics on stress and coping will be examined to assess the effectiveness of coping strategies. The utility of the SCCI as a guide for the development of interventions directed at reducing student stress requires investigation.

REFERENCES

Anderson, G. E. (1972). *College Schedule of Recent Experience.* Unpublished master's thesis, North Dakota State University.

Cohen, B. J. (1990). Assessing stress and coping in nursing students. In C. F. Waltz & O. L. Strickland (Eds.), *Measurement of nursing outcomes: Vol. 3. Measuring clinical skills and professional development in education and practice* (pp. 323–348). New York: Springer Publishing Company.

Jalowiec, A. (1988). Confirming factor analysis of the Jalowiec Coping Scale. In C. F. Waltz & O. L. Strickland (Eds.), *Measurement of nursing outcomes: Vol. 1. Measuring client outcomes* (pp. 287–308). New York: Springer Publishing Company.

Jalowiec, A., Murphy, S. P., & Powers, M. J. (1984). Psychometric assessment of the Jalowiec Coping Scale. *Nursing Research, 33*(3), 157–161.

Kirkland, M. L. (1998). Stressors and coping strategies among successful female African American baccalaureate nursing students. *Journal of Nursing Education 37*(1), 5–12.

Lazarus, R. S., & Folkman, S. (1984). *Stress, appraisal and coping.* New York: Springer Publishing Co.

Murphy, M. C. (1984). *The adjustment of rural high school students to a large, urban university: The identification of stressors and coping behaviors.* Unpublished doctoral dissertation, University of Texas at Austin.

Oermann, M. J. (1998). Differences in clinical experiences of ADN and BSN students. *Journal of Nursing Education, 37*(5), 197–201.

Parkes, K. R. (1984). Locus of control, cognitive appraisal and coping in stressful episodes. *Journal of Personality and Social Psychology, 46,* 655–668.

Sawatzky, J. A. (1998). Understanding nursing students' stress: A proposed framework. *Journal of Nursing Education Today, 18*(2), 108–115.

Speilberger, C. D., Gorsuch, R. L., Lushene, R., Vagg, P. R., & Jacobs, G. A. (1977). *The State-Trait Anxiety Inventory: Forms Y-1 and Y-2.* Palo Alto, CA: Consulting Psychologists Press.

Vicino, C. M. (1987). *Stress and coping modes of registered nurses returning to school for a baccalaureate degree.* Unpublished doctoral dissertation, Teachers College, Columbia University.

Zweig, N. B. (1988). *Stressful events and ways of coping of baccalaureate student nurses in clinical laboratory.* Unpublished doctoral dissertation, Teachers College, Columbia University.

STUDENT STRESS AND COPING INVENTORY

SECTION A: STRESSFUL SITUATIONS OR EXPERIENCES

STRESS IS DEFINED AS SOMETHING IN A PERSON'S ENVIRONMENT THAT HE/SHE BELIEVES OR FEELS IS UPSETTING, THREATENING, OR ENDANGERING TO HIM/HER.

The items in this section are divided into five areas of a student nurse's environment. These items describe situations or experiences which may be perceived as stressful. Please *circle one answer* indicating the level of stress that you have experienced.

In responding to these items you are to consider only the time period that has elapsed since the BEGINNING OF THIS SEMESTER.

III. NURSING	1 not at all stressful	2 slightly stressful	3 moderately stressful	4 extremely stressful
1. Excessive workload (e.g., amount of work, type of assignments, amount ofcontent covered)	1	2	3	4
2. Competition with other students	1	2	3	4
3. Preparing for examinations (e.g., focusing on textbook and/or lecture material)	1	2	3	4
4. Announcements of course requirements (e.g., hand-outs, syllabus)	1	2	3	4
5. Meeting the demands of more than one course (e.g., assignments, tests, too many credits)	1	2	3	4
6. Presentation of content in examinations (e.g., not sure what is being asked, manner in which questions are structured)	1	2	3	4
7. Attitude of faculty	1	2	3	4
8. Student participation in developing course content and requirements	1	2	3	4

	1	2	3	4
9. Due dates of assignments (e.g., negotiating dates with faculty, change of dates by faculty)	1	2	3	4
10. Course content *not* stimulating/challenging	1	2	3	4
11. Possibility of failure	1	2	3	4
12. Physical environment (length of classes, size of classes, seating, acoustics, temperature of room)	1	2	3	4
13. Availability of faculty for academic help	1	2	3	4
14. Receptiveness of faculty for academic help	1	2	3	4
15. Taking examinations	1	2	3	4
16. Asking questions/ speaking in class (e.g., language difficulty, public speaking)	1	2	3	4
17. Interactions with other students	1	2	3	4
18. Coordinating classes and clinical schedules				
19. Academic skills needed for level of work required	1	2	3	4
20. Meeting own expectations of academic performance	1	2	3	4

	1 not at all stressful	2 slightly stressful	3 moderately stressful	4 extremely stressful
II. NURSING CLINICAL EXPERIENCES				
1. Evaluation by instructor(s) (e.g., being observed)	1	2	3	4
2. Meeting own expectations in caring for clients	1	2	3	4
3. Availability of instructor(s) for assistance	1	2	3	4
4. Receptiveness of instructor(s) for assistance	1	2	3	4

5. Level of own competency (i.e., feeling of preparedness for client care)	1	2	3	4
6. Condition of clients assigned (e.g., dying, critically ill, disfigured clients)	1	2	3	4
7. Age of client	1	2	3	4
8. Sex of client (i.e., client of same sex/opposite sex)	1	2	3	4
9. Communicating with clients	1	2	3	4
10. Interaction with members of the health care team	1	2	3	4
11. The physical environment of the clinical agency (e.g., equipment, odor, sights)	1	2	3	4
12. Own abilities to meet requirements of clinical assignments	1	2	3	4
13. Exposure to experiences that will prepare me for nursing practice (e.g., level of assignment)	1	2	3	4
14. Possibility of making an error (e.g., medication, assessment of client)	1	2	3	4
15. Exposure to contagious disease/"catching" something from client(s)	1	2	3	4
16. Performing psychomotor skills	1	2	3	4
17. Being in an emergency situation	1	2	3	4
18. Organizational structure of clinical agency (e.g., channels of communication and authority)	1	2	3	4
19. Being in a new environment/ situation	1	2	3	4
20. Evaluation of performance by nursing staff	1	2	3	4
21. Preparing for clinical assignments	1	2	3	4

22. Traveling to clinical setting	1	2	3	4
23. Evaluation of performance by client(s)	1	2	3	4
24. Physical contact with a stranger	1	2	3	4

	1 not at all stressful	2 slightly stressful	3 moderately stressful	4 extremely stressful
III. OTHER (THAN NURSING) COLLEGE CLASSROOMS AND LABORATORIES				
1. Excessive workload (e.g., amount of work, type of assignments, amount of content covered)	1	2	3	4
2. Competition with other students	1	2	3	4
3. Preparing for examinations (e.g., focusing on textbook and/or lecture material)	1	2	3	4
4. Announcements of course requirements (e.g., handouts, syllabus)	1	2	3	4
5. Meeting the demands of more than one course (e.g., assignments, tests, too many credits)	1	2	3	4
6. Presentation of content in examinations (e.g., not sure what is being asked, manner in which questions are structured)	1	2	3	4
7. Attitude of faculty	1	2	3	4
8. Student participation in developing course content and requirements	1	2	3	4
9. Due dates of assignments (e.g., negotiating dates with faculty, change of dates by faculty)	1	2	3	4
10. Course content *not* stimulating/challenging	1	2	3	4

11. Possibility of failure	1	2	3	4
12. Physical environment (length of classes, size of classes, seating, acoustics, temperature of room)	1	2	3	4
13. Availability of faculty for academic help	1	2	3	4
14. Receptiveness of faculty for academic help	1	2	3	4
15. Taking examinations	1	2	3	4
16. Asking questions/speaking in class (e.g., language difficulty, public speaking)	1	2	3	4
17. Interactions with other students	1	2	3	4
18. Coordinating classes with clinical schedules	1	2	3	4
19. Academic skills needed for level of work required	1	2	3	4
20. Meeting own expectations of academic performance	1	2	3	4

	1 not at all stressful	2 slightly stressful	3 moderately stressful	4 extremely stressful
IV. COLLEGE ENVIRONMENT				
1. Change in major field of of study	1	2	3	4
2. Travel to college (e.g., time, distance)	1	2	3	4
3. Parking	1	2	3	4
4. Seeking and/or receiving academic counseling (college and department requirement)	1	2	3	4
5. Seeking and/or receiving student counseling (personal concerns)	1	2	3	4
6. Seeking and/or receiving tutorial assistance	1	2	3	4

		1	2	3	4
7.	Interactions with students in other disciplines	1	2	3	4
8.	Orientation to the college	1	2	3	4
9.	Registering for courses	1	2	3	4
10.	Library facilities (e.g., use and physical environment)	1	2	3	4
11.	Adding/dropping courses	1	2	3	4
12.	Purchasing textbooks and other course materials	1	2	3	4
13.	Registration process	1	2	3	4
14.	Involvement in campus extracurricular activities	1	2	3	4

		1 not at all stressful	2 slightly stressful	3 moderately stressful	4 extremely stressful
V.	SOCIAL/PERSONAL ENVIRONMENT IN RELATION TO ATTENDING SCHOOL				
1.	Holding a job while attending school	1	2	3	4
2.	Fatigue/energy level	1	2	3	4
3.	Ability to sleep	1	2	3	4
4.	Present financial status	1	2	3	4
5.	Child care	1	2	3	4
6.	Relationships/interactions with family members	1	2	3	4
7.	Relationships/interactions with friends	1	2	3	4
8.	Relationships/interactions with spouse	1	2	3	4
9.	Family responsibilities	1	2	3	4
10.	Insufficient time to do the things you want	1	2	3	4
11.	Physical status (e.g., weight, health)	1	2	3	4

SECTION B: COPING

COPING IS DEFINED AS THE ACTIONS OR THOUGHTS A PERSON USES TO ATTEMPT TO MANAGE, REDUCE, OR ALLEVIATE THE STRESS ASSOCIATED WITH A SITUATION OR EXPERIENCE.

The items in this section are ways that people respond or react to stressful situations or experiences. Considering the stresses that you have identified in the previous section, you are being asked to answer two questions for each of the items below.

1. Please CIRCLE ONE ANSWER that indicates the extent to which you have used/are using each response or reaction *SINCE THE BEGINNING OF THIS SEMESTER.*
2. For each item indicate the general area(s) for which you have used/are using that response or reaction. *CIRCLE AS MANY ANSWERS AS APPLY.* The examples used in each item are not all inclusive.

EXTENT TO WHICH
RESPONSE OR
REACTION USED

AREA(S) FOR WHICH USED

	not used	used a little	used moderately	used a great deal	Nursing classroom	Nursing clinical experience	Nonnursing class & laboratories	College environment	Social/personal environment
	1	2	3	4	1	2	3	4	5
1. Tried to deal directly with the situation (e.g., studied more, joined a study group, organized my time, hired a babysitter)	1	2	3	4	1	2	3	4	5
2. Tried to change the situation (e.g., changed my class schedule, dropped a class, changed my job)	1	2	3	4	1	2	3	4	5

3.	Sought out college services that might help me with my concern (e.g., Financial Aid Office, Office of Academic Advisement, Student Counseling Services)	1	2	3	4	1	2	3	4	5
4.	Discussed concern(s)/feelings with friends and/or classmates	1	2	3	4	1	2	3	4	5
5.	Lessened demands on myself by accepting the next best thing to what I wanted, do what is possible (e.g., I didn't need to get all A's)	1	2	3	4	1	2	3	4	5
6.	Thought of other ways of dealing with the situation by drawing on past experiences	1	2	3	4	1	2	3	4	5
7.	Sought out information about my concern so I could analyze and understand it better	1	2	3	4	1	2	3	4	5
8.	Did what is expected of me (e.g., set goals, prepared assignments)	1	2	3	4	1	2	3	4	5
9.	Accepted the situation	1	2	3	4	1	2	3	4	5
10.	Became depressed or worried	1	2	3	4	1	2	3	4	5
11.	Became involved in other activities to take my mind off things (e.g., exercised, read, watched television)	1	2	3	4	1	2	3	4	5
12.	Sleeping habits changed	1	2	3	4	1	2	3	4	5
13.	Eating habits changed	1	2	3	4	1	2	3	4	5
14.	Prayed or meditated	1	2	3	4	1	2	3	4	5
15.	Turned my concerns over to God, a higher power, or force	1	2	3	4	1	2	3	4	5
16.	Became angry, vented my feelings (e.g., yelled, cursed, released tension on others, cried)	1	2	3	4	1	2	3	4	5
17.	Postponed dealing with the situation temporarily (e.g., didn't go to class, tried to forget the whole thing)	1	2	3	4	1	2	3	4	5
18.	Changed my usual intake of alcohol, cigarettes, drugs	1	2	3	4	1	2	3	4	5
19.	Discussed concern(s)/feelings with family	1	2	3	4	1	2	3	4	5
20.	Realized I was not alone	1	2	3	4	1	2	3	4	5
21.	Tried to be optimistic, looked at the positive and/or humorous aspects of the situation	1	2	3	4	1	2	3	4	5
22.	If other people were involved, I talked to the individual who could do something about my concern(s) (e.g., faculty member)	1	2	3	4	1	2	3	4	5

SECTION C: BIOGRAPHICAL DATA

Please circle one answer for each item unless instructed otherwise.

1. Current level in college
   1. Freshman   3. Junior
   2. Sophomore   4. Senior

2. Current level in nursing program
   1. Freshman   3. Junior
   2. Sophomore   4. Senior

3. Year entered college _____

4. Transfer student: 1. Yes   2. No

5. If Yes, what year _____

6. Credit load for this semester:
   1. Less than 6 credits   3. 9–12 credits
   2. 6–8 credits   4. More than 12 credits

7. Your age:
   1. Under 18 years   6. 38–42 years
   2. 18–22 years   7. 43–47 years
   3. 23–27 years   8. 48–52 years
   4. 28–32 years   9. Over 52 years
   5. 33–37 years

8. Sex:
   1. Male   2. Female

9. Ethnicity:
   1. White, Non-Hispanic   4. Asian or Pacific Islands
   2. Hispanic   5. American Indian
   3. Black, Non-Hispanic   6. Other (specify)
                               _____

10. Country of Birth _____

11. Marital Status:
    1. Single   4. Separated
    2. Married   5. Living with
    3. Divorced   significant other

12. Number of *own* children under 21 years living in household
    1. none   4. three
    2. one   5. more than three
    3. two   (specify) _____

13. Number of children (over 21) living in household (your own)
    1. none   4. three
    2. one   5. more than three
    3. two   (specify) _____

14. Number of children under 21 years living in household
    who are *not* your own
    1. none   4. three
    2. one   5. more than three
    3. two   (specify) _____

15. Number of adults living in household other than yourself
    1. none   4. three
    2. one   5. more than three
    3. two   (specify) _____

16. Relationship of adults above (circle as many as appropriate)
        1. husband   5. friend
        2. wife   6. your adult child
        3. mother   7. other relative
        4. father
17. Total number of hours per week you are currently employed while attending college.
        1. less than 6   5. 25–30 hours
        2. 6–11 hours   6. 31–35 hours
        3. 12–18 hours   7. 36 hours or more
        4. 19–24 hours
18. Are you responsible for child care?
        1. Yes   2. No
19. Annual family income
        1. below $10,000   6. $30,000–$34,999
        2. $10,000–$14,999   7. $35,000 or more
        3. $15,000–$19,999
        4. $20,000–$24,999
        5. $25,000–$29,999
20. Are you currently a Registered Nurse?
        1. Yes   2. No
21. If yes, type of RN program attended
        1. Diploma   2. Associate Degree
22. If you are not an RN, have you ever worked in the health care field?
        1. Yes   2. No
23. If yes, what was your job? _____
24. Grade point average last semester _____

PLEASE ANSWER ALL THE QUESTIONS ON THIS PAGE
Thank you for your participation

Note: Used with permission of Barbara Jaffin Cohen.

21

Faculty Role Preparation
Self-Assessment Scale

Janet M. Burge

PURPOSE

The **Faculty Role Preparation Self-Assessment Scale** (Burge, 1990) measures the quality of programs preparing graduates for the faculty teaching role. It is designed to:

1. provide a means for graduates of master's programs in nursing to evaluate the quality of their programs in preparing them for the faculty teaching role, and
2. for new teachers and their employers to assess deficits in faculty teaching role preparation and structure on-the-job activities to decrease or eliminate deficits in performance in first employment in an academic environment.

INSTRUMENT DESCRIPTION

The conceptual basis for the tool is derived from concepts inherent in role and socialization theory (Biddle, 1979; Hardy & Conway, 1978) as it relates to and is applied to the preparation of faculty in nursing.

The instrument contains 53 items describing program attributes directly associated with curriculum development and implementation, methods and strategies of teaching, principles of evaluation, learning theory, and experiential learning through the use of teaching practicums. Four major indicators were developed to measure faculty teaching role preparation at the master's level. The first indicator—curriculum planning, implementation, and evaluation, has three independent components, and therefore represents three subscales containing a total of 34 items: 12 on the first subscale (planning), 9 on the second subscale (implementation), and 2 on the third (evaluation). The second indicator, general policies and procedures in a college of nursing, contains 14 items; the third indicator, general policies and procedures in a university, contains 3 items; and the fourth indicator, the socialization process in a university setting, contains 2 items. Content-related items were defined as those indicating specific information discussed or presented by either the teacher or graduate students within a formal classroom setting. Experience-related items were defined as those activities planned by the teacher or students to enhance or reinforce content taught in the classroom. These activities may have taken place within the classroom but usually occurred in a teaching practicum, small group work outside class time, or as planned, out-of-classroom observational experiences.

The instrument can be self-administered and used to direct a faculty member's own continuing education while employed in a first-time academic position. It may also be jointly used by an educational administrator with the faculty member to structure the additional activities and experiences needed in the first teaching experience. As noted, the instrument contains 53 items. Each item is rated on a 4-point, Likert-type scale: 1 point (poor), 2 points (fair), 3 points (good), and 4 points (excellent). A total score is obtained for each respondent by summing the ratings for all items. The summed score may range from 53 to 212. The following numerical range was developed for use in intrepreting the total score: 160 to 212 points indicate the student has rated at least 75% of the items as excellent in quality; 120 to 159 points indicate a rating of good quality; 80 to 119 points indicate a rating of fair quality; and 40 to 79 points indicate a rating of poor quality. The lower limit of each numerical range was determined on the basis of 75% of the items ($n = 40$) receiving a rating of 4 (excellent), 3 (good), 2 (fair) or 1 (poor), respectively. A copy of the Faculty Role Preparation Self-Assessment Scale is included at the end of the chapter.

RELIABILITY AND VALIDITY ASSESSMENT

The instrument was pilot tested for understanding and clarity of directions and items via seven graduate students who completed a sequence of three courses to prepare them for a faculty teaching role. No changes were indicated as a result of the pilot test. Content validity was determined by having two content experts rate the instrument for (a) relevancy of the items to the indicators, and (b) relevancy of the items to faculty–teaching-role preparation using a four-point scale of 1 (not relevant), 2 (somewhat relevant), 3 (quite relevant), and 4 (not relevant). Content validity indices used to quantify the results of the experts ratings were .92 (curriculum planning), .67 (curriculum implementation), .93 (policies and procedures in a college setting), 1.00 (policies and procedures in a university setting), 1.00 (socialization into an academic environment), and .94 for all items. Content experts held doctoral degrees, had teaching majors in their master's programs, and had a mean of 17 years of teaching experience.

Reliability was examined using test-retest procedures over a 2-week interval. Two different reliability testings were conducted. The first reliablity testing was implemented to establish whether two experienced faculty, over time, would rate the items as essential or not essential to faculty teaching at the master's level. Using Spearman rank correlations, an intrarater coefficient of .89 was obtained for one faculty member, and .76 was obtained for the second faculty member. Interrater coefficients between the two faculty members resulted in .80 for the test and .88 for the retest for items essential to faculty–teaching-role preparation.

Reliability was examined a second time employing a sample of 13 faculty members in their first academic positions in five different master's programs, who had been teaching one or two years and had a major or minor in faculty–teaching-role preparation in their master's program. Test-retest procedures over a 2-week interval, using Spearman rank correlation coefficients for intrarater reliability, resulted in coefficients ranging from .80 to .94 for total test scores. Coefficients for the four subscales ranged from .84 to .96 for curriculum planning, implementation, and evaluation; .78 to .82 for policies and procedures in a college of nursing; .64 to .88 for policies and procedures in a university setting; and .82 to .96 for socialization in an academic environment.

Future reliability and validity testing will include a larger number of master's programs to increase representativeness and to allow for generalizations to be made about the quality of master's educational preparation. Further validity issues to be addressed include: (a) determination of the usefulness of the instrument to educational administrators in planning and guiding structured experiences for new faculty members, and (b) examination of a shift of content and experiences into doctoral nursing programs related to faculty–teaching-role preparation that might invalidate the use of the tool at the master's level and provide direction for modifications for use at the doctoral level.

REFERENCES

Biddle, B. J. (1979). *Role theory: Expectations, identities, and behaviors*. New York: Academic Press.

Burge, J. M. (1990). Faculty teaching role preparation at the master's level. In C. F. Waltz & O. L. Strickland (Eds.), *Measurement of nursing outcomes: Vol. 3. Measuring clinical skills and professional development in education and practice* (pp. 311–322). New York: Springer Publishing Company.

Hardy, M. E., & Conway, M. E. (1978). *Role theory: Perspectives for health professionals*. New York: Appleton-Century-Crofts.

FACULTY ROLE PREPARATION SELF-ASSESSMENT SCALE

INDICATOR A: (SUBSCALE I)
CONTENT AND EXPERIENCES RELATED TO CURRICULUM PLANNING

	RATING SCALE			
ITEMS	Poor (1)	Fair (2)	Good (3)	Excellent (4)

1. There was *content* which reviewed and compared a variety of school of nursing philosophies.
2. There was *experience* in developing a school of nursing philosophy.
3. There was *content* related to conceptual framework(s) including identification of vertical and horizontal strands.
4. There was *content* related to the relationship of terminal, level, and course objectives for a nursing curriculum.
5. There was *experience* in writing terminal, level, course objectives and for a nursing curriculum.
6. There was *content* related to various curriculum designs and sequencing of nursing courses.
7. There was *experience* in developing a curriculum design including sequencing of nursing courses.
8. There was *content* related to pre-requisite, support, and elective courses in a curriculum design.
9. There was *content* related to a variety of learning theories with application to nursing education.
10. There was *content* related to state board of nursing criteria for approving schools of nursing.
11. There was *experience* provided in reviewing and conducting a critique of curriculum reports prepared by a school of nursing seeking or having obtained approval of a state board of nursing.
12. There was *content* related to NLN criteria of accrediting schools of nursing.

INDICATOR A: (SUBSCALE II)
CONTENT AND EXPERIENCES RELATED TO CURRICULUM
IMPLEMENTATION

ITEMS	RATING SCALE			
	Poor (1)	Fair (2)	Good (3)	Excellent (4)
13. There was a variety of *classroom* teaching strategies/methods discussed and demonstrated.				
14. There was a variety of *clinical* teaching strategies/methods discussed and/or demonstrated.				
15. There was a variety of *college laboratory* teaching strategies/methods discussed and/or demonstrated.				
16. There was *content* related to effective teaching styles and behaviors.				
17. There was *content* related to the development of course syllabi.				
18. There was *experience* in developing a course syllabus.				
19. There was *experience* in *classroom teaching* as a portion of a teaching practicum course.				
20. There was *experience* in *clinical teaching* as a portion of a teaching practicum course.				
21. There was *experience* in assisting in a *college laboratory* session as a portion of a teaching practicum.				

INDICATOR A: (SUBSCALE III)
CONTENT AND EXPERIENCES RELATED TO CURRICULUM EVALUATION

ITEMS	RATING SCALE			
	Poor (1)	Fair (2)	Good (3)	Excellent (4)
22. There was *content* related to admission, progression, and retention, policies governing student nurses.				
23. There was *content* related to general theories of evaluation.				
24. There was *content* related to specific testing methods used in the *classroom*.				
25. There was *experience* in developing/ writing test items for use in the *classroom*.				
26. There was *content* related to specific testing methods used in *clinical practice*.				
27. There was *content* related to test item analysis including discrimination index and level of difficulty.				

28. There was *experience* in developing, administering, and analyzing test items.
29. There was *content* related to various methods of faculty record-keeping of student performance in the *classroom* and/or *clinical practice.*
30. There was *experience* in using various methods of record-keeping of student performance in the *classroom* and/or *clinical practice.*
31. There was *content* related to the academic appeals/grievance process for students.
32. There was *content* related to the role of students in planning, revising, and evaluating a nursing curriculum.
33. There was *content* related to the process of conducting program evaluation.
34. There was *experience* in developing a model/plan for program evaluation.

INDICATOR B:
CONTENT AND EXPERIENCES RELATED TO POLICIES AND PROCEDURES IN A COLLEGE OF NURSING

	RATING SCALE			
ITEMS	Poor (1)	Fair (2)	Good (3)	Excellent (4)

35. There was *content* related to negotiating teaching contracts in an academic environment.
36. There was *content* related to faculty workload policies.
37. There was *content* related to organizational structures of schools of nursing including structure and functions of school committees.
38. There was *experience* in observing meetings of selected school of nursing committees.
39. There was *experience* provided for reviewing and/or comparing selected school of nursing faculty handbooks regarding policies of the school such as release time criteria, leave of absences, etc.
40. There was *content* related to the process of preparing of faculty dossiers when faculty seek reappointment, promotion, and tenure.

41. There was *experience* in reviewing prepared faculty dossiers.
42. There was *content* related to letters of agreement or contracts with agencies providing clinical practice sites for student learning.
43. There was *experience* provided for reading and comparing selected letters of agreement or contracts used with agencies.
44. There was *content* related to the process and procedures used for peer evaluation among faculty groups.
45. There was *content* related to purposes and methods of conducting student evaluations of faculty teaching effectiveness.
46. There was *content* related to administrative expectations and evaluation of faculty.
47. There was *content* related to the service expectations of faculty.
48. There was *content* related to the research and scholarly expectations of faculty.

INDICATOR C:
CONTENT AND EXPERIENCES RELATED TO POLICIES AND PROCEDURES IN A UNIVERSITY

	RATING SCALE			
ITEMS	Poor (1)	Fair (2)	Good (3)	Excellent (4)

49. There was *content* related to a university's organizational structure and governance system including faculty senate and standing university committees.
50. There was *experience* provided for reading and reviewing a university *faculty handbook* for policies associated with personnel issues, promotion and tenure criteria, and appeals/grievance procedures for faculty.
51. There was *content* related to policies and documents contained in the American Association of University Professors (AAUP) guidelines governing faculty and institutional behavior.

INDICATOR D:
CONTENT AND EXPERIENCES RELATED TO THE SOCIALIZATION
PROCESS INTO AN ACADEMIC ENVIRONMENT

	RATING SCALE			
ITEMS	Poor (1)	Fair (2)	Good (3)	Excellent (4)
52. There was *content* related to purpose and methods of conducting effective orientation programs for new faculty in a school of nursing.				
53. There was *content* related to stressors and sources of conflict in an academic environment.				

22

Assertiveness Behavior Inventory Tools

Paulette Freeman Adams and Linda Holbrook Freeman

PURPOSE

The purpose of the **Assertive Behavior Inventory Tool** (ABIT) is to measure assertive behavior in registered nurses.

INSTRUMENT DESCRIPTION

Drawing on the work of Alberti and Emmons (1970), assertive behavior is viewed as "(a) acting in one's own best interest, (b) standing up for oneself, (c) expressing honest feelings, and (d) exercising one's rights without denying the rights of others" (Adams & Freeman, 1988, p. 223).

Adams and Freeman (1988) had previously developed the Assertiveness Inventory, which measured assertive, nonassertive, and aggressive behaviors. Since their goal was to measure only assertive behavior in the instrument being developed, they submitted 44 items with definitions of the three types of behaviors included to judges ($n = 23$) and asked them to link each item with a behavior. On the basis of the judges' review, 25 items met the criteria of a minimum 70% agreement of assertive behavior.

The revised instrument was named the Assertiveness Behavior Inventory Tool (ABIT) (Adams & Freeman, 1988). It is a paper-and-pencil measure with items grouped into categories of where the behaviors occurred: at work or away from work. Each item is a complete sentence worded in first person. Respondents use a 5-point, Likert-type scale (0 = don't know; 1 = almost never; 2 = seldom; 3 = often; and 4 = almost always. Item scores are summed to provide a total score. The maximum score that can be achieved is 96 (24 × 4). A copy of the ABIT is included at the end of the chapter.

RELIABILITY AND VALIDITY ASSESSMENT

Test-retest reliability was estimated from two administrations of the ABIT to 45 registered nurses from an urban acute care agency within a 2-week interval. The reliability coefficient obtained was .78.

Content validity was estimated by two judges using the technique as described by Waltz, Strickland, & Lenz (1991). The construct validity index obtained from these ratings was .92. One item was dropped, resulting in a total of 24 items in the ABIT.

The developers used the ABIT in a quasi-experimental design. Scores of registered nurses working in a for-profit acute care agency who participated in a single-session, assertiveness training program ($n = 27$) were compared with those of registered nurses also working in for-profit acute care agencies in another city ($n = 35$). There were no statistically significant differences between scores for the two groups at baseline or at 4 months post-intervention. The developers concluded that the single session assertiveness training program was ineffective in producing behavior change.

Use of the instrument in larger samples, estimation of internal consistency reliability, and work on construct validity are recommended. Adding a three-session assertiveness training program to the single-session and control groups for further comparisons is also suggested.

The authors have further revised the ABIT, which is now named the Behavior Inventory Tool II (BIT II). A single-sentence instruction asking the respondents to check the box best describing themselves has been added. The BIT II still contains 24 items, although six of the items were reworded so that they must now be reverse scored. Five additional statements were added at the end of the instrument to further address validity of the measure. These include four distractor items as well as the focal item "I am assertive." The response format offers four response options (strongly agree to strongly disagree). A copy of the BIT II is included at the end of the chapter.

The BIT II was administered to 300 registered nurses. The estimate of internal consistency was .75. The correlation of the "strongly agree" response on the item "I am assertive" and the total score on the BIT II was not statistically significant.

Scores on the BIT-II and the Nurses Assertiveness Inventory (Michelson, Molcan, & Poorman, 1986) were compared to estimate concurrent validity in another study of assertive behavior in registered nurses. The correlation coefficient between these scores was $r = .58$; $p < .001$ (Freeman & Adams, 1999).

REFERENCES

Adams, P. F., & Freeman, L. H. (1988). Measuring assertive behavior in registered nurses as an outcome of a continuing education program. In O. L. Strickland & C. F. Waltz (Eds.), *Measurement of nursing outcomes: Vol. 2. Measuring nursing performance: Practice, education and research* (pp. 221–229). New York: Springer Publishing Company.

Alberti, R., & Emmons, M. (1970). *Your perfect right.* San Luis Obispo, CA: Impact.

Freeman, L. H., & Adams, P. F. (1999). Comparative effectiveness of two training programmes on assertive behavior. *Nursing Standard, 13*(33), 32–35.

Michelson, L., Molcan, K., & Poorman, S. (1986). Development and psychometric properties of the Nurses' Assertiveness Inventory. *Behavioral Research and Therapy, 24,* 77–81.

Waltz, C. F., Strickland, O. L., & Lenz, E. R. (1991). *Measurement for nursing research.* (2nd ed.). Philadelphia: F. A. Davis.

BEHAVIOR INVENTORY II

Please check the box that best describes you.

AT WORK:	ALMOST ALMOST	OFTEN	SELDOM	ALMOST NEVER	NOT APPLICABLE
I tell others of my special skills.	/ /	/ /	/ /	/ /	/ /
I suggest new policies, procedures, and solutions.	/ /	/ /	/ /	/ /	/ /
I tell co-workers in a calm and reasonable way when I disagree	/ /	/ /	/ /	/ /	/ /
with their opinions.	/ /	/ /	/ /	/ /	/ /
I tell co-workers when they have done a good job.	/ /	/ /	/ /	/ /	/ /
I let co-workers know in a calm, reasonable way when they have done something wrong.	/ /	/ /	/ /	/ /	/ /
I express anger at work without being "out of control."	/ /	/ /	/ /	/ /	/ /
I express my ideas when serving on a committee.	/ /	/ /	/ /	/ /	/ /
I ask the doctor any question I have about a patient.	/ /	/ /	/ /	/ /	/ /
I ask my co-workers in a very direct way for help.	/ /	/ /	/ /	/ /	/ /
I take work assignments that I do not want to do.	/ /	/ /	/ /	/ /	/ /

AWAY FROM WORK:	ALMOST ALMOST	OFTEN	SELDOM	ALMOST NEVER	NOT APPLICABLE
I hide my feelings from my family.	/ /	/ /	/ /	/ /	/ /
I tell friends when I think they are being unfair.	/ /	/ /	/ /	/ /	/ /

AWAY FROM WORK *(continued)*:	ALMOST ALWAYS	OFTEN	SELDOM	ALMOST NEVER	NOT APPLICABLE
I let other persons introduce themselves first when I enter the room.	/ /	/ /	/ /	/ /	/ /
I speak up in a line at the store when I am next to be waited on and someone tries to get in front of me.	/ /	/ /	/ /	/ /	/ /
	/ /	/ /	/ /	/ /	/ /
I say "yes" to family members when I really want to say "no."	/ /	/ /	/ /	/ /	/ /
I request my family members to help with household chores.	/ /	/ /	/ /	/ /	/ /
I tell a salesperson "no" when I'm shown something I don't want.	/ /	/ /	/ /	/ /	/ /
I make good decisions about everyday life issues.	/ /	/ /	/ /	/ /	/ /
I compliment family members.	/ /	/ /	/ /	/ /	/ /
I let family members know, without becoming angry, that I disagree with their opinion.	/ /	/ /	/ /	/ /	/ /
I say "yes" to requests when I really want to say "no."	/ /	/ /	/ /	/ /	/ /
I express my preferences for an evening of entertainment to my friends.	/ /	/ /	/ /	/ /	/ /
I prevent other people from expressing their opinions when I disagree.	/ /	/ /	/ /	/ /	/ /
I maintain eye contact when talking to people.	/ /	/ /	/ /	/ /	/ /

IN GENERAL:	ALMOST ALWAYS		OFTEN		SELDOM		ALMOST NEVER		NOT APPLICABLE	
I am an introvert.	/	/	/	/	/	/	/	/	/	/
I am outgoing.	/	/	/	/	/	/	/	/	/	/
I am assertive.	/	/	/	/	/	/	/	/	/	/
I am aggressive.	/	/	/	/	/	/	/	/	/	/
I am compliant.	/	/	/	/	/	/	/	/	/	/

PART III
Measuring Professionalism

23

Nursing Activity Scale

Karen Kelly

PURPOSE

The **Nursing Activity Scale** (NAS) was developed to measure professional autonomy in nurses. The NAS is a revision of the Schutzenhofer Professional Nursing Autonomy Scale (SPNAS) (Schutzenhofer, 1987, 1988; Schutzenhofer & Musser, 1994).

INSTRUMENT DESCRIPTION

As nursing roles change in an evolving health care system (Bellack & O'Neil, 2000), continued attention to the professional autonomy of nurses will be an important focus. The conceptual framework of the SPNAS and later NAS is feminist theory (Ashley, 1976). The working definition of professional autonomy used in the scales was "the practice of one's occupation in accordance with one's education, with members of that occupation governing, defining, and controlling their own activities in the absence of external controls" (Schutzenhofer, 1988, p. 3).

There were several stages undertaken in developing the SPNAS. First, using information from a survey of deans, directors of nursing, and clinical nurse specialists in a metropolitan area, as well as the nursing literature, 29 items were generated. These items were reviewed for relevance to the measuring of professional autonomy by a panel of doctorally prepared nurses; 20 items were retained. Next, a panel of nursing faculty reviewed these items to rate the extent to which each reflected professional autonomy: low, medium, or high. A 12-item instrument resulted that was later revised into a 30-item instrument, which was named the SPNAS (Schutzenhofer, 1987). The items are brief descriptions of situations that are not specific to any one clinical area in which a nurse must take some action requiring the exercise of professional nursing judgment.

The SPNAS is a paper-and-pencil, self-report measure that is self-administered. In addition to the 30 items actually scored, it also contains five experimental items that represent the same categories of nursing action, but reflect dependent, deferent, or self-effacing outcomes. These experimental items (numbers 9, 21, 32, 34, 35) may be omitted when using the scale. Alternatively, scores from these experimental items may be correlated with item numbers that are scored as shown in Table 23.1.

Users of the scale are asked to send raw data from administration(s) of the experimental items to the author.

The response format is a 4-point, Likert-type scale with 1 = very unlikely of me to act in this manner; 2 = unlikely of me to act in this manner; 3 = likely of me to act in this manner; and 4 = very likely of me to act in this manner. Responses are weighted to reflect three levels of autonomy, from 1 = low level of autonomy to 3 = high level of autonomy. To achieve the weighting, each respondent's numerical item score is multiplied by the weight of each item as specified below:

Items 1–6, 12–13, 19, and 30; use weight of 3.
Items 7, 11, 14, 17, 20, 22, 23, 25, 26, and 29; use weight of 2.
Items 8, 10, 15, 16, 18, 24, 27–28, 31, 33; use weight of 1.

The adjusted item scores are then summed so that total scores produced can range from 60 to 240. Levels of autonomy reflected by the scores are: (a) 60 to 120 = lower level of autonomy; (b) 121 to 180 = mid-level of professional autonomy; and (c) 181 to 240-higher level of professional autonomy (Schutzenhofer, 1988). Copies of the SPNAS and NAS are included at the end of the chapter.

RELIABILITY AND VALIDITY ASSESSMENT

Instrument testing was done with female nurse respondents because female socialization is considered an important factor in the development and exercise of professional autonomy, as identified in the conceptual frame-

TABLE 23.1 Correlations of Experimental and Scale Items

Experimental item	Scale item
9	30
21	31
32	8
34	19
35	25

work for the study. Only work with the 30-item version is reported here as the Guttman scaling response format of the initial 12-item instrument proved unworkable (Schutzenhofer, 1983).

Data from a mailed administration of the SPNAS to a random sample of 500 female registered nurses in a midwestern state were used to estimate internal consistency. A question was included with the demographic questions to ascertain that the respondent was currently working. Only data from working nurses were considered to ensure familiarity with contemporary nursing practice and issues ({Kelly}Schutzenhofer, 1988). Respondents were primarily diploma graduates who had worked an average of 14 years; mean age was 38.2 years. These respondents used a 5-point rating scale to indicate how autonomous a nurse had to be (1 = low level of professional autonomy to 5 = very high level of professional autonomy). They were also given the working definition of professional autonomy used in developing the instrument, because earlier work had indicated low levels of understanding of professional autonomy. The alpha value obtained was .92.

Data from two administrations of the SPNAS at a 4-week interval were used to estimate test-retest reliability. Respondents were primarily diploma graduates employed an average of 6.3 years since graduation; 95% were female. The correction coefficient obtained was $r = .79$.

Content validity (Issac & Michaels, 1995) was assessed by review by doctorally prepared nursing faculty to ensure a range of autonomous behavior. Grounding in the nursing literature was also reported as a priori evidence of content validity.

Future use of the SPANS was recommended in research on professional autonomy of registered nurses to include behavioral and personal characteristics of nurses with high and low levels of autonomy.

Note

The current version of the instrument has been reformatted and labeled the Nursing Activity Scale (NAS). It contains 35 items with the four Likert-scale response options. The instrument has been widely used.

REFERENCES

Ashley, J. (1976). *Hospitals, paternalism, and the role of the nurse.* New York: Teacher's College Press.

Bellack, J. P. & O'Neil, E. H. (2000). Recreating nursing practice for a new century: Recommendations and implications of the Pew Health Professions Commission's final report. *Nursing Health Care Perspectives, 21*(1), 14–21.

Isaac, S. & Michael, W. B. (1995). *Handbook in research and evaluation (3rd ed.). San Diego, CA: EdITS.*

Schutzenhofer, K. K. (1983). Guttman scale analysis of professional autonomy in the attitudes of female nurses. *Unpublished doctoral dissertation, Southern Illinois University at Edwardsville.*

Schutzenhofer, K. K. (1987). The measurement of professional autonomy. Journal of Professional Nursing, 3, *278–283.*

Schutzenhofer, K. K. (1988). *Measuring professional autonomy in nurses. In O. Strickland & C. F. Waltz (Eds.),* Measurement of nursing outcomes: Vol. 2. Measuring nursing performance: Practice, education, and research *(pp. 3–18). New York: Springer Publishing Company.*

Schutzenhofer, K. K., & Musser, D. B. (1994). *Nurse characteristics and professional autonomy.* Image: The Journal of Nursing Scholarship, 26*(3),* 201–205.

Schutzenhofer Professional
Nursing Autonomy Scale

The following items describe situations in which a nurse must take some action that requires the exercise of professional nursing judgment. You are asked to respond to each item according to how likely you would be to carry out the action in each item. Please respond to *each item* even if you have not encountered such a situation before. Use the following scale in responding to the items.

1 = Very unlikely of me to act in this manner
2 = Unlikely of me to act in this manner
3 = Likely of me to act in this manner
4 = Very likely of me to act in this manner

Circle the number after each situation that best describes how you would act as a nurse. There are no right or wrong answers.

Code Number _____

	Very unlikely	Unlikely	Likely	Very likely	Do not make in this space
1. Develop a career plan for myself and regularly review it for achievement of steps in the plan.	1	2	3	4	_____
2. Consider entry into independent nursing practice with the appropriate education and experience.	1	2	3	4	_____
3. Voice opposition to any medical order to discharge a patient without an opportunity for nursing follow-up if my teaching plan for the patient is not completed.	1	2	3	4	_____
4. Initiate clinical research to investigate a recurrent clinical nursing problem.	1	2	3	4	_____
5. Refuse to administer a contraindicated drug despite the physician's insistence that the drug be given.	1	2	3	4	_____
6. Consult with the patient's physician if the patient is not responding to the treatment plan.	1	2	3	4	_____

7. Depend upon the profession of   1   2   3   4 _____
    nursing and not on physicians for the
    ultimate determination of what I do
    as a nurse.

8. Evaluate the hospitalized patient's   1   2   3   4 _____
    need for home nursing care and
    determine the need for such a referral
    without a medical order.

9. Accept a temporary assignment to a   1   2   3   4 _____
    unit even if I lack the education and
    experience to work in that unit.

10. Propose changes in my job description   1   2   3   4 _____
    to my supervisor in order to develop
    the position further.

11. Answer the patient's questions about   1   2   3   4 _____
    a new medication or a change in
    medication before administering a
    drug, whether or not this has been
    done previously by the physician.

12. Institute nursing rounds.   1   2   3   4 _____

13. Withhold a medication that is   1   2   3   4 _____
    contraindicated for a patient despite
    pressure from nursing peers to carry
    out the medical order.

14. Consult with other nurses when a   1   2   3   4 _____
    patient is not responding to the
    plan of nursing care.

15. Routinely implement innovations in   1   2   3   4 _____
    patient care identified in the current
    nursing literature.

16. Initiate a request for a psychiatric   1   2   3   4 _____
    consult with the patient's physician if
    my assessment of the patient indicates
    such a need.

17. Promote innovative nursing activities,   1   2   3   4 _____
    like follow-up phone calls to recently
    discharged patients, to evaluate the
    effectiveness of patient teaching.

18. Assess the patient's level of understanding 1   2   3   4 _____
    concerning a diagnostic procedure and
    its risks before consulting with the
    patient's physician if a patient has
    questions about the risks of the
    procedure.

19. Assume complete responsibility for   1 2 3 4 _____
    my own professional actions without
    expecting to be protected by the
    physician or hospital in the case of a
    malpractice suit.

20. Develop effective communication   1 2 3 4 _____
    channels in my employing institution
    for nurses' input regarding the policies
    that affect patient care.

21. Make appropriate in-house referrals   1 2 3 4 _____
    to social service and dietary only after
    obtaining a medical order.

22. Develop and refine assessment tools   1 2 3 4 _____
    appropriate to my area of clinical
    practice.

23. Record in the chart the data from my   1 2 3 4 _____
    physical assessment of the patient to
    use in planning and implementing
    nursing care.

24. Initiate discharge planning concerning   1 2 3 4 _____
    the nursing care of the patient, even in
    the absence of medical discharge
    planning.

25. Report incidents of physician
    harassment to the appropriate manager   1 2 3 4 _____
    or administrator.

26. Offer input to administrators   1 2 3 4 _____
    concerning the design of a new nursing
    unit or the purchase of new equipment
    to be used by nurses.

27. Complete a psychosocial assessment   1 2 3 4 _____
    on each patient and use this data in
    formulating nursing care.

28. Adapt assessment tools from other   1 2 3 4 _____
    disciplines to use in my clinical area.

29. Carry out patient care procedures   1 2 3 4 _____
    utilizing my professional judgment to
    meet the individual patient's needs
    even when this means deviating from
    the "cookbook" description in the
    hospital procedure manual.

30. Decline a temporary reassignment to   1 2 3 4 _____
    a specialty unit when I lack the
    education and experience to carry out
    the demands of the assignment.

31. Initiate referrals to social service   1   2   3   4   _____
    and dietary at the patient's request.
32. Assess needs of patient for home nursing   1   2   3   4   _____
    care only under order of physician.
33. Write nursing orders to increase   1   2   3   4   _____
    the frequency of vital signs of a patient
    whose condition is deteriorating even in
    the absence of a medical order to
    increase the frequency of such monitoring.
34. Administer a medication to which a   1   2   3   4   _____
    patient reports an allergy if the physician
    will assume responsibility for my actions.
35. Assume all blame for any conflicts or   1   2   3   4   _____
    problems I have with physicians.

Scoring Instructions for the Schutzenhofer Professional Nursing Autonomy Scale

Of the 35 items in the instrument, only 30 are scored. Five items (nos. 9, 21, 32, 34, and 35) are nonscored items that are used in comparison with five scale items for continuing measures of internal consistency. You may omit these items when using the scale. If you include these items in your use of the scale, please send the results to me (either the raw data or the correlation scores). The items that are compared are listed below:

Experimental items	Scale items
9	30
21	31
32	8
34	19
35	25

The table below gives the weight for each scale item. A weight of 1 indicates a low level of autonomy; a weight of 3 indicates a high level.

Item	Weight	Item	Weight	Item	Weight
1	3	12	3	23	2
2	3	13	3	24	1
3	3	14	2	25	2
4	3	15	1	26	2
5	3	16	1	27	1
6	3	17	2	28	1
7	2	18	1	29	2
8	1	19	3	30	3
10	1	20	2	31	1
11	2	22	2	33	1

Multiply the respondent's score on each item by the weight of the item. Total these adjusted scores. Scores can range from 60 to 240 with the following break-down for approximate levels of autonomy:

60 to 120 = lower level of professional autonomy
121 to 180 = mid level of professional autonomy
181 to 240 = higher level of professional autonomy

Code #_____

NURSING ACTIVITY SCALE

The following items describe situations in which a nurse must take some action that requires the exercise of some degree of professional nursing judgment. You are asked to respond to each item according to how likely you would be to carry out the action in each item. *Please respond to each item even if you have not encountered such a situation before.* Use the following scale in responding to the items.

1 = Very unlikely of me to act in this manner
2 = Unlikely of me to act in this manner
3 = Likely of me to act in this manner
4 = Very likely of me to act in this manner

Circle the number after each situation that most accurately describes how you would act as a nurse. There are *no* right or wrong answers, just *different* ways of responding to a situation. Please do not add qualifying statements to the items to justify your answer. Answer the items as stated.

1.	Develop a career plan for myself and regularly review it for achievement of steps in the plan.	1	2	3	4
2.	Consider entry into independent nursing practice with the appropriate education and experience.	1	2	3	4
3.	Voice opposition to any medical order to discharge a patient without an opportunity for nursing follow-up if the teaching plan for the patient is not completed.	1	2	3	4
4.	Initiate nursing research to investigate a recurrent clinical nursing problem.	1	2	3	4
5.	Refuse to administer a contraindicated drug despite the physician's insistence that the drug be given.	1	2	3	4
6.	Consult with the patient's physician if the patient is not responding to the treatment plan.	1	2	3	4
7.	Depend upon the profession of nursing and not on physicians for the ultimate determination of what I do as a nurse.	1	2	3	4
8.	Evaluate the hospitalized patient's need for home nursing care and determine the need for such a referral without waiting for a physician's order.	1	2	3	4

9. Propose changes in my job description to my supervisor in order to develop the position further.	1	2	3	4	
10. Answer the patient's questions about a new medication or change in medication before administering drug, whether or not this has been done previously by the physician.	1	2	3	4	
11. Institute nursing rounds on the patient unit.	1	2	3	4	
12. Withhold a medicine that is contraindicated for a patient despite pressure from nursing peers to carry out the medical order.	1	2	3	4	
13. Consult with other nurses when a patient is not responding to the plan of nursing care.	1	2	3	4	
14. Routinely implement innovations in patient care identified in the current nursing literature.	1	2	3	4	
15. Initiate a request for a psychiatric consult with the patient's physician if my assessment of the patient indicated such a need.	1	2	3	4	
16. Promote innovative nursing activities, like follow-up phone calls to recently discharged patients, to evaluate the effectiveness of patient teaching.	1	2	3	4	
17. Assess the patient's level of understanding concerning a diagnostic procedure and its risks before consulting with the patient's physician if a patient has questions about the risks of the procedure.	1	2	3	4	
18. Assume complete responsibility for my own professional actions without expecting to be protected by the physician or hospital in the case of a malpractice suit.	1	2	3	4	
19. Develop effective communication channels in my employing institution for nurses' input regarding the policies that affect patient care.	1	2	3	4	
20. Develop and refine assessment tools appropriate to my area of clinical practice.	1	2	3	4	
21. Record in the chart the data from my physical assessment of the patient to use in planning and implementing nursing care.	1	2	3	4	
22. Initiate discharge planning concerning the nursing care of the patient, even in the absence of discharge planning by the physician.	1	2	3	4	

23. Report a physician who harasses me to the appropriate manager or administrator.	1	2	3	4	
24. Offer input to administrators concerning the design of a new nursing unit or the purchase of new equipment to be used by nurses.	1	2	3	4	
25. Complete a psychosocial assessment on each patient and use this data in formulating nursing care.	1	2	3	4	
26. Adapt assessment tools from other disciplines to use in my clinical practice.	1	2	3	4	
27. Carry out patient care procedures utilizing my professional judgment to meet the individual patient's needs even when this means deviating from the "cookbook" description in the hospital procedure manual.	1	2	3	4	
28. Decline a temporary reassignment to a specialty unit when I lack the education and experience to carry out the demands of the assignment.	1	2	3	4	
29. Initiate referrals to social service and dietary at the patient's request even in the absence of a physician's order.	1	2	3	4	
30. Write nursing orders to increase the frequency of vital signs of a patient whose condition is deteriorating even in the absence of a medical order to increase the frequency of such monitoring.	1	2	3	4	
31. Accept a temporary assignment to a specialty unit even if I lack the education and experience to work there.	1	2	3	4	
32. Make appropriate in-house referrals to social service and dietary only if I have a physician's order.	1	2	3	4	
33. Assess the needs of a patient for home nursing care only if ordered by physician.	1	2	3	4	
34. Administer a medication to which a patient reports an allergy if the physician agrees to be responsible for my actions.	1	2	3	4	
35. Assume all the blame or fault for any incidents of nurse-physician conflict in which I am involved.	1	2	3	4	

Scoring Instructions for the Nursing Activity Scale

Of the 35 items in the instrument, only 30 are scored. Five items (nos. 31, 32, 33, 34, and 35) are nonscored items that are used in comparison with five scale items for continuing measurement of internal consistency. You may omit these items when using the scale. If you include these items in your use of the scale, please send the results to me (either the raw data or the correlation scores). The items that are compared are listed below:

Experimental items	Scale items
31	28
32	29
33	8
34	18
35	23

The table below gives the weight for each scale item. A weight of 1 indicates a low level of autonomy; a weight of 3 reflects a high level.

Item	Weight	Item	Weight	Item	Weight
1	3	11	3	21	2
2	3	12	3	22	1
3	3	13	2	23	2
4	3	14	1	24	2
5	3	15	1	25	1
6	3	16	2	26	1
7	2	17	1	27	2
8	1	18	3	28	3
9	1	19	2	29	1
10	2	20	2	30	1

Multiply the respondent's score on each item by the weight of the item. Total these adjusted scores. Scores can range from 60 to 240 with the following breakdown for approximate levels of autonomy:

    60 to 120   = lower level of professional autonomy
    121 to 180 = mid level of professional autonomy
    181 to 240 = higher level of professional autonomy

Questions regarding scoring should be sent to: Karen Kelly, EdD, RN, CNAA, 305 Schwarz Meadow Court, O'Fallon, IL 62269-6707. Phone: 618-624-3468. Fax: 618-624-2116. E-mail: kkellys@aol.com.

24

Nursing Care Role Orientation Scale

Jacqueline Stemple

PURPOSE

The purpose of the **Nursing Care Role Orientation Scale** is to measure orientation to the nursing care role on the part of nurses.

INSTRUMENT DESCRIPTION

The development of nursing roles and one's orientation to those roles begins in an individual's basic professional nursing program in carefully planned formal and informal learning experiences such as those described by Tracy, Samarel, & DeYoung (1995). Role models can be key players in how this development is shaped, particularly in the learning of clinical aspects of the role. Measuring the competence of role models (Lynn, 1995) as well as the orientation to the nursing care role of the nurse (Stemple, 1988) offers further dimensions to the study of the resulting nursing role care orientation.

The conceptual basis of the Nursing Care Role Orientation Scale was derived from various nurse theorists including Harmer (1922), Harmer & Henderson (1955), Kinlein (1977), Nightingale (1859), Orem (1971, 1980), and Smith (1981). Additional sources used included Lysaught's (1981) work on characteristics of a profession as well as the West Virginia University School of Nursing (1984) conceptual framework.

The original 20-item version of the Nursing Care Role Orientation Scale was developed at the West Virginia University School of Nursing drawing on literature related to the nursing care role and in particular, self-care aspects of the school's conceptual framework. This instrument was refined through several revisions. A total of 24 items (10 original items, 7 revised items, and 7 new items) comprise the Nursing Care Role Orientation Scale, which is a norm-referenced, paper-and-pencil measure.

Items are statements for which two response options are possible. Respondents use a 5-point, Likert-type scale (1 = low nursing care role orientation to 5 = high nursing care role orientation) to indicate their response. Numerical responses are summed for each of the 24 items to provide a total score; the maximum score possible is 120. Some items require reverse scoring. A copy of the original instrument is found at the end of the chapter.

RELIABILITY AND VALIDITY

Data from a mailed administration of the Nursing Care Role Orientation Scale as part of a larger study were used to estimate reliability and validity. Respondents ($N = 241$) were registered nurses with associate ($n = 53$), baccalaureate ($n = 78$), or master's ($n = 100$) degrees from a southeastern state. The mean total score was 96.8 ($S.D. = 10$).

Internal consistency reliability was estimated using coefficient alpha; the value obtained was .83. Most of the items (19 of 24) had item-to-total correlations above .40. Items 1, 10, 18, and 23 had coefficients below .30. When these items were deleted from the analysis, the alpha value increased to .87.

Content validity was estimated via review of the instrument by two undergraduate program faculty members and two graduate program faculty members. They were asked to link each item with the program competency it best reflected. There was 54% agreement from the undergraduate faculty raters and 79% agreement from the graduate faculty raters.

Hypothesis testing was used to estimate construct validity. The first hypothesis tested was that there would be a significant difference in scores of AD versus BSN graduates. This hypothesis was supported ($p = .003$). The second hypothesis was that there would be a significant difference between scores of BSN versus master's prepared nurses; this hypothesis was also supported ($p < .001$). The third hypothesis tested was that there were four factors of professional role orientation: collaboration, research, nurse/client, and autonomy. This hypothesis was partially supported by factor analysis. First, an eight-factor solution was produced, accounting for 60% of the variance; however, the factors were not interpretable. A rotated four-factor solution, accounting for 42% of the variance, revealed factors of autonomy/research, nurse/client, health goals/care, and collaboration. When coefficient alpha values were computed for these factors as subscales, the respective alpha values obtained were .75, .60, .80, and .34, respectively.

Recommendations for future work included attention to items with low item-total correlations (items 1, 10, 18, and 23) and use of the instrument with larger regional groups of nursing students in the various types of programs preparing registered nurses. Stemple (1988) also suggested that generalizability theory may be useful in addressing reliability of the Nursing Care Role Orientation Scale.

Low item-to-total correlations of items 1, 10, 18, and 23 in the above study led to revisions of these items. The Nursing Scale Role Orientation Scale Revised was also used in a 1994 study of the relationship between nursing care role orientation and health promotion behaviors of registered professional nurses in one state. Mailed responses were received from 529 nurses; 56 of these had doctoral degrees, 255 had master's degrees, and 218 had baccalaureate degrees. The coefficient alpha for this administration was .87 with item-to-total correlations improved for revised items as follows: item 1, .17 to .39; item 10, .29 to .35; item 18, .11 to .71; and item 23, .21 to .64.

A copy of the revised instrument is found at the end of the chapter following the original instrument.

REFERENCES

Harmer, B. (1922). *Textbook of the principles and practice of nursing.* New York: Macmillan.

Harmer, B. & Henderson, V. (1955). *Textbook of the principles and practice of nursing* (5th ed.). New York: Macmillan.

Kinlein, L. (1977). *Independent nursing practice with clients.* Philadelphia: J. B. Lippincott.

Lynn, M. R. (1995). Development and testing of the nursing role model competence scale (NRMCS). *Journal of Nursing Measurement, 3*(2), 93–108.

Lysaught, J. P. (1981). *Action in affirmation toward an unambiguous profession of nursing.* New York: McGraw-Hill.

Nightingale, F. (1859). *Notes on nursing: What it is and is not.* London: Harrison.

Orem, D. E. (1971). *Nursing concepts of practice.* New York: McGraw-Hill.

Orem, D. E. (1980). *Nursing concepts of practice* (2nd ed.). New York: McGraw-Hill.

Smith, M. C. (1979). Proposed metaparadigm for nursing research the theory development. *Image, 11*(3), 75–79.

Stemple, J. (1988). Measuring nursing care role orientation. In O. L. Strickland & C. F. Waltz (Eds.), *Measurement of nursing outcomes: Vol. 2. Measuring nursing performance: Practice, education and research* (pp. 19–31). New York: Springer Publishing Company.

Stemple, J. (1981). *Self-care orientations of associate degree and baccalaureate degree and baccalaureate degree students: Test of a causal model.* Unpublished doctoral dissertation, West Virginia University, Morgantown.

Tracy, J., Samarel, N., & DeYoung, S. (1995). Professional role develop-
    ment in baccalaureate nursing education. *Journal of Nursing Education,*
    34(4), 180–182.
West Virginia University School of Nursing (WVUSN). (1984). *Conceptual*
    framework. Unpublished document, Morgantown, WV, West Virginia
    University.

NURSING CARE ROLE ORIENTATION SCALE

CONCEPT MEASUREMENT

I am conducting a survey of nurses' perception of concepts in nursing. The purpose is to determine the relationship between nurses' conceptualization of nursing from different educational programs and practice settings.

Your participation in the project is voluntary. All information will be kept confidential and will not be used in any way to identify specific individuals. Thank you very much for your cooperation.

Please circle   Please record
Highest Academic Degree: AD BSN MSN   Date of Birth _____
Present Practice Setting: Primary Care Acute Care Long-Term Care

Example:

The major function of
teaching is to

        assist the student
        in developing skills
        in critical thinking.   <u>1 2 3 4 5</u>   present nursing content.

1. Indicates you *strongly agree* with (assist the student in developing skills in critical thinking is the major function).

2. Indicates that you *agree* with (assist the student in developing skills in critical thinking is the more important function).

3. Indicates that you *agree* with both (assist the student in developing skills in critical thinking and present nursing content are equally important functions).

4. Indicates that you *agree* with (present nursing content as the major function).

5. Indicates that you *strongly agree* with (present nursing content as the major function).

Directions:

Circle the number that best expresses your view on the following statements.
1. Health care for the client (community, family, individual) in most situations is most efficiently performed
through health team   through nursing
collaboration.   <u>1 2 3 4 5</u>   care only.

2. The nursing care goals of Client X are determined mostly by the consideration of the client
needs.   1 2 3 4 5   physicians' orders.

3. Nursing is best defined at what point on the following continuum?
Assisting the client in his   Administering
self-care practices.   1 2 3 4 5   therapeutic measures.

4. The quality of health care for the client is increased through nurses'
collaboration with the   careful attention to
nursing team.   1 2 3 4 5   their technical skills.

5. It is more important to nursing that the nurse
document client   record data for
outcomes.   1 2 3 4 5   physician's record.

6. The assessment of the client's problem should begin with
where the client is in
understanding.   1 2 3 4 5   complaints and tests.

7. Most nursing practices should be based upon
research by others.   1 2 3 4 5   research by nurses.

8. Nursing practice is best described by the nurse's
concepts used in practice.   1 2 3 4 5   activities performed.

9. The client in most situations, if given an understanding of his
health state, can make   still requires
appropriate decisions   judgmentand advice
regarding his health   regardinghealth
practices.   1 2 3 4 5   practices.

10. Most individuals' contacts with a nurse for nursing care should be
through the physician.   1 2 3 4 5   direct.

11. Strategies for meeting the health goals of the client are best done
by collaboration with the   identifying the nature
client.   1 2 3 4 5   of the health problem.

12. Most of the nurse-client interactions should be based on
client needs.   1 2 3 4 5   physicians' orders.

13. The primary data source for health assessment of the client should
be obtained from the client's
behavior and responses.   1 2 3 4 5   Kardex and chart.

14. The health history of the client should be directed toward
helping the client identify   identifying symptoms
and express health needs.   1 2 3 4 5   of illness.

15. The identification of health goals of the client is best done by
assessment of nature of   collaboration with the
illness.   1 2 3 4 5   client.

16. The quality of nursing care is increased more through
technical skills of nurse.   1 2 3 4 5   nursing research.

17. The nurse's purpose in performing a physical exam should be to
gain data to assist the
client to understand   diagnose the client's
his health state.   1 2 3 4 5   illness.

18. The effective program on nutrition for the client could best be developed through
collaboration with the nutritionist. <u>1 2 3 4 5</u> use of extensive literature review.

19. The obligation of the nurse should be to which of the following?
Mainly physician. <u>1 2 3 4 5</u> Mainly client.

20. The lifestyle data should be used
to request the physician to discuss causes of heart disease. <u>1 2 3 4 5</u> to educate the client about health promotion activities.

21. The specific dimensions of nursing care and the specific dimensions of medical care
are very different. <u>1 2 3 4 5</u> similar.

22. Blood pressure data should be used
to educate the client about change in status. <u>1 2 3 4 5</u> by the doctor in health assessment.

23. The effective program on drug abuse for the client could be best developed through
collaboration with the pharmacist. <u>1 2 3 4 5</u> use of extensive literature review.

24. The best nursing care is determined by nurse and
client. <u>1 2 3 4 5</u> doctor.

NURSING CARE ROLE ORIENTATION SCALE REVISED

Example:

The major function of teaching is to

assist the student in developing skills in critical thinking. <u>1 2 3 4 5</u> present nursing content.

1. Indicates you *strongly agree* with
(assist the student in developing skills in critical thinking is the major function).

2. Indicates that you *agree* with
(assist the student in developing skills in critical thinking is the more important function).

3. Indicates that you *agree* with both
(assist the student in developing skills in critical thinking and present nursing content are equally important functions).

4. Indicates that you *agree* with
(present nursing content as the major function).

5. Indicates that you *strongly agree* with
(present nursing content as the major function).

Directions:

Circle the number that best expresses your view on the following statements.

1. Health care for the client (community, family, individual) in most situations is performed best
    through health team   through nursing care
    collaboration.   1 2 3 4 5 only.
2. The nursing care goals of Client X are determined mostly by the consideration of the
    client needs.   1 2 3 4 5 physicians' orders.
3. Nursing is best defined at what point on the following continuum?
    Assisting the client in his   Administering
    self-care practices.   1 2 3 4 5 therapeutic measures.
4. The quality of health care for the client is increased through nurses' collaboration with the   careful attention to
    nursing team.   1 2 3 4 5 their technical skills.
5. It is more important to nursing that the nurse
    document   record data for
    client outcomes.   1 2 3 4 5 physician's record.
6. The assessment of the client's problem should begin with where the client is in
    understanding.   1 2 3 4 5 complaints and tests.
7. Most nursing practices should be based upon
    research by others.   1 2 3 4 5 research by nurses.
8. Nursing practice is best described by the nurse's
    concepts used in practice. 1 2 3 4 5 activities performed.
9. The client in most situations, if given an understanding of his health state,
    can make appropriate   still requires judgment
    decisions regarding his   and advice regarding
    health practices.   1 2 3 4 5 health practices.
10. Most clients' contacts with a nurse for nursing care should be
    through the physician.   1 2 3 4 5 direct.
11. Strategies for meeting the health goals of the client are best done
    by collaboration with the   identifying the nature
    client.   1 2 3 4 5 of the health problem.
12. Most nurse-client interactions should be based on
    client needs.   1 2 3 4 5 physicians' orders.
13. The primary data source for health assessment of the client should be obtained from the client's
    behavior and responses.   1 2 3 4 5 Kardex and chart.
14. The health history of the client should be directed toward
    helping the client identify   identifying symptoms
    and express health needs. 1 2 3 4 5 of illness.

15. The identification of health goals of the client is best done by assessment of nature of illness. <u>1 2 3 4 5</u> collaboration with the client.

16. The quality of nursing care is increased more through technical skills of nurse. <u>1 2 3 4 5</u> nursing research.

17. The nurse's purpose in performing a physical exam should be to gain data to assist the client to understand his health state. <u>1 2 3 4 5</u> diagnose the client's illness.

18. The effective program on nutrition for the client could best be developed through collaboration with the health team. <u>1 2 3 4 5</u> use of extensive literature review.

19. The obligation of the nurse should be to which of the following? Mainly physician. <u>1 2 3 4 5</u> Mainly client.

20. The lifestyle data should be used to request the physician to discuss causes of heart disease. <u>1 2 3 4 5</u> to educate the client about health promotion activities.

21. The specific dimensions of nursing care and the specific dimensions of medical care arc very different. <u>1 2 3 4 5</u> similar.

22. Blood pressure data should be used to educate the client about change in status. <u>1 2 3 4 5</u> by the doctor in health assessment.

23. The effective program on drug abuse for the client could be best developed through collaboration with the health team. <u>1 2 3 4 5</u> use of extensive literature review.

24. The best nursing care is determined by nurse and client. <u>1 2 3 4 5</u> doctor.

25

Justification of Moral Judgment and Action Tool*

Sara T. Fry

PURPOSE

The purpose of the **Justification of Moral Judgment and Action** (JMJA) tool is to measure moral answerability of a practicing nurse in general nursing practice relevant to moral standards contained in the tool.

INSTRUMENT DESCRIPTION

Nurses in nearly every area of practice encounter moral challenges. Examples include: (a) end-of-life decisions (Riley, Mahoney, Fry, & Field, 1999); (b) pediatric ambulatory care (Butz, Redman, Fry, & Kolodner, 1998); and (c) diabetes education (Redman & Fry, 1996, 1998). The JMJA allows for the measurement of moral answerability of nurses in the highly dynamic arena of professional nursing practice.

The definition of moral answerability used in instrument development was "providing an explanation (giving an account) for one's moral judgment and action in terms of moral standards (such as moral rules, principles, and theories) that serve as the individual's reason(s) for the moral judgment and/or action" (Fry, 1990, p. 169). Moral answerability is conceptually distinct from moral responsibility which is a particular form of moral accountability.

The conceptual basis used in developing the JMJA was moral philosophy (Beauchamp, 1982). The focus is on explaining judgments and actions. This may be an internal process using an established system of thought

---

* The tool may be obtained from Sara T. Fry, School of Nursing, Boston College, Chestnut Hill, Massachusetts.

or an external process of considering beliefs and principles as a basis for morality.

The JMJA focuses on internal justification from a criterion-referenced framework with three categories of answerability: (a) no answerability (absence of justification); (b) low answerability (internal justification according to the level of generality of rules); and (c) high answerability (internal justification according to the levels of generality of theories and/or principles) (Fry, 1990).

Content of the JMJA was derived from analysis of 137 situations involving moral conflict that were self-reported by nurses. Eleven types of moral conflict were identified: (a) obligations to do good and avoid harm; (b) nursing authority vs. patient authority to determine patient welfare; (c) obligations to benefit individual patients and society; (d) limits to the obligation to benefit patients; (e) allocation of nursing resources; (f) overriding of patient autonomy (paternalism); (g) lying to the patient (veracity); (h) lying to cover up mistakes (veracity); (i) obligation to protect patient confidentiality; (j) avoiding direct/indirect killing of the patient; and (k) foregoing life-sustaining treatments (food and water).

Each of these types of moral conflict was written into two parallel case situations requiring the nurse to make a moral judgement or to carry out of a moral action. An example of a typical case is provided at the end of the chapter.

Item characteristics described in the stimulus attributes for the JMJA are as follows:

Part A
1. Each hypothetical case situation requires the nurse to make a moral judgment or carry out a moral action.
2. The moral judgment (action) made (carried out) is one that falls within the decision-making capacity and authority of the nurse.
3. All case situations involve routine medical/surgical nursing care and *not* specialty care (such as psychiatric/mental health nursing, etc.).

Part B
4. All conceivable reasons for the judgment (action) described in Part A are solicited and considered for moral standards and levels of generality that constitute internal justification (Fry, 1990).

The response attributes of the JMJA follow:

Part A
1. The judgment (action) described by the respondent represents the judgement (action) that he/she would most likely make (carry out) in a similar case situation.

2. Any judgment (action) described constitutes what the nurse believes to be a moral judgment or action.

Part B

3. All reasons stated for the moral judgment (action) in Part A are considered.
4. Levels of generality will be indicated by statements encompassing ethical rules, principles, and/or theories (Fry, 1990).

The levels of moral standards (generality) that are contained in the response attributes are provided at the end of the chapter.

The JMJA is scored by identifying the levels of generality (moral standards) that appear in the reasons for the moral judgment or action the nurse included in the reasons given for the moral judgment. To allow for the possibility that respondents have different answerability scores for various types of moral actions, the paired case situations (11 parallel situations) are scored separately as the Case Answerability Score. The Case Answerability Scores are summed to produce a total score referred to as the Answerability Index Score.

Degrees of answerability are quantified by assigning numbers to the levels of generality indicated in the subject's responses as follows: theories = 4; principles = 3; rules = 2; none = 1. There is no cut-score established for the instrument. However, three levels of answerability are identified as follows: (a) high answerability—two levels of generality (ethical principles and/or theories); (b) low answerability—internal justification involving one level of generality (ethical rules); and (c) no answerability—no internal justification.

RELIABILITY AND VALIDITY ASSESSMENT

Reliability of the JMJA will be estimated using P_o and Cohen's K to assess the stability using the parallel forms of the measure. Work on classifying responses to Part B during pilot testing resulted in levels of interrater agreement ranging from 59% to 86.3%.

Content validity of the 22 case situations on the JMJA (11 content domains with two questions each) was estimated by five content specialists in ethics. Future work on accruing evidence for the validity of the instrument includes construct validity and decision validity using the contrasted groups technique. A sample of first-year baccalaureate nursing students (low answerability) and a sample of baccalaureate graduates with more than 3 years of employment (high answerability) will be used.

REFERENCES

Beauchamp, T. L. (1982). *Philosophical ethics: An introduction to moral philosophy.* New York: McGraw-Hill.

Butz, A. M., Redman, B. K., Fry, S. T., & Kolodner, K. (1998). Ethical conflicts experienced by certified pediatric nurse practitioners in ambulatory settings. *Journal of Pediatric Health Care, 12*(4), 183–190.

Fry, S. T. (1981). Accountability in research: The relationship of scientific and humanistic values. *Advances in Nursing Science, 4,* 1–13.

Fry, S. T. (1990). Measurement of moral answerability in nursing practice. In C. F. Waltz & O. L. Strickland (Eds.), *Measurement of nursing outcomes: Vol. 3. Measuring clinical skills and professional development in education and practice* (pp. 169–180). New York: Springer Publishing Company.

Redman, B. K., & Fry, S. T. (1996). Ethical conflicts reported by registered nurse/certified diabetes educators. *The Diabetes Educator, 22*(3), 219–224.

Redman, B. K., & Fry, S. T. (1998). Ethical conflicts reported by registered nurse/certified diabetes educators: A replication. *Journal of Advanced Nursing, 28*(6), 1320–1325.

Riley, J. M., Mahoney, M. A., Fry, S. T., & Field, L. (1999). Factors related to decision making about withholding or withdrawing nutrition and/or hydration. *The Online Journal of Knowledge Synthesis for Nursing [On line serial], 6*(3).

EXAMPLE OF TYPICAL CASE SITUATION OF THE JMJA

Case #1.1

The nurses on a surgical care unit had been under a great deal of stress
from very ill patients, a high census, and frequent staff illnesses during a
two-week period. On one particular evening, two nurses recognized that
they were developing the symptoms of an upper respiratory infection that
had been affecting other members of the staff. Since they had three postoperative patients needing one-to-one care and were receiving another
admission from the emergency room, they wondered if they could solicit
medication from the house staff in order to suppress their symptoms and
"keep going." This would allow them to remain on the unit and would
not contribute to an already critical staffing situation. Yet they also recognized that they might be causing more harm by communicating their
illnesses to already vulnerable patients and by the mistakes they might
make under the influence of medications (antihistamines). If you were
one of these nurses, what would you do?

Part A

Describe the moral action you would carry out in this situation.

Part B

Write *all* of the reasons why you would carry out the action described in
Part A.

LEVELS OF GENERALITY IN RESPONSE
ATTRIBUTES OF THE JMJA

Level of Rules

Specific do's and don'ts related to the judgment (action) described; indicate that actions of a certain kind ought (or ought not) to be done.
   (*Example:* The nurse should always tell the truth; The nurse should
never lie to a patient.)

Level of Principles

More general than rules; sometimes serve as the reasons for accepting
rules; abstract reasons for actions.
   (*Example #1:* The nurse ought to do more good than harm whenever
he/she can: the nurse is obligated to balance disbenefits whenever he/she
can: the nurse should strive to promote the self-determined choices of

the patient; the nurse ought to treat patients in a fair and just manner; the nurse is obliged to respect the privacy of patients.)

(*Example #2:* The nurse ought to accept or confirm the patient (receptiveness); the nurse ought to relate to the patient as another human being (relatedness); the nurse ought to be committed to the patient (responsiveness). All of these responses may be construed as "care" or "caring.")

Level of Theoretical Propositions

Bodies of moral principles and rules, more or less systematically related that indicate how what is good or bad, right or wrong, is interpreted.

(*Example: Consequentialist theories* interpret what is good/bad, right/wrong according to outcomes; thus, what is good/bad, right/wrong is determined by the consequences of acts. *Nonconsequentialist theories* interpret what is good/bad, right/wrong according to characteristics inherent in the act itself; thus, what is good/bad, right/wrong is independent of consequences. Consequentialist reasons for judgments/actions follow: the nurse ought to do 'x' because it would make the patient happy; *not* doing 'x' would make the patient lose trust in the nurse; or because it would, in the long run, be easiest for the patient. Nonconsequentialist reasons for judgments/actions follow: the nurse ought to do 'x' because there is something wrong about lying to patients; because breaking confidentiality is prohibited by the code for nurses; or because a person ought always to keep the promises they have made.

26

Reliability and Validity of the Nursing Role Conceptions Instrument

Gretchen Reising Cornell

PURPOSE

The purpose of the **Nursing Role Conceptions Instrument** (Pieta, 1976) is to measure the outcome of professional socialization of nursing students and/or nurses in various roles.

INSTRUMENT DESCRIPTION

Strategies for facilitating professional socialization in nursing proliferate for students (e.g., Coudret, Fuch, Roberts, Suhrheinrich, & White, 1994; Nichols & Lachat, 1994), and nurses (e.g., Allen, 1998). The Nursing Role Conceptions Instrument provides a measure of this nursing outcome.

Role theory and role development (Corwin, 1961) provided the conceptual basis for the Nursing Role Conceptions Instrument. It was adapted by Pieta (1976) from Corwin's role conception scale by means of changing the items that were questions into statements. In addition, new situation descriptions were developed (Cornell, 1990).

Three aspects of the nursing role are addressed: bureaucratic (12 items), professional (10 items), and service role conceptions (12 items). The situational statements are considered as subscales. The bureaucratic subscale focuses on loyalty to the employing institution, those in authority, and following administrative rules and routines. The professional subscale focuses on loyalty to the profession of nursing, involvement in professional organizations, commitment to practice standards, a scientific basis for practice, and use of professional judgment in decision making (Ketefian,

1985). The service subscale addresses loyalty or allegiance to patient welfare (Pieta, 1976).

As a self-report, paper-and-pencil measure, the Nursing Role Conceptions Instrument lists 34 statements descriptive of nursing situations. Respondents use a 5-point, Likert-type scale to respond to two questions following each statement. The first addresses the respondent's perception of the ideal situation and the second, their perception of actual nursing practice (Ketefian, 1985). Since each statement has two questions following it, there are actually 68 items.

A 5-point, Likert-type scale is used as the response format with 1 = strongly agree to 5 = strongly disagree (Ketefian, 1985). This is the reverse of the schema used by Pieta (1976). The most "socialized" response is indicated by responses of "strongly agree" to both the actual and ideal situations (Cornell, 1990).

Scoring is achieved by separately summing the numerical responses for the ideal and actual statements for each subscale as follows:

Ideal Bureaucratic Role	— Items 1, 13, 15, 17, 29, 31, 35, 37, 39, 49, 51, 59
Actual Bureaucratic Role	— Items 2, 14, 16, 18, 20, 32, 36, 38, 40, 50, 52, 60
Ideal Service Role	— Items 3, 5, 9, 11, 21, 29, 33, 47, 53, 57, 61, 67
Actual Service Role	— Items 4, 6, 10, 12, 22, 30, 24, 48, 54, 58, 62, 68
Ideal Professional Role	— Items 7, 23, 25, 27, 41, 53, 45, 55, 63, 65
Actual Professional Role	— Items 8, 24, 26, 28, 42, 54, 46, 56, 64, 66

This schema allows for calculation of a discrepancy score which is the difference between "actual" and "ideal" scores. Both Pieta (1976) and Ketefian (1985) used this discrepancy score, which could be either positive or negative, in their research. Cornell (1990) used only the magnitude of the direction in positive numbers. A copy of the instrument is included at the end of the chapter.

RELIABILITY AND VALIDITY ASSESSMENT

Internal consistency of the three subscales on the Nursing Role Conceptions Instrument was estimated by Pieta (1976) who obtained alpha values ranging from .58 to .84. Separate estimates of internal consistency for the ideal and actual responses for the three subscales were reported by Forrester (1983), who obtained alpha values ranging from .61 to .69. Pieta (1976) also reported estimates of test-retest reliability, with coefficients ranging from .83 to .92.

Cornell (1990) administered the Nursing Role Conceptions Instrument in a classroom setting to baccalaureate nursing students ($N = 260$). The Six-Dimension Scale (Schwirian, 1981), a measure of perceived role performance and competence, was also administered (Ward & Fetler, 1979). The students included freshmen through seniors. They ranged in age from 18 to 37 years; all but three were female and all but one was white. A random sample of responses ($n = 47$) was used to estimate internal consistency. The alpha values obtained ranged from .52 to .96; only the Ideal Professional Role and Ideal Service Role estimates were below .72. Test-retest reliability was estimated with coefficients ranging from .85 to .96.

Individual item alphas were calculated. All were at least .70 with the exception of items 21, 29, 33, 53, 57, 61, and 67 (Ideal Service Role) and items 7, 23, 27, 43, 55, and 65 (Ideal Professional Role).

Another estimate of internal consistency reliability was obtained by subscale item-to-item correlation. Significant correlations were found within three categories: Actual Professional Role, Actual Service Role, and Ideal Bureaucratic Role. There were six items (2, 14, 16, 36, 60, and 51) on the Actual Bureaucratic Role with no significant within-category correlations. In addition, in this category, there was a significant negative correlation between items 50 and 52. In the Ideal Professional and Ideal Service Role categories, each had two items (41 and 55 and 3 and 61) with no significant within-subscale correlations.

Correlation between scores on Actual and Ideal categories were examined. In freshman and sophomore students ($n = 114$), seven positive values and six negative correlations were obtained that were significant at the $p < .05$ level. In junior and senior students ($n = 146$), there were 12 such significant correlations (Cornell, 1990).

Content validity of the Nursing Role Conceptions Instrument was first estimated by a panel of six nurse experts who sorted items into subscales; 75% of these experts agreed that the 34 statements measured the respective role conceptions of the bureaucratic, professional, or service role subscales (Pieta, 1976).

Cornell (1990) again estimated content validity of the Nursing Role Conceptions Instrument for use with undergraduate nursing students. Two judges with expertise in nursing education and professional socialization rated the relevance of items to current nursing roles, the subscale assigned, and use with undergraduate nursing students. The content validity index obtained was .68. Subscale estimates were: (a) Professional Role, 1.0; (b) Bureaucratic, .33; and (c) Service, .75. Item-to-subscale congruence was confirmed. These judges made recommendations for item revision and addition of new items.

Construct validity was estimated by Ketefian (1985) using the known groups technique. She administered the Nursing Role Conceptions Instrument to undergraduate nursing students and practicing nurses. A detectable difference in scores was observed, with those of nursing students being lower.

Evidence for concurrent criterion validity was obtained in data from Cornell's (1990) total sample with the negative correlation found between scores on the Actual Bureaucratic subscale and the Six-Dimension Scale. Further, in junior students ($n = 75$), grade point average was significantly correlated with scores on the Ideal Bureaucratic Role. In the group of juniors and seniors ($n = 146$), grade point average, age, and class were significantly correlated with at least one of the subscales.

Predictive validity was estimated by comparing scores of nurse faculty with those of nurse administrators. Faculty scores were higher on professional role conception and administrators were higher on bureaucratic role conceptions (Pieta, 1976).

The issues revealed in Cornell's estimates of reliability and validity of the Nursing Role Conceptions Scale may be partially explained by factors such as: (a) the homogeneity of the respondent group and a possible response bias to respond as expected; (b) manner of scoring (i.e., "A" = "1" or strongly agree); (c) length of the instrument; and (d) the dynamic nature of the concept of professional socialization. Future revision of the instrument is warranted, particularly due to the ability to measure the difference between perceived ideal and ideal situations (Cornell, 1990).

REFERENCES

Allen, D. W. (1998). How nurses become leaders: Perceptions and beliefs about leadership development. *Journal of Nursing Administration, 28*(9), 15–20.

Cornell, G. R. (1990). Measuring undergraduate nursing student professional socialization. In C. F. Waltz & O. L. Strickland (Eds.), *Measurement of nursing outcomes: Vol. 3. Measuring clinical skills and professional development in education and practice* (pp. 281–298). New York: Springer Publishing Company.

Corwin, R. G. (1961). Professional employee: A study in conflict in nursing roles. *American Journal of Sociology, 66*, 604–615.

Coudret, N. A., Fuch, P. L. Roberts, C. S., Suhrheinrich, J. A., & White, A. H. (1994). *Journal of Professional Nursing, 10*(6), 342–349.

Forrester, D. A. (1983). *The relationship between sex-role identity and perceptions of nurse role discrepancy among professional nurses employed in hospital settings.* Unpublished doctoral dissertation, New York University.

Ketefian, S. (1985). Professional and bureaucratic role conceptions and moral behavior among nurses, *Nursing Research, 34*, 248–253.

Nichols, M. R., & Lachat, M. F. (1994). Senior-led groups: a strategy for professional development. *Nurse Educator, 19*(6), 46–48.

Pieta, B. A. (1976). *A comparison of role conceptions among nursing students and faculty from associate degree, baccalaureate degree, and diploma nursing programs and head nurses.* Unpublished doctoral dissertation, State University of New York, Albany.

Schwirian, P. M. (1981). Toward an explanatory model of nursing performance. *Nursing Research, 30,* 247–253.

Ward, M. J., & Fetler, M. E. (1979). *Instruments for use in nursing education research.* Boulder, CO: Western Interstate Commission for Higher Education.

NURSING ROLE CONCEPTIONS INSTRUMENT*

Instructions: This section consists of 34 situations in which a nurse might find herself. You are asked to indicate both:

(A) The extent to which you think the situation *actually exists* in the hospital.

(B) Notice that *two* statements require answers for each situation. Consider the statements of what *should be* the case and of what *is actually* the case separately; try not to let your answer to one statement influence your answer to the other statement. Give your opinions; there are no "wrong" answers. Indicate the degree to which you agree or disagree with the statement by marking one of the alternative answers ranging from: STRONGLY AGREE (A), AGREE (B), UNDECIDED (C), DISAGREE (D), AND STRONGLY DISAGREE (E).

STRONGLY AGREE (A)　　indicates that you agree with the statement with *almost no exceptions.*

AGREE (B)　　indicates that you agree with the statement with *some exceptions.*

UNDECIDED (C)　　indicates that you could either "agree" or "disagree" with the statement with about an equal number of exceptions in either case.

DISAGREE (D)　　indicates that you disagree with the statement with *some exceptions.*

STRONGLY
DISAGREE (E)　　indicates that you disagree with the statement with *almost no exceptions.*

HERE IS AN EXAMPLE:

Registered nurses in Hospital Z consider the patient's physical, social, and psychological needs when developing a plan of nursing care.

1. This is the way nurses *should* plan nursing care. _____
2. This is the way nurses *actually* do plan nursing care. _____

BE SURE TO PLACE A MARK AFTER *BOTH* STATEMENTS FOR EACH SITUATION ACCORDING TO YOUR DEGREE OF AGREEMENT WITH IT.

STRONGLY AGREE (A)
AGREE (B)
UNDECIDED (C)
DISAGREE (D)
STRONGLY DISAGREE (E)

---

* Developed by Barbara A. Pieta, RN, EdD. Reprinted with permission.

Situation

One head nurse at Hospital F insists that all procedures be performed as described in the procedure manual.
1. This is what a head nurse *should do*.   _____
2. This is what a head nurse *actually does*.   _____

Registered nurses at Hospital W are encouraged to discuss with patients as much about their conditions as the nurse believe would be best for the patient to know.
3. This is what nurses *should do*.   _____
4. This is what nurses *actually do*.   _____

One registered nurse at Hospital Y modified the hospital routines and procedures to meet the needs of the patients.
5. This is what nurses *should do*.   _____
6. This is what nurses *actually do*.   _____

The nursing staff at Hospital O are encouraged to read new drug and treatment brochures and memoranda.
7. This is what nurses *should do*.   _____
8. This is what nurses *actually do*.   _____

Mrs. B was to have a quart of a high protein liquid drink during a 24-hour period. The registered nurse spaced this treatment to provide the patient with small amounts during the daytime so that Mrs. B. would not be disturbed during the night.
9. This is what nurses *should do*.   _____
10. This is what nurses *actually do*.   _____

At Hospital A the rules state that registered nurses are to report for duty at least 10 minutes before the hour. One registered nurse cannot report until five after the hour because of the schedule of the bus she must ride to work. Because she is always late, she is not being considered for promotion.
13. This is what *should be done*.   _____
14. This is what *actually is done*.   _____

Situation

Preparing work schedules of staff is the responsibility of the supervisor of Hospital G. Registered nurses are given the opportunity to request their working hours and days but the hospital's needs always take precedence.
15. This is the way it *should be*.   _____
16. This is the way it *actually is*.   _____

At hospital B the rules clearly state that patients may only take showers in the morning. The registered nurses enforce this rule even when the patients request otherwise.

17. This is what nurses *should do.* _____

18. This is what nurses *actually do.* _____

Head nurses and supervisors at Hospital A when evaluating registered nurses for promotion consider the nurse's length of experience on the job to be important.

19. This is what *should be* considered important. _____

20. This is what *actually* should be important. _____

In Hospital Y a physician ordered a patient to sit up in a wheelchair twice a day. The registered nurse caring for the patient believed that the patient was not ready to sit up in the wheelchair. The nurses discussed the patient's condition with the physician.

21. This is what nurses *should be.* _____

22. This is what nurses *actually* do. _____

Registered nurses from Hospital M attend conferences outside of the hospital to learn about new techniques and to increase their knowledge of various topics.

23. This is what nurses *should be.* _____

24. This is what nurses *actually do.* _____

The head nurses and supervisors at Hospital R, when evaluating registered nurses for promotion, consider the nurses' membership in the professional association to be important.

25. This is what *should be* considered important. _____

26. This is what *actually* is considered important. _____

Conferences conducted at Hospital N with the nursing staff to review new techniques and procedures.

27. This is what *should* happen. _____

28. This is what *actually* happens. _____

SITUATION

The head nurses and supervisors at Hospital U, when evaluating registered nurses for promotion, consider the nurses' ability to plan nursing care based upon the patient's needs to be the most important.

29. This is what *should be* considered most important. _____

30. This is what *actually* is considered most important. _____

A registered nurse in Hospital E, although she administers excellent nurs-

ing care, is not being considered for promotion because she does not carry out hospital routines as established.
31. This is the way it *should be.*   _____
32. This is the way it *actually is.*   _____

In Hospital X patient B was scheduled for a physical therapy treatment at 9 A.M. The patient experienced some abdominal discomfort after eating breakfast so the registered nurse rescheduled the treatment.
33. This is what nurses *should do.*   _____
34. This is what nurses *actually do*   _____

One registered nurse at Hospital K follows all hospital routines even though she disagrees with several of them.
35. This is the way a nurse *should* function.   _____
36. This is the way most nurses *actually do* function.   _____

The regulations at Hospital D state that patients are to be transported to their cars via wheelchair upon discharge. Patient Y had been walking about for several days prior to being discharged but the registered nurse had the nurse's aide transport him to his car in a wheelchair.
37. This is what the nurse *should do.*   _____
38. This is what a nurse *actually does.*   _____

Registered nurses at Hospital H may only assign duties to the practical nurse, nurse's aide, and orderly that are described in their respective job descriptions.
39. This is what nurses *should do.*   _____
40. This is what nurses *actually do.*   _____

SITUATION

Hospital Q attempted to recruit and employ only registered nurses who were educated in programs sponsored by a college or university which is equipped to teach the supportive biological and social science courses as well as the nursing science courses.
41. This is what hospitals *should do.*   _____
42. This is what hospitals *actually do.*   _____

Registered nurses in Hospital O subscribe to and read professional journals and other professional material to keep abreast of new techniques and knowledge.
43. This is what nurses *should do.*   _____
44. This is what nurses *actually do.*   _____

Registered nurses at Hospital L attend inservice meetings at the hospital

even when they are not required to attend.
45. This is what nurses *should do.* _____
46. This is what nurses *actually do.* _____

Mrs. K. had difficulty sleeping during the night so the registered nurse allowed her to sleep in the morning even though, according to the hospital routine at Hospital Z, Mrs. K. should have been awakened at 7 A.M.
47. This is what a nurse *should do.* _____
48. This is what a nurse would *actually do.* _____

The policies at Hospital C state that any violation of hospital regulations must be reported. Head Nurse A observed registered nurse X violating a hospital regulation and reported the incident to the supervisor.
49. This is what a head nurse *should do.* _____
50. This is what a head nurse would *actually do.* _____

Registered nurses at Hospital J place a high priority on maintaining the patient's record, completing requisitions, and ordering supplies.
51. This is what nurses *should do.* _____
52. This is what nurses *actually do.* _____

SITUATION

Registered nurses in Hospital V are respected by their peers for taking the time to talk with patients in an attempt to allay any of the patient's anxieties which could affect the patient's recovery.
53. This is what nurses *should do.* _____
54. This is what nurses *actually do.* _____

The head nurses at Hospital F when evaluating registered nurses place considerable emphasis on the nurses' ability to make decisions based upon scientific principles.
55. This is what head nurses *should do.* _____
56. This is what head nurses *actually do.* _____

Registered nurses at Hospital X spend the majority of their time administering direct care to the patients.
57. This is what nurses *should do.* _____
58. This is what nurses *actually* do. _____

Regulations at Hospital K state that all patients must have their baths and treatments completed by 10 A.M. Registered nurses who complete their assignments in this time are considered valued employees.

59. This is the way it *should be*.   _____

60. This is the way it *actually is*.   _____

One registered nurse at Hospital T, while distributing dinner trays to the patients, approached Mrs. J. who began to cry. The nurse got another nurse to distribute the trays, pulled the curtain around the bed, and sat down and talked to Mrs. J.

61. This is what nurses *should do*.   _____

62. This is what nurses *actually do*.   _____

Registered nurses in Hospital M are active members of their professional nursing association.

63. This it the way it *should be*.   _____

64. This is the way it *actually is*.   _____

SITUATION

The registered nurses at Hospital Q demonstrate their ability to relate nursing practice to the scientific principles which they learned in school.

65. The is the way it *should be*.   _____

66. This is the way it *actually is*.   _____

The registered nurses at Hospital W work with the patients in developing the plan of care to be used by the nursing staff.

67. This is what nurses *should do*.   _____

68. This is what nurses *actually do*.   _____

27

Attitudes Toward Physically Disabled College Students

Patricia R. Messmer, Alice Conway,
Janice Giltinan, and Kathy Stroh

PURPOSE

The purpose of the **Attitudes Toward Physically Disabled College Students** (ATPDSC) instrument is to measure the attitudes of nursing students toward physically disabled college students.

INSTRUMENT DESCRIPTION

Sanchez et al. (2000) found that perceived accessibility appeared to be based on simple physical access rather than on the real needs and issues of persons with mobility impairments. As the perspectives of disabled persons become more widely known in studies (e.g., Pierce, 1998), the implications for nurses and other health care providers (Treloar, 1999) become better articulated for inclusion in curricula.

The conceptual basis for this instrument is identified as the theory of stigma as articulated by Goffman (1963), who described stigmatized people as persons possessing some characteristic that tends to turn people away. He posited that normal people carry out various types of discrimination toward the stigmatized. This perspective was confirmed by Werner-Beland (1980), who added that in interpersonal interactions, the visably disabled individual becomes a negative stimulus object.

The earliest measure of attitudes toward the disabled was the Attitude Toward Disabled Persons Scale (ATDP) developed by Yuker, Block, and Campbell (1960). Moving the focus somewhat, Rice (1979) developed the Attitudes of Able-Bodied College Students Toward Physically Handicapped College Students questionnaire (ATPDSC). This measure served as a starting point for this effort to study attitudes of nursing students.

A panel of experts selected items in Rice's (1979) work with interrater agreement reported at .968; test-retest reliability from two administrations in a random sample of college students was reported at .75. Messmer's (1990) adaptation of the ATPDSC consisted of substituting the word "disabled" for "handicapped" and "nondisabled" for "nonhandicapped."

The adapted ATPDSC contains two sections. The first part consists of ten questions that request demographic information. The second part contains 47 items that are statements. Three categories of items are considered: (a) attitudes related to in-class academic experiences (items 13, 15, 27–35, 38, 40, 42, 43, and 47–53); (b) attitudes related to out-of-class experiences (items 12, 16, 39, 44–46, and 57); and (c) attitudes related to mainstreaming the disabled into a collegiate setting (items 11, 14, 17–26, 36, 37, 41, and 54–56). Positively and negatively worded items are interspersed to help minimize response bias. Nine items require reverse scoring (items 14, 18, 23, 29, 36, 38, 49, 51, and 57).

The ATPDSC is a paper-and-pencil instrument allowing for self-administration. Respondents are instructed to use a 5-point response scale to indicate their extent of agreement with each statement (1 = strongly agree to 5 = strongly disagree). Item scores within a category are summed to produce a subscale score. The range of possible scores for these subscale scores is: (a) for in-class academic, 38 (most favorable) to 94 (least favorable); (b) for out-of-class, 11 (most favorable) to 31 (least favorable); and (c) mainstreaming, 34 (most favorable) to 74 (least favorable). Item scores, or the three subscale scores, can also be summed to create a total attitude score; the possible range of this score is 83 (most favorable) to 189 (least favorable). The lower the score, the more favorable the attitude toward disabled students. A copy of the ATPDCS is included at the end of the chapter.

RELIABILITY AND VALIDITY ASSESSMENT

Messmer's adaptation of the ATPDSC was administered to 47 senior nursing students at a small college at the beginning and end of a course that entailed theoretical- and clinical-focused rehabilitation concepts. The mean age of the respondents was 21.5 years and an average of 1.89 had worked at the campus Office for Disabled Students program. Only one student respondent self-identified as disabled with a hearing impairment. The estimates of internal consistency reliability obtained were .78 and .80 for the total instrument. Subscale alpha values were: (a) in-class (22 items), .70; (b) out-of-class (7 items), .47; and (c) mainstreaming (18 items), = .78. In addition, item-to-total correlations were all positive and statistically significant at $p < .05$. Over the course of the semester, total scores did not change significantly.

Content validity of the adapted ATPDSC was addressed in a review by a five-member panel of experts. Two of the experts were experienced in rehabilitation counseling and three in nursing. Their ratings provided an interrater agreement of .95, and face validity was reaffirmed by the author. Evidence of construct validity was identified in the ability to detect differences in scores by student age as well as by grade point average.

Users of the ATPDCS should be aware that the specific focus is on attitudes toward the physically disabled rather than disabled people in general. Results of this project suggest further work on the out-of-class subscale items to enhance internal consistency. If the instrument were to be used with other health care providers as respondents, further work on reliability and validity of the measure would be necessary.

On July 21, 2000, the ATPDCS was administered a second time to 22 nursing students in the last semester of their senior year to ascertain if attitudes toward the disabled had changed since the 1990 study. This group was older with a mean age of 28.62 years and a higher grade point average. None of these students self-identified as having a disability or having worked at the campus Office for Disabled Students. The mean score was 123.82. There were no relationships found between scores and either grade point average or age. The author urges that nursing curricula more fully address attention to the needs of the disabled.

REFERENCES

Goffman, E. (1963). *Stigma: Notes in the management of spoiled identity.* Englewood Cliffs, NJ: Prentice Hall.

Messmer, P. R. (1990). Nursing students' attitudes toward physically disabled college students. In C. F. Waltz & O. L. Strickland (Eds.), *Measurement of nursing outcomes: Vol. 3. Measuring clinical skills and professional development in education and practice* (pp. 203–219). New York: Springer Publishing Company.

Pierce, L. L. (1998). Barriers to access: Frustrations of people who use a wheelchair for full-time mobility. *Rehabilitation Nursing, 23*(3), 120–125.

Rice, D. (1979). *An investigation of the attitudes of the able-bodied college student toward the physically handicapped college student in the competitive academic setting.* Unpublished doctoral dissertation, University of Pittsburgh.

Sanchez, J., Byfield, G., Brown, T., LaFavor, K., Murphy, D., & Laud, P. (2000). Perceived accessibility versus actual physical accessibility of healthcare facilities. *Rehabilitation Nursing, 25*(1) 6–9.

Treloar, L. L. (1999). People with disabilities—the same, but different: Implications for health care practice. *Journal of Transcultural Nursing, 10*(4), 358–364.

Werner-Beland, J. A. (1980). *Grief responses to long-term illness and disability.* Reston, VA: Reston Publishing Co.

Yuker, H., Block, J., & Campbell, W. (1960). *A scale to measure attitudes toward disabled persons.* Albertson, NY: Human Resources Center.

Attitudes Toward Physically Disabled College Studesnts
(ATPDCS)

I. Background information
    Please mark the appropriate response or fill in the blank with the
    answer that best describes you.

    1. Age: _____

    2. Do you have a physical disability which limits one or more of
       your life's major activities (e.g., walking, talking, seeing, or
       hearing)?
       _____Yes   _____No

    3. Have you ever worked for pay for the handicapped college student?
       _____Yes   _____No

    4. If your response to item #3 is yes, how many semesters have you
       worked for the disabled?

       _____

    5. Have you ever been in an academic class with a disabled student?
       _____Yes   _____No

    6. If your response to item #5 is yes, how many classes?

       _____

    7. What is your current quality point average as of the end of the
       last academic semester?

       _____

    8. What year in school are you?
       _____Freshman
       _____Sophomore
       _____Junior
       _____Senior

    9. Have you ever attended a party with a disabled student?
       _____Yes   _____No

    10. Have you ever dated a disabled student?
        _____Yes   _____No

II. Please circle the number that best describes your belief for each
    statement
    For each statement's response use:
    (1) strongly agree
    (2) agree
    (3) undecided
    (4) disagree
    (5) strongly disagree

11. If one sees a disabled student who needs help (e.g., opening the door, or putting on a coat) one should always offer to help.   1 2 3 4 5

12. In any situation, it is all right for nondisabled students to be seen socially with disabled students on the same campus.   1 2 3 4 5

13. Most disabled college students are more dependable than nondisabled students in carrying out what they promised to do in the academic classroom.   1 2 3 4 5

14. Disabled students appear to be less happy at college than nondisabled students.   1 2 3 4 5

15. Disabled students appear to be more open and less set in their ways than nondisabled students in the academic classroom.   1 2 3 4 5

16. If qualified for membership, disabled students should be welcomed into a sorority, fraternity, or club.   1 2 3 4 5

17. Whenever a nondisabled student sees a disabled student who needs help, he should wait until the disabled person asks for help before offering assistance.   1 2 3 4 5

18. Disabled students should not be expected to meet the same admission standards to college as non disabled students.   1 2 3 4 5

19. Disabled students should be expected to meet the same academic standards in college as nondisabled students.   1 2 3 4 5

20. Disabled students should be provided more financial aid than nondisabled students in order to defray their costs for extra services (e.g. personal care, van transportation, meal aid, and academic aid).   1 2 3 4 5

21. Disabled students should be enrolled on campus even if they are unable to be totally independent in taking care of their personal and/or academic needs.   1 2 3 4 5

22. Disabled students should have meal aids in the cafeteria to bring them their food, help them eat, and return their trays.   1 2 3 4 5

23. Disabled students should live in separate housing facilities from nondisabled students on campus.   1 2 3 4 5

24. Disabled students should be provided   1   2   3   4   5
    transportation about the campus even
    though non-disabled students do not
    have access to transportation on the
    college campus.

25. Disabled students who are unable to   1   2   3   4   5
    walk or see should, without exception,
    be provided transportation about the
    campus even when nondisabled students
    do not have access to campus transportation.

26. Transportation should be provided to   1   2   3   4   5
    the disabled student only during inclement
    weather (e.g., heavy snow or rain).

27. Special academic services (e.g., note takers,   1   2   3   4   5
    tutors, readers, and other special equipment)
    should be provided to disabled students
    regardless of the severity of the disability.

28. Disabled students should be provided   1   2   3   4   5
    tutors when their grades fall below C for
    any academic class.

29. Disabled students should not have academic   1   2   3   4   5
    aids in the classroom if they are able to write.

30. All special services (e.g., interpreters,   1   2   3   4   5
    readers, and library aids) should be
    provided to the disabled student at no extra
    cost to the student.

31. Hearing impaired students should be   1   2   3   4   5
    permitted to have interpreters and/or
    electronic equipment in any class-related
    activity regardless of cost to the college.

32. Disabled students should be permitted   1   2   3   4   5
    more time than nondisabled students in
    completing tests and other in-class
    assignments when disabled students have
    problems with their hands.

33. As means of helping the disabled student,   1   2   3   4   5
    the student should be able to arrange with
    the professor for oral tests, tests outside of
    the classroom, extra time for tests, and
    test aids.

34. Disabled students should be permitted   1   2   3   4   5
    more time than nondisabled students in
    completing short-term, out-of-class
    assignments.

35. Libraries (campus) should, at their expense, provide readers, visual aid equipment, magnifying devices, recorders, and library aids for the disabled to use within the library for class-related activities.　　1　2　3　4　5

36. The college should develop a quota system to limit the number of disabled students on the campus.　　1　2　3　4　5

37. The college should actively recruit disabled students to enroll in college on a full-time basis.　　1　2　3　4　5

38. Faculty members are being unfair to disabled students when they expect the same of disabled students as of nondisabled students.　　1　2　3　4　5

39. In general, disabled students should not have their own clubs, sororities, or fraternities.　　1　2　3　4　5

40. Disabled students stimulate nondisabled students to do better in the academic classroom.　　1　2　3　4　5

41. I believe that the disabled student has as much ability to succeed in college as does the nondisabled student.　　1　2　3　4　5

42. In the classroom where a nondisabled student and a disabled student could work on a class project together, I would choose the nondisabled student over the disabled student in almost every situation.　　1　2　3　4　5

43. Disabled students appear to have no greater difficulty learning than do nondisabled students in the academic classroom.　　1　2　3　4　5

44. I feel nervous or uncomfortable when I am near a disabled student.　　1　2　3　4　5

45. It is not difficult for me to study when a disabled student is nearby in the dormitory, the library, or the classroom.　　1　2　3　4　5

46. I would be willing to live with a disabled student if scheduled to do so by the dormitory housing office.　　1　2　3　4　5

47. Disabled students usually turn in higher quality work than do nondisabled students in the academic classroom.　　1　2　3　4　5

48. Disabled students deserve all of the   1   2   3   4   5
    academic aid necessary to help them
    compete on an equal basis with the
    nondisabled student.

49. Most disabled students have difficulty   1   2   3   4   5
    in totally adapting to classroom procedures.

50. If I had a choice between a nondisabled   1   2   3   4   5
    and a disabled student to sit next to in class,
    I would choose the nondisabled student.

51. Disabled students are less cooperative than   1   2   3   4   5
    nondisabled students in carrying out their
    classroom assignments and other class-related
    group projects.

52. Disabled students are as capable as   1   2   3   4   5
    nondisabled students to carry out their
    classroom assignments and other
    class-room activities.

53. Disabled students do not have any more   1   2   3   4   5
    difficulty than do nondisabled students in
    adapting to classroom activities.

54. Disabled students should be provided   1   2   3   4   5
    tuition, room and board, book, and supplies,
    and other college costs through tax dollars
    (e.g., the Bureau of Vocational Rehabilitation,
    or the Office of the Visually Handicapped)
    so that they can attend college with
    nondisabled students.

55. Disabled students should meet the same   1   2   3   4   5
    academic and grade criteria as do
    nondisabled students on campus.

56. Academically qualified disabled students   1   2   3   4   5
    have the right to enroll in the college of
    their choice regardless of the level of their
    personal and/or academic care.

57. It is unwise for nondisabled students to   1   2   3   4   5
    be seen socially with disabled students
    because they will be looked down upon
    by other groups of nondisabled students
    (e.g., fraternities, sororities, and clubs).

Thank you for your consideration and your cooperation.

28

Organizational Climate Descriptive Questionnaire

Q. Kay Branum

PURPOSE

The purpose of the **Branum Organizational Climate Descriptive Questionnaire** (OCDQ) is to measure a single aspect of organizational climate: "collective perception of group and leader behaviors among members of a given group" (Branum, 1990, p. 263).

INSTRUMENT DESCRIPTION

Effective leadership in contemporary nursing by definition must include engaging people, building learning communities (Simpson, 2000), and harnessing the collective resources and talents of interdisciplinary teams needed to achieve desired outcomes (Bell, 2000).

This instrument is an adaptation of the original OCDQ (Halpin & Croft, 1963) as modified by Margulies (1965). The conceptual basis for this instrument is the work of Halpin and Croft (1963), which was conducted in the context of educational settings. In seeking to describe leader and group behaviors promoting both social needs satisfaction, which is key to group cohesiveness, and social control, needed to achieve goals, they developed the original 64-item OCDQ. Factor analysis of their data resulted in identification of four group behaviors (disengagement, hindrance, esprit, and intimacy) and four leader behaviors (aloofness, production emphasis, thrust, and consideration). This model evolved from the testing of the OCDQ that followed.

Halpin and Croft (1963) used data from the OCDQ to conceptualize a continuum of six organizational climate prototypes ranging from closed to open. The types of organizational climates identified are: closed, paternal, familiar, controlled, autonomous, and open.

Branum (1990) adapted a later version of the OCDQ (Margulies, 1965) by revising terms used in the items to move the focus from educational settings to hospitals. The following substitutions were made: "teacher" became "nurse" or "staff nurse"; "principal" became "head nurse"; and "school" became "hospital". The 64 items on the Branum adaptation of the OCDQ are statements. Respondents use a 5-point, Likert-type scale to indicate the extent of their agreement (1 = strongly agree; 2 = agree; 3 = neither agree nor disagree; 4 = disagree; 5 = strongly disagree) with each statement. The OCDQ is administered as a paper-and-pencil instrument to all group members.

Scoring involves several steps. First, each individual respondent's ratings are double standardized (Broverman, 1962). Then these individual scores are grouped together to produce a "climate profile." To do this, group scores are placed in a matrix of the eight behaviors (four group and four leader) by the six organizational climate prototypes (closed to open). To determine the organizational climate prototype, absolute differences are summed between each dimension for each climate prototype. The climate taxon(omy) assigned to the group is the prototype with the smallest absolute difference (Halpin & Croft, 1963). A copy of the modified OCDQ is included at the end of the chapter.

RELIABILITY AND VALIDITY ASSESSMENT

To estimate reliability and validity of the adaptation of the OCDQ, the author (1990) collected data via mail from nurses ($N = 366$) in five hospitals in southeastern states that varied in size, mission, acuity, and organizational/financial bases. Respondents were over 99% RNs; the remainder were LPNs. Mean age was 36 years. Respondents had worked on their respective units an average of 3 to 8 years.

Internal consistency reliability estimates of the eight dimensions (four group and four leader behaviors) reported as subscales were: disengagement (.7277), hindrance (.5006), esprit (.7443), intimacy (.6149), aloofness (.2743), production emphasis (.2212), thrust (.9080), and consideration (.7421). These estimates were compared to split-half coefficients corrected by the Spearman-Brown formula as reported by Halpin & Croft (1963). Estimates of disengagement, esprit, thrust, and consideration compare favorably with data from the original study.

Hypothesis testing was used to estimate construct validity. The first hypothesis was "factor analysis of responses to the OCDQ will result in eight factors that are similar to the eight dimensions factored in the original study" (Branum, 1990, p. 267). This hypothesis was conditionally supported with a rotated eight-factor solution explaining 45.2% of the variance. In this solution, the first four factors—thrust, disengagement, esprit, and intimacy—explained 34.9% of the variance. A rotated three-factor solution of social needs, social control, and esprit explained 66.2 % of the variance; and a rotated two-factor solution (social needs and social control) explained 54.6% of the variance.

The second hypothesis tested was "group assignment based on discriminant analysis of dimensions of the OCDQ for subjects and units will match true group membership more than 50% of the time" (Branum, 1990, p. 267). Support for this hypothesis was reported as mixed. The extent of correct assignments varied by how the analyses were conducted. The overall correct assignment was 33%. When the grouping variable used was the hospital, the rate of correct assignment was 36%. However, when only units from the same hospital were included in the analysis, correct assignment improved and ranged from 48% to 100%. Using units having at least four participants produced an inconclusive analysis.

The third hypothesis was "there will be no difference between the climate taxon assigned by the Halpin and Croft method and the taxon assigned by the openness continuum" (Branum, p. 271). An alternative method of scoring of the OCDQ was used to produce scores for testing of this hypothesis. The openness score is "calculated by adding the double-standardized scores for thrust and esprit and subtracting disengagement (Thrust + Esprit – Disengagement)" (Branum, 1990, p. 264) with a range of 0 to 20. The hypothesis was supported: taxon assignments were not significantly different from each other (z = .9683; p = .3329) and were significantly correlated (Spearman's correlation coefficient = .9253; p = .000).

Instrument refinement and item revision should be undertaken to strengthen reliability and validity estimates. The author advocates the use of the openness score in this work and points to the need for further study on describing climate in nursing with attention to other variables such as effects of physical environment and type of nursing care delivery. As work continues in the study of organizational climates in nursing, additional key variables such as nurse job satisfaction (Keuter, Byrne, Voell, & Larson, 2000) and patient outcomes (Seago, 1997; Shortell et al., 1994) are being considered.

REFERENCES

Bell, P. (2000). Creating a career: Realizing a dream. *Reflections on Nursing LEADERSHIP, 1st Quarter,* 6–10.

Branum, Q. K. (1990). Assessing organizational climate. In C. Waltz & O. L. Strickland (Eds.), *Measurement of nursing outcomes: Vol. 3. Measuring clinical skills and professional development in education and practice* (pp. 259–278). New York: Springer Publishing Company.

Broverman, D. M. (1962). Normative and ipsative measurement in psychology. *Psychological Review, 69*(4), 295–305.

Halpin, A. W., & Croft, D. B. (1963). *The organizational climate of schools.* Chicago: University of Chicago.

Keuter, K. Byrne, E., Voell, J., & Larson, E. (2000). Nurses' job satisfaction and organizational climate in a dynamic work environment. *Applied Nursing Research, 13*(1), 46–49.

Margulies, N. (1965). *A study of organizational culture and the self-actualizing process.* Unpublished doctoral dissertation, University of California.

Seago, J. A. (1997). Organizational culture in hospitals: Issues in measurement. *Journal of Nursing Measurement, 5*(2), 165–178.

Shortell, S. M., Zimmerman, J. E., Rousseau, D. M., Gillies, R. R., Wagner, D. P., Draper, E. A., Knaus, W. A., & Duffy, J. (1994). The performance of intensive care units: Does good management make a difference? *Medical Care, 32*(5), 508–525.

Simpson, B. (2000). Evolution of a leader. *Reflections on Nursing LEADERSHIP, 1st Quarter,* 6–10.

Modified Organizational Climate
Descriptive Questionnaire

The head nurse shares ideas with staff nurses.	1	2	3	4	5
The head nurse explains reasons for criticism.	1	2	3	4	5
The head nurse goes out of her way to help staff nurse.	1	2	3	4	5
Nurses interrupt each other in group meetings.	1	2	3	4	5
The head nurse contacts staff nurses every day.	1	2	3	4	5
Staff nurses leave the unit whenever possible.	1	2	3	4	5
Nurses in this unit keep to themselves.	1	2	3	4	5
The head nurse runs group meetings in a formal way.	1	2	3	4	5
Nurses talk about their personal life to other nurses.	1	2	3	4	5
There is a minority group of nurses who always oppose the majority.	1	2	3	4	5
The head nurse uses constructive criticism.	1	2	3	4	5
Staff nurses go about their work with great vim, vigor, and pleasure.	1	2	3	4	5
Group meetings are mainly management report meetings.	1	2	3	4	5
The head nurse helps staff nurses settle any differences.	1	2	3	4	5
The head nurse tries to get better salaries for staff nurses.	1	2	3	4	5
Nurses seek special favors from the head nurse.	1	2	3	4	5
Nurses spend time after work with other nurses who have problems.	1	2	3	4	5
The head nurse talks a great deal.					
The head nurse makes all work-related decisions.	1	2	3	4	5
Nurses socialize together in small select groups.	1	2	3	4	5
The morale of nurses in this unit is high.	1	2	3	4	5
The head nurse corrects the mistakes of staff nurses.	1	2	3	4	5
The head nurse sets an example by working hard herself.	1	2	3	4	5
Group meetings are organized with a strict agenda.	1	2	3	4	5

Nurses know the family background of other nurses.	1	2	3	4	5
The head nurse helps staff nurses solve personal problems.	1	2	3	4	5
The head nurse ensures that staff nurses work to their fullest capacity.	1	2	3	4	5
Nurses exert group pressure on nonconforming workers.	1	2	3	4	5
Nurses work together when doing routine duties.	1	2	3	4	5
Nurses have fun socializing together during working hours.	1	2	3	4	5
The head nurse encourages staff nurses to improve their weaknesses.	1	2	3	4	5
The head nurse stays after work to finish my uncompleted work.	1	2	3	4	5
Routine duties interfere with our primary jobs.	1	2	3	4	5
Nurses usually eat lunch by themselves.	1	2	3	4	5
Nurses ask senseless questions in group meetings.	1	2	3	4	5
The mannerisms of nurses in this unit are annoying.	1	2	3	4	5
The head nurse exchanges ideas with staff nurses.	1	2	3	4	5
Nurses in this unit have a good deal of loyalty.	1	2	3	4	5
Staff nurses are informed of the reasons for a supervisor's visit.	1	2	3	4	5
The head nurse looks out for the personal welfare of staff nurses.	1	2	3	4	5
Assistance from other units is readily available when needed.	1	2	3	4	5
Nurses prefer to work by themselves.	1	2	3	4	5
Extra materials are available for job use.	1	2	3	4	5
The head nurse is usually well prepared at group meetings.	1	2	3	4	5
There is considerable laughter when nurses gather informally.	1	2	3	4	5
Sufficient instruction is available for the operation of equipment.	1	2	3	4	5
Too much time is spent in meetings.	1	2	3	4	5
The head nurse is easy to understand.	1	2	3	4	5

The head nurse checks on the capability of all staff nurses.	1	2	3	4	5
Administrative paperwork is burdensome in this hospital.	1	2	3	4	5
The rules set by the nursing service are never questioned.	1	2	3	4	5
Sufficient time is given to prepare administrative reports and nurses' notes.	1	2	3	4	5
Procedures in this hospital are bothersome.	1	2	3	4	5
Supplies are quickly available.	1	2	3	4	5
Nurses in this unit talk about leaving the hospital.	1	2	3	4	5
The head nurse does personal favors for her staff nurses.	1	2	3	4	5
In group meetings there is the feeling of "let's get things done."	1	2	3	4	5
Nurses help select jobs to be worked on and patient assignments.	1	2	3	4	5
Nurses invite other nurses to visit them at home.	1	2	3	4	5
Nurses ramble on when they talk in group meetings.	1	2	3	4	5
Most nurses accept the faults of their co-workers.	1	2	3	4	5
The head nurse is on the job before other nurses arrive.	1	2	3	4	5
Staff nurses' closest friends are other nurses of this unit.	1	2	3	4	5
The head nurse schedules work for all nurses.	1	2	3	4	5

Note. From *The Organizational Climate of Schools* (pp.), by A. W. Halpin and D. B. Croft, 1963, Chicago: Midwest Administration Center. Adapted with permission.

29

Blaney/Hobson Nursing Attitude Scale

Doris R. Blaney, Charles J. Hobson,
and Anna B. Stepniewski

PURPOSE

The purpose of the **Blaney/Hobson Nursing Attitude Scale** is to measure attitudes of nurses toward cost effectiveness in nursing practices and procedures.

INSTRUMENT DESCRIPTION

Emphasis on cost effectiveness spans the nursing literature in education (McBride, Neiman, & Johnson, 2000), practice (Lessner, Organek, Shah, William, Bruttomesso, 1994), and research (Duren-Winfield, Berry, Jones, Clark, & Sevick, 2000). The close linkages between nursing attitudes and behavior posited by Fishbein and Ajzen (1972, 1975) continue to make nursing attitudes toward cost effectiveness an important outcome.

The conceptual framework for development of the Blaney/Hobson Nursing Attitude Scale (BHNAS) was the attitude model of Fishbein and Ajzen (1972, 1975), which posits that attitudes can be developed and changed by focusing on beliefs about the attitude objects. Further, attitudes and behavior are closely linked. Thus, to promote cost effective behavior by nurses, efforts need to be directed toward development of a favorable attitude toward cost effectiveness and focusing on positive and personally relevant beliefs concerning cost effectiveness in nursing (Blaney & Hobson, 1988). To form and change attitudes, five mechanisms (participation in decision making, position discrepancy, fear reduction, fear arousal, and providing new information [Steers, 1984]) were incorporated into a continuing education seminar. The BHNAS was developed to evaluate this program.

The BHNAS is a 10-item questionnaire; each item is a statement dealing with the issue of cost effectiveness in nursing practices and procedures. Five of the statements are positively worded and five are negatively worded. Respondents are instructed to use a 5-point, Likert-type scale to indicate the extent of their agreement (strongly disagree to strongly agree) by circling the appropriate response abbreviation (SD, D, N, A, and SA).

The BHNAS is a paper-and-pencil instrument designed for self-administration. Numeric scores are assigned to each response option with 1 = strongly disagree and 5 = strongly agree. The five negatively worded statements require reverse scoring. Summing the 10 item scores produces a total score with a possible range of 10 to 50. The higher the score, the more positive the attitude of respondents toward cost effectiveness in nursing. The instrument was administered to a pilot sample of students. Results indicated the need for revision of two items. This was done and the revision of the original instrument is found at the end of this chapter (Instrument A) (Blaney & Hobson, 1988).

RELIABILITY AND VALIDITY ASSESSMENT

In the above pilot administration of the BHNAS to 85 university students, the estimate of internal consistency obtained was alpha = .82. In using the scale to evaluate a continuing education program aimed at improving nursing attitudes toward cost effectiveness, a pretest/posttest design was used. Participants consisted of 156 nurses. Most (96%) of the sample were female with the largest percentage (29.1%) aged 20 to 24 years. Most (79.5%) were graduates of associate degree programs with just over half (50.3%) having 1 to 4 years of work experience in nursing. Over 87% worked 30 or more hours/week. The average pretest score was 33.19 (*SD* 6.13). The estimate of internal consistency obtained on the pretest administration was .75. Two months later when the posttest was administered, there were 135 participants. The alpha value obtained was .80.

Test-retest reliability was estimated by correlating the pretest scores of the control group ($n = 67$) with their posttest scores obtained approximately two months later. The reliability coefficient obtained was .43. Explanations offered for this finding were: (a) hospital and nursing cost effectiveness were very evident in national and local news; (b) attitudes were fluctuating during the period; and (c) the 2-month period was much longer than the usual recommended time for test-retest estimates. A second test-retest analysis was carried out with a separate sample of 54 nurses. The time interval between administrations was 2 weeks. The reliability coefficient obtained was .81.

Hypothesis testing was used to estimate construct validity. The first hypothesis tested was that the training program given to improve nursing attitudes toward cost effectiveness would result in program participants having: (a) more positive attitudes at the end of the program than at base-line, and (b) more positive attitudes than those of participants in the control group who did not attend the program. In the experimental group of nurses (n = 68), the mean score was 32.79 at baseline, and after the program, 36.13. This difference was statistically significant at $p < .001$. In addition, the mean posttest score of the program participants was 36.13, while the mean for the control participants was 33.43 ($p < .01$). Thus, both parts of the hypotheses were supported.

A second hypothesis tested was that attitudes toward cost effectiveness in nursing would positively correlate with cost-effective nursing behaviors as reported by head nurses of those participating in the continuing education program to improve attitudes toward cost effectiveness in nursing. Using information from staff and head nurses as well as nursing administrators, behaviorally anchored rating scales (BARS) were developed for three aspects of nursing practice. These were 9-point scales with specific behavioral anchors or examples to represent the 2, 5, and 8 levels (Schwab, Heneman, & Decotiis, 1975). The three areas addressed by BARS were supply utilization practices, patient goal setting, and patient scheduling. The BARS used had a test-retest reliability of .68 in a sample of 75 nurses with administrations separated by a 2-month period. The correlation of the behavior ratings obtained from adding the scores on the three BARS and total scores on the BHNAS was $r = .15$, $p < .05$. When mean scores on the BARS were compared for the participants who had the continuing education program between baseline and post-program scores, there was significant improvement ($p < .001$), and BARS ratings of participants were higher ($p < .001$) than those of controls after the continuing education program. Copies of the three BARS used in this hypothesis testing are found at the end of the chapter (Instrument B) (Blaney & Hobson, 1988).

In subsequent work, the BHNAS was expanded to 20 items. Ten statements were added using the same response format and response options. Total scores can range from 20 to 100; higher scores reflect more positive attitudes toward cost effectiveness in nursing practice. The reformatted instrument appears at the end of this chapter (Blaney, Hobson, & Stepniewski, 1990).

The current 20-item version of the BHNAS was given one time to nurses in a midwestern hospital ($N = 110$). Of these randomly selected respondents, 44% were staff nurses, 40% were head nurses, and 16% were senior administrators. The estimate of internal consistency reliability from this administration was alpha = .93.

A quasi-experimental approach to the contrasted groups method of estimating construct validity was used in testing for differences in scores of the three groups of respondents, with the hypothesis being that senior administrators would have the most positive (highest) scores, followed by head nurses, and then staff nurses. Analysis of variance (ANOVA) was used to test this hypothesis; the result was $F = 14.36$, $p = < .01$. Scheffe post hoc comparisons revealed that mean scores of senior administrators and head nurses were significantly different from the mean score of staff nurses. Group norms established for the three groups appear in Table 29.1.

To estimate criterion validity, stepwise multiple regression using seven demographic variables to predict total BHNAS scores resulted in a multiple R of .45, $p < .01$. Only one variable, position held, was a statistically significant single predictor of the BHNAS score.

TABLE 29.1 Group Norms

Group	Scale Mean	SDs
Senior nursing administrators	90	7.75
Head nurses	85.73	7.76
Staff nurses	76.85	12.85

REFERENCES

Blaney, D. R., & Hobson, C. J. (1988). Measuring attitudes towards cost-effectiveness in nursing. In O. L. Strickland & C. F. Waltz (Eds.), *Measurement of nursing outcomes: Vol. 2. Measuring nursing performance: Practice, education, and research* (pp. 178–190). New York: Springer Publishing Company.

Blaney, D. R., Hobson, C. J., & Stepniewski, A. B. (1990). Measuring nursing attitudes toward cost-effectiveness: Further development and psychometric evaluation of the Blaney/Hobson Scale. In C. F. Waltz & O. L. Strickland (Eds.), *Measurement of nursing outcomes: Vol. 3. Measuring clinical skills and professional development in education and practice* (pp. 181–191). New York: Springer Publishing Company.

Duren-Winfield, V., Berry, M. J., Jones, S. A., Clark, D. H., & Sevick, M. A. (2000). Cost-effectiveness analysis for the REACT study. *Western Journal of Nursing Research, 22*(4), 460–474.

Fishbein, M., & Ajzen, I. (1972). Attitudes and opinions. *Annual Review of Psychology, 23*, 487–544.

Fishbein, M., & Ajzen, I. (1975). *Belief, attitude, intention, and behavior: An introduction to theory and research.* Reading, MA: Addison-Wesley.

Lessner, M. W., Organek, N. S., Shah, H. S., Williams, C. A., & Bruttomesso, K. A. (1994). Orienting nursing students to cost-effective clinical practice. *Nursing and Health Care, 15*(9), 458–462.

McBride, A. B., Neiman, S., & Johnson, J. (2000). Responsibility-centered management: A 10-year nursing assessment. *Journal of Professional Nursing, 16*(4), 201–209.

Schwab, D. P., Heneman, H. G., & Decotiis, T. A. (1975). Behaviorally
   anchored rating scales: A review of the literature. *Personnel Psychology*,
   28, 549–562.
Steers, R. M. (1984). *Introduction to organizational behavior* (2nd ed.).
   Glenview, IL: Scott, Foresman.

Blaney/Hobson Nursing Attitude Scale*

TOP

Directions: Please respond to the following statements dealing with the issue of cost-effectiveness in nursing practices and procedures by indicating the extent to which you disagree or agree with each one. Please *circle* your response.

		Strongly Disagree	Disagree Some-what	Neither Agree Nor Disagree	Agree Some-what	Strongly Agree
1.	The introduction and use of cost-effective practices and procedures will improve overall nursing effectiveness.	SD	D	N	A	SA
2.	The introduction and use of cost-effective nursing practices and procedures will benefit me personally.	SD	D	N	A	SA
3.	Operating a nursing unit in order to make a profit is wrong.	SD	D	N	A	SA
4.	I look forward to the introduction and use of cost-effective practices and procedures in nursing.	SD	D	N	A	SA
5.	The introduction and use of cost-effective nursing practices and procedures will result in a decrease in the quality of patient care.	SD	D	N	A	SA
6.	The introduction and use of cost-effective practices and procedures will benefit the nursing profession as a whole.	SD	D	N	A	SA

7. The thought of intro   SD   D   N   A   SA
    ducing "cost-effective-
    ness" into nursing
    makes me uneasy.

8. Hospital nursing   SD   D   N   A   SA
    units should not be
    concerned with making
    or losing money.

9. The introduction and   SD   D   N   A   SA
    use of cost-effective
    nursing practices and
    procedures will benefit
    patients.

10. Nurses should not be   SD   D   N   A   SA
    obligated to provide
    patient care in a cost-
    effective manner.

11. I look forward to   SD   D   N   A   SA
    learning more about
    cost-effectiveness
    in nursing.

12. Cost-effectiveness   SD   D   N   A   SA
    goes against the basic
    principles of good
    nursing.

13. The whole idea of   SD   D   N   A   SA
    cost-effectiveness in
    nursing upsets me.

14. Cost effectiveness   SD   D   N   A   SA
    is bad for nursing.

15. I feel good when   SD   D   N   A   SA
    I save the hospital
    money.

16. I welcome the new   SD   D   N   A   SA
    emphasis on cost
    effectiveness in nursing.

17. Cost effectiveness   SD   D   N   A   SA
    programs only mean
    more work for nurses.

18. Cost effectiveness   SD   D   N   A   SA
    programs are a hassle
    for nurses.

19. Learning more about   SD   D   N   A   SA
    cost-effectiveness will
    help me be a better
    nurse.

20. I fully agree with the   SD   D   N   A   SA
    need to improve cost
    effectiveness in nursing.

---

* Copyright 1985 by Doris R. Blaney and Charles J. Hobson.

INSTRUMENT A
Blaney/Hobson Nursing Attitude Scale*

Revised Nursing Questionnaire

Directions: Please respond to the following statements dealing with the issue of cost-effectiveness in nursing practices and procedures by indicating the extent to which you disagree or agree with each one. Please *circle* your response.

	Strongly Disagree	Disagree Some-what	Neither Agree Nor Disagree	Agree Some-what	Strongly Agree
1. The introduction and use of cost-effective practices and procedures will improve overall nursing effectiveness.	SD	D	N	A	SA
2. The introduction and use of cost-effective nursing practices and procedures will benefit me personally.	SD	D	N	A	SA
3. Operating a nursing unit in order to make a profit is wrong.	SD	D	N	A	SA
4. I look forward to the introduction and use of cost-effective practices and pro-cedures in nursing.	SD	D	N	A	SA
5. The introduction and use of cost-effective nursing practices and procedures will result in a decrease in the quality of patient care.	SD	D	N	A	SA
6. The introduction and use of cost-effective practices and procedures will benefit the nursing profession as a whole.	SD	D	N	A	SA

7. The thought of   SD   D   N   A   SA
    introducing cost-
    effectiveness into
    nursing makes me
    uneasy.

8. Hospital nursing   SD   D   N   A   SA
    units should not be
    concerned with
    making or losing
    money.

9. The introduction   SD   D   N   A   SA
    and use of cost-
    effective nursing
    practices and
    procedures will
    benefit patients.

10. Cost-effectiveness   SD   D   N   A   SA
    should not influence
    the way in which
    nurses provide
    patient care.

INSTRUMENT B
BEHAVIORALLY ANCHORED RATING SCALE

PERFORMANCE DIMENSION: GOAL SETTING AND PATIENT CARE PLAN

Nurse's Name: _____

best ____ 9

____ 8   Nearly always develops and actively utilizes a patient care plan consisting of explicit overall discharge objectives, along with specific daily goals.

____ 7

____ 6

average ____ 5   Generally attempts to develop and utilize a patient care plan with overall discharge objectives and specific daily goals; however, occasionally the patient care plan lacks explicit overall objectives or specific daily goals and is not actively utilized.

____ 4

____ 3

____ 2   Nearly always fails to develop or utilize an effective patient care plan with overall objective patient care plan with overall objectives and specific daily goals.

worst ____ 1

PERFORMANCE DIMENSION: EFFICIENT SUPPLY UTILIZATION

Nurse's Name: _____

best ——— 9

——— 8 Consistently aware of the cost of supplies used in providing patient care and nearly always utilizes these supplies in an efficient, nonwasteful manner.

——— 7

——— 6

average ——— 5 Generally aware of the cost of supplies used in providing patient care and attempts to utilize supplies efficiently; however, cases occasionally occur in which supplies are utilized in an inefficient and wasteful manner.

——— 4

——— 3

——— 2 Consistently unaware of the cost of supplies used in providing patient care and nearly always utilizes these supplies in an inefficient, wasteful manner.

worst ——— 1

PERFORMANCE DIMENSION: OPTIMAL SCHEDULING

Nurse's Name: _____

best   9

          8   Nearly always schedules patient tests, procedures, and preparations in an efficient, logical manner resulting in timely processing and discharge.

          7

          6

average   5   Generally attempts to schedule patient tests, procedures, and preparations in an efficient, logical manner; however, occasionally scheduling is done in an inefficient, illogical manner resulting in unnecessary delays and untimely discharge.

          4

          3

          2   Nearly always schedules patient tests, procedures, and preparations in an inefficient, illogical manner resulting in unnecessary delays and untimely discharge.

worst   1

PART IV
Research and Evaluation

30

Research Appraisal Checklist

Mary E. Duffy

PURPOSE

The purpose of the **Research Appraisal Checklist** (RAC) is to develop a mechanism for assessing the value of published research reports.

INSTRUMENT DESCRIPTION

The importance of systematic evaluation of research reports in nursing is evident in studies such as that reported by Brown (1990) in which 47 studies relating to diabetes patient education were reviewed; using the RAC to measure the quality of the studies, scores ranged widely from 34 to 95. Recently, Lohr and Carey (1999) reported that 12 Association of Health Care Policy and Research funded evidence-based practice centers used a variety of tools for "grading" studies and further stressed the need for systematic evaluation.

Research appraisal is viewed as being focused on the research process and the outcome of the process. Research appraisal is concerned with what research is, how it should be conducted, and the credibility and value of the outcome. Little information is available on how to do this, with most of the published literature focusing on questions to be asked as part of a research appraisal. The checklist format for the RAC (Duffy, 1988) was selected a priori; it serves as a reminder to the appraiser of elements to be addressed.

The first step in instrument development was a review of all nursing research texts and articles addressing the parts of the research process. This comprehensive list of criteria for research appraisal was subjected to content analysis. Three research colleagues reviewed the 49 resulting items. Some re-wording was done and the addition of two more items brought the total number of items to 51 in 10 categories.

In the next step, members of the American Nurses' Association Council of Nurse Researchers were selected via stratified random sampling to receive a mailed copy of the criteria items. Raters ($n = 156$) were asked to rate each item for its importance in appraising research reports using a 5-point summated rating scale (1 = not important to 5 = extremely important). Mean importance ratings ranged from 4.01 to 4.86. Minor item revisions were done for clarity.

Using ratings from the above review process, items were classified into four categories by importance. For items in category 1 (25 items), 90% or more of the sample rated them as greatly important or extremely important, which were the two highest ratings. For category 2 (17 items), this percentage was 80% to 90%; for category 3 (6 items), 70% to 80%; and for category 4 (3 items), less than 70%.

The 51 items were placed in checklist format, each with three response options: fully met, partially met, or not met. A weighting scheme based on the category of importance and whether the criteria was fully, partially, or not met was developed for use in scoring. This schema was used by 11 doctoral students; they each appraised the same article with the checklist. While the students had positive comments about the helpfulness of the RAC in the appraisal process, issues with the complexity of the scoring system prompted a revision of the scoring process. The result was that weighting was dropped. Instead, respondents use a 6-point rating scale to indicate the extent to which each criterion item is met in the report being reviewed (1 or 2 = not met; 3 or 4 = partially met; and 5 or 6 = completely met). An NA option is available if the criterion is not applicable.

The RAC is a paper-and-pencil measure. It is designed to be used during the review process of a report of a quantitative research study.

Summated scores are computed for each of the 10 categories of criteria (title, abstract, problem, review of the literature, subjects, instruments, design, data analysis, discussion, and form and style). The number of items per category ranges from three to seven. Category scores are added to produce a total score. If the NA response is used one or more times, instructions are provided for adjusting the total score as follow: (a) count the number of times the rating was given; (b) multiply the scale values of 2, 4, and 6 by the number to arrive at three numbers; (c) subtract the lowest of those three numbers from the highest number in the below average range, the second of those numbers in the highest number in the average range, and the highest of those three numbers in the superior range; and (d) revise the grand total score range scores to reflect this systematic decrease of the NA items (Duffy, 1985).

In this summated scoring schema, the highest possible score is 306 (i.e., 51×6). Scores between 205 and 306 are considered superior; scores between 103 and 204 are considered average; and scores from zero to 102 are considered below average. In addition, the RAC instructions ask the user to list strengths and weaknesses in the research report being reviewed to amplify the appraisal process. A copy of the checklist is included at the end of the chapter.

RELIABILITY AND VALIDITY ASSESSMENT

Interrater reliability of the 10 categories in which the RAC's 51 criteria/items were placed was estimated by independent reviews of a research report carried out by the author and a research assistant who was a doctoral candidate. Correlation coefficients for categories ranged from $r = .50$ to 1.00, with the coefficient for the total instrument, $r = .94$.

The RAC was administered in classes to 44 nursing students at different points in nursing education programs. The first group ($n = 20$) were in an undergraduate research course and the second group ($n = 24$) were master's students in their first research course.

Considering each of the 10 categories on the RAC as subscales, estimates of internal consistency (Cronbach's alpha) ranged from .48 (data analysis, 4 items) to .87 (abstract, 4 items). The alpha value for the total RAC was .91. All item-to-total correlations were reported as statistically significant at least at the .05 level.

Hypothesis testing was used to estimate construct validity. The hypothesis tested follows: PhD students' rating of the research report using the RAC criteria would be closer to an expert's ratings than would beginning master's students' ratings of the same report.

The category and total RAC scores of each group's summed mean scores were then subtracted from those of the expert rater who was doctorally prepared with a track record as a teacher of research as well as publication of research. Using one-tailed t-tests for independent groups, no statistically significant differences were found except on the data analysis category ($p = .05$). There was a trend (seven categories and total) of the differences between the scores of the PhD students and the expert rater being smaller than those of the master's students. In three categories (title, problem, and form and style), the differences from the expert rater's scores were approximately equal for the two groups.

Yet to be done is the testing of the constructed-response section of the RAC where the respondent lists strengths and limitations of the study being reviewed. The author suggests that work with the weighted scoring system used in the original version of the instrument might be fruitful. Development of a glossary of terms relating to the criteria to ensure interrater reliability as well as further work on estimating construct validity are also suggested.

REFERENCES

Brown, S. A. (1990). Quality of reporting in diabetes patient education research: 1954–1986. *Research in Nursing and Health, 13*(1), 53–62.

Duffy, M. E. (1985). A research appraisal checklist for evaluating nursing research reports. *Nursing and Health Care, 6*, 538–547.

Duffy, M. E. (1988). The research appraisal checklist: Appraising nursing research reports. In O. L. Strickland & C. F. Waltz (Eds.), *Measurement of nursing outcomes: Vol. 2. Measuring nursing performance: Practice, education and research* (pp. 420–437). New York: Springer Publishing Company.

Lohr, K. N., & Carey, T. S. (1999). Assessing "best evidence": Issues in grading the quality of studies for systematic reviews. *Joint Commission Journal of Quality Improvement, 25*(9), 470–479.

RESEARCH APPRAISAL CHECKLIST

Instructions: The Research Appraisal Checklist (RAC) contains 51 criteria that have been ordered under eight major research categories. The RAC is designed to assist you to carefully and systematically assess the worth of a written quantitative research report.

In appraising a research report, you are asked to give only one rating to each criterion. Circle the number you think best describes the degree to which each criterion is met in the research report. The numbers in the rating scale range from "1," meaning "Not Met," to "6," meaning "Completely Met." If you rate a category less than a 5 or 6, indicating that you believe it to be Partially or Not Met, write a very brief note summarizing your thoughts about that portion of the report. At the end of each category, sum the numbers circled beside the appropriate criteria and place these numbers in the boxes provided at the end of the category.

After completing the ratings of the 51 criteria, sum the category scores and enter them in the appropriate Total Score box. Then, sum scores for all categories and enter the score in the Grand Total box. Finally, write a brief summary citing the major strengths and limitations of the report.

<u>Criteria</u>	<u>Appraisal Rating</u>	<u>Comments</u>
I. TITLE		
1. Title is readily understood.	1 2 3 4 5 6 NA	
2. Title is clear.	1 2 3 4 5 6 NA	
3. Title is clearly related to content.	1 2 3 4 5 6 NA	

> CATEGORY SCORE

II. ABSTRACT		
4. Abstract states problem and, where appropriate, hypotheses clearly and concisely.	1 2 3 4 5 6 NA	
5. Methodology is identified and described briefly.	1 2 3 4 5 6 NA	
6. Results are summarized.	1 2 3 4 5 6 NA	
7. Findings and/or conclusions are stated.	1 2 3 4 5 6 NA	

> CATEGORY SCORE

Criteria	Appraisal Rating	Comments

III. PROBLEM

8. The general problem of the study is introduced early in the report.   1 2 3 4 5 6 NA

9. Questions to be answered are stated precisely.   1 2 3 4 5 6 NA

10. Problem statement is clear.   1 2 3 4 5 6 NA

11. Hypotheses to be tested are stated precisely in a form that permits them to be tested.   1 2 3 4 5 6 NA

12. Limitations of the study can be identified.   1 2 3 4 5 6 NA

13. Assumptions of the study can be identified.   1 2 3 4 5 6 NA

14. Pertinent terms are/can be operationally defined.   1 2 3 4 5 6 NA

15. Significance of the problem is identified.   1 2 3 4 5 6 NA

16. Research is justified.   1 2 3 4 5 6 NA

> CATEGORY SCORE

IV. REVIEW OF LITERATURE

17. Cited literature is pertinent to research problem.   1 2 3 4 5 6 NA

18. Cited literature provides rationale for the research.   1 2 3 4 5 6 NA

19. Studies are critically examined.   1 2 3 4 5 6 NA

20. Relationship of problem to previous research is made clear.   1 2 3 4 5 6 NA

21. A conceptual framework/ theoretical rationale is clearly stated.   1 2 3 4 5 6 NA

22. Review concludes with a brief summary of relevant literature and its implications to the research problem under study.   1 2 3 4 5 6 NA

> CATEGORY SCORE

Criteria	Appraisal Rating	Comments

V. METHODOLOGY

A. Subjects

23. Subject population (sampling frame) is described. 1 2 3 4 5 6 NA

24. Sampling method is described. 1 2 3 4 5 6 NA

25. Sampling method is justified (especially for nonprobability sampling). 1 2 3 4 5 6 NA

26. Sample size is sufficient to reduce Type II error. 1 2 3 4 5 6 NA

27. Possible sources of sampling error can be identified. 1 2 3 4 5 6 NA

28. Standards for protection of subjects are discussed. 1 2 3 4 5 6 NA

CATEGORY SCORE

B. Instruments

29. Relevant previous reliability data are presented. 1 2 3 4 5 6 NA

30. Reliability data pertinent to the present study are reported. 1 2 3 4 5 6 NA

31. Relevant previous reliability data are presented. 1 2 3 4 5 6 NA

32. Validity data pertinent to present study are reported. 1 2 3 4 5 6 NA

33. Methods of data collection are sufficiently described to permit judgment of their appropriateness to the present study. 1 2 3 4 5 6 NA

CATEGORY SCORE

C. Design

34. Design is appropriate to study questions and/or hypothesis. 1 2 3 4 5 6 NA

35. Proper controls are included where appropriate. 1 2 3 4 5 6 NA

36. Confounding/moderating variables are/can be identified. 1 2 3 4 5 6 NA

37. Description of design is explicit enough to permit replication. 1 2 3 4 5 6 NA

CATEGORY SCORE

Criteria	**Appraisal Rating**	**Comments**

VI. DATA ANALYSIS

38. Information presented is   1 2 3 4 5 6 NA
    sufficient to answer research
    questions.

39. Statistical tests used are   1 2 3 4 5 6 NA
    identified.

40. Reported statistics are   1 2 3 4 5 6 NA
    appropriate for hypotheses/
    research questions.

41. Tables and figures are   1 2 3 4 5 6 NA
    presented in an easy-to-
    understand, informative way.

> CATEGORY SCORE

VI. DISCUSSION

42. Conclusions are clearly stated.   1 2 3 4 5 6 NA
43. Conclusions are substantiated   1 2 3 4 5 6 NA
    by the evidence presented.
44. Methodological issues in study   1 2 3 4 5 6 NA
    are identified and discussed.
45. Findings of study are   1 2 3 4 5 6 NA
    specifically related to
    conceptual/theoretical
    basis of study.
46. Implications of the findings   1 2 3 4 5 6 NA
    are discussed.
47. Results are generalized only   1 2 3 4 5 6 NA
    to population on which study
    is based.
48. Recommendations are made   1 2 3 4 5 6 NA
    for further research.

> CATEGORY SCORE

VIII. FORM & STYLE

49. Report is clearly written.   1 2 3 4 5 6 NA
50. Report is logically organized.   1 2 3 4 5 6 NA
51. Tone of report displays an   1 2 3 4 5 6 NA
    unbiased, impartial, scientific
    attitude.

> CATEGORY SCORE

GRAND TOTAL: _____

FINAL SUMMARY OF MAJOR STRENGTHS AND LIMITATIONS

STRENGTHS: LIMITATIONS:

Enter Grand Total Score in Appropriate Category:

_____ Superior   (205–306 Points)

_____ Average   (103–204 Points)

_____ Below Average   (0–102 Points)

31

Knowledge of Research Consumerism Instrument

Cheryl B. Stetler and E. Ann Sheridan

PURPOSE

The purpose of the **Knowledge of Research Consumerism Instrument** (KRCI) (Stetler & Sheridan, 1988) is to measure basic understanding of the research process needed by nursing students or newly graduated nurses to be able to read, understand, and evaluate scientific aspects of reports of research studies.

INSTRUMENT DESCRIPTION

With the growing emphasis on evidence-based practice, research is fundamental to promoting and sustaining innovative practice (Hynes, 2000), the outcome of nursing understanding of the research process remains key. Research consumerism continues to be fostered in strategies such as a graduate student research practicum (Howard, Beauchesne, Shea, & Meservey, 1996) and a research utilization forum (Stetler, Bautista, Verale-Hannon, & Foster, 1995).

The criterion-referenced framework used in instrument development was selected to be consistent with the goal of whether the respondent has the requisite level of understanding to be a research consumer.

The conceptual basis for this instrument draws on the model of "applicability of research findings to practice" by Stetler and Marram (1976) as well as subsequent work by Stetler (1984) and Van Servellan (Marram) and Stetler (1986). This hierarchical model posits three levels of knowledge: (a) validation—the ability to critique research reports, which is foundational to; (b) comparative evaluation—consideration of the findings of research reports for application to practice; and (c) decision making as to whether to use the findings in practice. The KRCI addresses validation, the most basic level of this model. Additional work has been initiated by Stetler and Grady that addresses competencies related to evidence-based practice, including but not limited to comparative evaluation and decision making. The KRCI is a self-report tool that has been updated and includes both essential knowledge for use of evidence and related behaviors. Items cover basic, intermediate, and advanced levels of competence, as well as sequential categories of utilization beginning with exploration and ending with evaluation.

Because the wide variation during a review of the literature by the authors made it impossible to identify standardized content regarding basic knowledge of nursing research, they selected a widely used nursing research text (Polit & Hungler, 1983b) to further define the domain. Chapters in the text focus on seven areas that serve as subdomains: (a) scientific research process; (b) preliminary research steps; (c) types of research approaches and research design considerations; (d) data collection methods; (e) measurement and sampling; (f) analysis of data; and (g) communication in the research process.

The KRCI was developed with two parts. Items in Part I consisted of 207 questions in a multiple-choice response format from the instructor's manual (Polit & Hungler, 1983a) accompanying the nursing research text. These items encompassed objectives related to knowledge and interpretation. The 30 items for Part II were developed to focus on objectives related to problem solving/evaluation. Also in multiple-choice response format, these items related to three "hypothetical research abstracts" created by the test developer. These 237 items were reviewed for content validity by six nursing faculty with a minimum of a master's degree, who were currently teaching research in a baccalaureate program. They rated each item for relevancy and congruency with subdomain specifications, as well as for technical construction factors. As a result of this rating, the number of items on the instrument was reduced by more than half to 126. The average percentage of items retained for Part I was 53%; for Part II, it was 80%.

The instrument is administered as a paper-and-pencil test. The response to each item on both parts of the instrument is scored correct or incorrect. Then the number of correct responses divided by the number of items for the respective section of the instrument (for Part I, 102 items; for Part II, 24 items), as well as for the total instrument (126 items), is calculated to create three separate percentage scores: Part I, Part II, and Total.

The cut score, or level at which respondents would be considered as having mastered research content contained in the instrument, was established with use of a modification of Angoff's (1971) standard setting method. This method seeks to identify the point at which a respondent on the border between acceptable/nonacceptable knowledge of research consumerism would perform. Six judges individually rated each item as to the percentage of minimally competent nurses who are Phase I consumers of research will answer this item correctly. They were told to use no more than three contiguous percentages in this process. The individual judges then discussed their ratings within their group; some judges adjusted their ratings at this point. The resulting ratings were averaged for each item for each of the two parts of the instrument and for the total instrument. The resulting scores were: Part I, 62.7%; Part II, 64.3%; and Total, 63.5%. A copy of the tool is included at the end of the chapter.

RELIABILITY AND VALIDITY ASSESSMENT

The Kuder-Richardson formula 20 was used to estimate reliability. Estimates obtained were: Part I, .826, Part II, .575, and Total, .854 ($N = 165$).

Content validity was estimated during the instrument development process as described above and used to reduce the number of items on the instrument. Face validity was addressed in a pretest with nine new graduate baccalaureate nurses.

Validity testing was conducted with two groups of respondents. One group, considered to be "instructed" ($n = 129$), was made up of baccalaureate students or new graduates from four schools of nursing who had research content. The other group, considered to be "uninstructed" ($n = 36$), was comprised of RNs having had no research coursework during the previous five years. These uninstructed respondents were either working in a large medical teaching center or current students in an RN-to-BSN program. The educational preparation of the uninstructed group varied, and included ADN (6.5%), diploma (64.5%), BSN (64.5%), and MA (3.2%).

Given concerns about the wisdom of combining data from various schools of nursing as well as combining data from two different types of uninstructed respondents, the authors examined differences in scores among as well as between groups of respondents. Scores on the KRCI were significantly higher in the instructed group than in the uninstructed group. Within the instructed group, scores of respondents having research coursework integrated into the curriculum rather than a separate course were significantly lower than those having a separate course. The scores of these "integrated" respondents also approximated the average scores of the uninstructed group. Within the uninstructed group, scores of respondents from the RN-to-BSN program were higher than those of respondents from the medical center.

At the item level, several analyses were conducted. Item difficulty (proportion of correct responses/item) was calculated using chi-square on raw numbers. Significant test statistics were found for 35% of items in at least one of the group comparisons made, and for 23% in two or more. Item discrimination (proportion of correct responses in each instructed group minus the proportion of correct responses in the uninstructed group) was done with 43% of the items with a criterion groups difference index (CGDI) of ≥.20 in at least half of the group comparisons. Item discrimination was calculated with 50% of items having a K_{max} of ≥.20. In comparisons of the proportion of respondents correctly classified as masters (decision validity), percentages varied from 5% to 60%. In all cases, uninstructed respondents were classified as nonmasters.

Work on reducing the number of items on the KRCI has begun along with explication of criteria being used. Calculation of test-rest reliability, using only instructed respondents, is needed. Pre-testing and post-testing of respondents relative to research content in courses and the exploration of an empirically set cut score are other examples of evidence required to further substantiate validity of the instrument.

REFERENCES

Angoff, W. (1971). Scales, norms, and equivalent scores. In R. L. Thorndike (Ed.), *Educational measurement* (pp. 508–600). Washington, DC: American Council on Education.

Howard, E. P., Beauchesne, M. A., Shea, C. A., & Meservey, P. M. (1996). Research practicum: Linking education to practice. *Nurse Educator, 21*(6), 33–37.

Hynes, D. M. (2000). Research as a key to promoting and sustaining innovative practice. *Nursing Clinics of North America, 35*(2), 453–459.

Polit, D., & Hungler, B. (1983a). *Instructor's manual for nursing research: Principles and methods* (2nd ed.). Philadephia: J. B. Lippincott.

Polit, D., & Hungler, B. (1983b). *Nursing research: Principles and methods* (2nd ed.). Philadephia: J. B. Lippincott.

Stetler, C. (1984). *Nursing research in a service setting: Massachusetts General Hospital, Department of Nursing.* Reston, VA: Reston Publishing.

Stetler, C. B., Bautista, C., Vernale-Hannon, C., & Foster, J. (1995). Enhancing research utilization by clinical nurse specialists. *Nursing Clinics of North America, 30*(3), 457–473.

Stetler, C., & Marram, G. (1976). Evaluating research findings for applicability in practice. *Nursing Outlook, 24*, 559–563.

Stetler, C. B., & Sheridan, E. A. (1988). Measuring knowledge of research consumerism. In O. L. Strickland & C. F. Waltz (Eds.), *Measurement of nursing outcomes: Vol. 2. Measuring nursing performance: Practice, education and research* (pp. 438–451). New York: Springer Publishing Company.

Van Servellen, G. M., & Stetler, C. (1986). Utilization of research: Critiquing research for practice. In A. M. Lieske (Ed.), *Clinical nursing research* (pp. 231–242). Rockville, MD: Aspen Systems.

KNOWLEDGE OF RESEARCH CONSUMERISM INSTRUMENT

Instructions: This questionnaire is designed to assess your current level of knowledge about nursing research. It consists of two sections:

> Part I: A series of multiple-choice questions that focus on various aspects of research.
>
> Part II: Abstracts of two research studies, each followed by a series of multiple-choice questions about the content of the abstracted study.
>
>   For each question in Part I and Part II, select the ONE BEST answer (a, b, c, or d) and indicate your choice on the answer sheet provided. Please use a No. 2 lead pencil and *completely* fill in the circled number on the answer sheet that corresponds to the *letter* which you believe indicates the right answer. Please answer ALL of the test questions.

Part I

1.   The majority of studies at midcentury focused on
     a.   consumer satisfaction
     b.   clinical problems
     c.   health promotion
     d.   educational issues
2.   Inductive reasoning is the process of
     a.   verifying assumptions that are part of our heritage
     b.   developing scientific predictions from general principles
     c.   empirically testing observations that are made known through our sense organs
     d.   forming generalizations from specific observations
3.   Empiricism refers to the process of
     a.   making generalizations from specific observations
     b.   deducing specific predictions from generalizations
     c.   gathering evidence rooted in objective reality
     d.   verifying the assumptions upon which the study was based
4.   The concept of generalization refers to
     a.   the ability to go beyond the specifics of the situation at hand
     b.   the confidence that a researcher has in the outcomes of the investigation
     c.   whether the study has been linked to a theory
     d.   the belief that all phenomena have antecedent causes

5. The purpose of an operational definition is to
   a. assign numerical values to variables
   b. specify how a variable will be defined and measured
   c. state the expected relations between the variables under investigation
   d. designate the overall plan by which the research will be conducted
6. Of the following, the most appropriate example of an attribute variable is
   a. maternal-infant bonding
   b. method of teaching
   c. nurse-client teaching
   d. blood type
7. The dependent variable(s) in the study "Is the job performance of nurses affected by salary or perceived job autonomy?" is (are)
   a. job performance
   b. salary
   c. perceived job autonomy
   d. both salary and perceived job autonomy
8. The overall plan developed by the researcher to obtain answers to the questions being studied is called
   a. analysis of the data
   b. operationally defining the variables
   c. problem statement
   d. research design
9. Individuals who participate in a study are referred to as the
   a. data
   b. target population
   c. subjects
   d. probability statistics
10. Representativeness in a sample refers to
    a. how well the sample reflects the characteristics of the population in terms of the variables being studied
    b. the possibility of a particular person from the population being included in the study
    c. the use of random procedures in selecting sample units
    d. the sampling technique employed to obtain subjects from the population
11. The following are all examples of descriptive statistics except
    a. criterion measures
    b. frequencies
    c. means
    d. percentages

12. Developing a research problem from a theory or conceptual framework requires the logical reasoning process of
    a. critical thinking
    b. deduction
    c. induction
    d. conceptualization

13. Which of the following statements best describes the problem statement "to what extent do health policies influence the health of American citizens"?
    a. acceptable as stated
    b. not a research problem because it addresses a moral issue
    c. not acceptable as stated because it lacks an independent variable
    d. not acceptable because of the vagueness of the concepts

14. A primary source for literature review may be defined as
    a. a description of an investigation written by the researcher who conducted the study
    b. a summarization of relevant research that has been conducted on the topic of interest
    c. a thesaurus that directs the reader to a subject heading germane to the topic
    d. any retrieval mechanism that helps to locate articles on the area of interest

15. Sources for literature review include all the following *except*
    a. bibliographies
    b. books
    c. computer searches
    d. personal experience

16. A set of logically interrelated propositions is associated with
    a. statistical model
    b. conceptual framework
    c. theory
    d. schematic model

17. The power of theories lies in their ability to
    a. capture the complexity of human nature by the richness of the operational definitions associated with the variables
    b. minimize the number of words required to explain phenomena and thereby eliminate semantic problems
    c. prove conclusively that relations exist among the phenomena studied
    d. specify the nature of the relations that exist among phenomena

18. The purpose of a theory is to
    a. make scientific findings meaningful and generalizable
    b. explain relations that exist among variables as well as the nature of the relation

    c. stimulate the generation of hypotheses that can be empirically tested

    d. summarize the accumulated facts

19. The building blocks for theory are
    a. concepts
    b. empirical testing
    c. hypothesis
    d. models

20. The major similarity between theories and conceptual frameworks i is that both
    a. use concepts as their building blocks
    b. use the deductive reasoning process almost exclusively
    c. contain a set of logically interrelated propositions
    d. provide a mechanism for developing new propositions from the original propositions

21. A research hypothesis
    a. is a set of logically interrelated propositions
    b. is usually more general in scope than a problem statement
    c. predicts the nature of the relation between two or more variables
    d. predicts the absence of a relation between two or more variables

22. The following are all purposes of the research hypothesis *except*
    a. proving the validity of a theory
    b. extending human knowledge
    c. linking the abstract and conceptual with the concrete and observable
    d. providing direction to the research design

23. A research hypothesis predicts the nature of the relationship between
    a. the functional and causal nature of the variables
    b. a theoretical framework and observable phenomena
    c. a presumed cause and a presumed effect
    d. statistical testing and the assumption of innocence

24. Deductive hypotheses are almost always
    a. testable
    b. researchable
    c. complex
    d. directional

25. The term randomization may be defined as
    a. assignment of subjects to a group in such a way that neither the subject nor the researcher knows who is receiving the treatment
    b. each subject having an equal chance of being selected for any group
    c. the assurance that systematic bias will be present in the selection of subjects into groups
    d. the matching of subjects' attributes that are likely to affect the outcome

26. Which of the following must be present in quasi-experimental research?
    a. a comparison group
    b. manipulating a variable
    c. matching of subjects
    d. randomization

27. The term internal validity refers to
    a. the elimination of competing explanations that could account for any of the observed differences
    b. making an inference that the experimental intervention resulted in any observed differences
    c. the nonequivalence of groups before the treatment
    d. the occurrence of events external to the treatment that could affect the manipulation

28. Which of the following research designs is *weakest* in terms of the researcher's ability to establish causality?
    a. experimental
    b. ex post facto
    c. pre-experimental
    d. quasi-experimental

29. In an ex post facto study, compared to an experimental study, the researcher forfeits control of
    a. the independent variables(s)
    b. the dependent variable
    c. the criterion variable
    d. the attribute variable

30. A study that followed, over a 20-year period, users and nonusers of oral contraceptives to find long-term effects would be called a
    a. prediction study
    b. retrospective study
    c. prospective study
    d. univariate descriptive

31. If a researcher wanted to describe the frequency with which nursing students performed breast self-examination, the study would be classified as
    a. descriptive correlational
    b. prospective
    c. retrospective
    d. univariate descriptive

32. Which of the following types of nonexperimental research would probably require the longest data collection period?
    a. descriptive correlational
    b. prospective
    c. retrospective
    d. univariate descriptive

33. In survey research, the approach that typically yields the highest response rate is
    a. personal interviews
    b. telephone interviews
    c. home-delivered questionnaires
    d. mailed questionnaires
34. One of the advantages of the case study method is the
    a. ease with which the data can be analyzed
    b. facility with which the findings can be generalized
    c. objectivity that can be maintained by the researcher
    d. in-depth nature of the data collected
35. Data collected before the institution of a treatment are sometimes referred to as
    a. posttest data
    b. baseline data
    c. case study data
    d. secondary data
36. How many hypotheses can be tested in a two-factor design?
    a. 1
    b. 2
    c. 3
    d. 4
37. The most effective method of controlling extraneous variables is by
    a. analysis of covariance
    b. matching
    c. randomized control group
    d. repeated measures design
38. Suppose a researcher conducted a study using clients in a rehabilitation facility as subjects. The researcher does the study again. However, for the second study, clients in a general hospital became the subjects. The process refers to the concept of
    a. counterbalancing
    b. precision
    c. variability
    d. replication
39. Research projects that collect data at one point in time are referred to as
    a. cohort studies
    b. cross-sectional studies
    c. cross-sequential studies
    d. panel studies

40. A researcher used hemoglobin levels as an index of the likelihood that a person would develop a pressure sore. Hemoglobin levels are classified as what type of physiological measure?
    a. physical
    b. chemical
    c. microbial
    d. cytological

41. The concept of objectivity for physiological measures refers to the
    a. lack of interactions that generally accompany their use
    b. unobtrusive nature of their presence
    c. precision with which they measure the target concept
    d. agreement of two independent observers of the observed measurement

42. Which of the following topical areas would be most conducive to study by observational methods?
    a. attitude toward preventive health practices
    b. knowledge of the danger signals of cancer
    c. interactions in a psychiatric crisis center
    d. effectiveness of support groups for drug abusers

43. When the researcher uses a self-report technique but specifies neither the questions nor the response alternatives in advance, the interview is referred to as
    a. standardized
    b. structured
    c. unstructured
    d. face-to-face

44. A data collection technique that quantifies a person's attitude along a bipolar dimension is called a
    a. cafeteria checklist
    b. checklist
    c. graphic rating scale
    d. rank-order question

45. A major purpose of a pre-test is to
    a. detect inadequacies in an interview/schedule/questionnaire
    b. obtain some preliminary results on the research problem
    c. assess the adequacy of the research design
    d. evaluate whether a structured or unstructured schedule is preferable

46. On a 7-point Likert scale, the response "undecided" would be scored as
    a. 0
    b. 1
    c. 4
    d. 7

47. On a 20-item Likert scale with five response categories, the range of possible scores is
    a. 0 to 100
    b. 20 to 80
    c. 20 to 100
    d. 0 to 50
48. Which of the following scaling procedures is an example of a cumulative scale?
    a. Thurstone scale
    b. Likert scale
    c. Guttman scale
    d. Semantic differential scale
49. Which of the following techniques *cannot* be administered by mail?
    a. critical incidents technique
    b. Delphi technique
    c. sentence completion process
    d. psychodrama
50. Suppose a researcher wants to forecast future priorities for research in obstetrical nursing. The participants will be nurse midwives. Which of the following techniques would most probably be employed?
    a. content analysis
    b. projective technique
    c. Delphi procedure
    d. Thematic Apperception Test
51. The technique that is least susceptible to response set bias is
    a. interviews
    b. Delphi procedure
    c. questionnaires
    d. projective measures
52. A bias that may be present in the use of records is known as
    a. acquiescence bias
    b. extreme response bias
    c. selective deposit bias
    d. social desirability bias
53. Another term for universe is
    a. sample
    b. population
    c. true scores
    d. set of rules
54. The level of measurement that classifies and ranks objects in terms of the degree to which they possess an attribute of interest is
    a. nominal
    b. ordinal
    c. interval
    d. ratio

55. Religion is measured on the
    a. nominal scale
    b. ordinal scale
    c. interval scale
    d. ratio scale
56. The most primitive and least precise level of measurement is
    a. nominal scale
    b. ordinal scale
    c. interval scale
    d. ratio scale
57. Keeping a record of fluid intake, in ounces, of a postsurgical
    patient is an example of which level of measurement?
    a. nominal scale
    b. ordinal scale
    c. interval scale
    d. ratio scale
58. Which level of measurement permits the researcher to add,
    subtract, multiply, and divide?
    a. nominal scale
    b. ordinal scale
    c. interval scale
    d. ratio scale
59. The difference between a true score and an obtained score is
    referred to as
    a. internal consistency
    b. discriminability
    c. response sampling
    d. error of measurement
60. One source of measurement error is
    a. response set bias
    b. inefficiency
    c. speed
    d. absence of validity
61. The Spearman-Brown prophecy formula is applied after using
    a. K-R 20
    b. split-half technique
    c. Cronbach's alpha
    d. multitrait-multimethod matrix
62. Cronbach's alpha is used to determine which of the following
    instrument attributes
    a. internal consistency
    b. stability
    c. criterion validity
    d. construct validity

63. The aspect of reliability for which interobserver reliability is appropriate is
    a. stability
    b. internal consistency
    c. equivalence
    d. criterion related

64. If a Cronbach's alpha was computed to be .80, the coefficient would respresent
    a. the true variability in scores
    b. the observed variability in scores
    c. the variability associated with random error
    d. the proportion of true to obtained variability

65. A perfect correlation between two variables would be represented by a coefficient of
    a. 0.00
    b. −1.00
    c. 2.00
    d. 100.00

66. The type of validity that employs only logical rather than empirical procedures in its assessment is
    a. content
    b. concurrent
    c. predictive
    d. construct

67. Suppose a researcher were interested in assessing the adequacy of an instrument to measure the theoretical conceptualization of territorial space. The type of validation procedure would most probably be
    a. content
    b. concurrent
    c. predictive
    d. construct

68. Which of the following terms does not belong with the other three?
    a. content validity
    b. criterion-related validity
    c. predictive validity
    d. concurrent validity

69. Sampling may be defined as the
    a. set of elements used for selecting the sample
    b. process of selecting a subset of the population to represent the entire population
    c. aggregation of subjects who meet a designated set of criteria for inclusion in the study
    d. technique used to ensure that every element in the population has an equal chance of being included in the study

70. Bias in sampling refers to
    a. systematic overrepresentation or underrepresentation of some segment of the population on the attribute of interest
    b. lack of heterogeneity in the population on the attribute of interest
    c. sample selection in nonprobability-type sampling designs
    d. the margin of error in the data obtained from samples
71. Strata are incorporated into the design of which of the following types of samples?
    a. systematic
    b. purposive
    c. quota
    d. simple random
72. The type of sampling design that is most likely to obtain a representative sample is
    a. stratified random
    b. snowball
    c. purposive
    d. quota
73. Which of the following types of samples is considered to be the weakest in sampling design?
    a. accidental
    b. quota
    c. purposive
    d. systematic
74. Suppose a nurse researcher subdivided a list of nurses obtained from the board of registration in nursing according to type of nursing position held and then randomly selected 50 nurses from each position listed. The type would be
    a. stratified random
    b. cluster
    c. systematic
    d. simple random
75. If the bulk of scores from a test occurred at the upper end of the distribution, the distribution would be described as
    a. normal
    b. bimodal
    c. positively skewed
    d. negatively skewed
76. A parameter is a characteristic of
    a. a population
    b. reliability
    c. a sample
    d. validity

77. The standard deviation is an index of
   a. bivariate relationships
   b. central tendency
   c. skewness
   d. variability
78. The measure of variability that takes into account the actual score values is the
   a. mean
   b. median
   c. range
   d. standard deviation
79. The degree of relationship between two variables is best expressed by a
   a. correlation coefficient
   b. mean
   c. standard deviation
   d. univariate statistic
80. The most appropriate measure of central tendency to use with the variable "pulse rate" is the
   a. mode
   b. median
   c. mean
   d. correlation coefficient
81. Which of the following is an example of a bivariate descriptive statistic?
   a. frequency distribution
   b. mean
   c. semiquartile range
   d. correlation coefficient
82. One of the characteristics of a normal distribution is that
   a. it is bimodal
   b. 68% of the values are within two standard deviations from the mean
   c. semiquartile range
   d. correlation coefficient
83. The symbol X represents
   a. the sum of
   b. the mean
   c. the number of cases
   d. an individual score
84. The symbol (represents
   a. the sum of
   b. the mean
   c. the number of cases
   d. an individual score

85. The use of inferential statistics permits the researcher to
    a. generalize to a population based on information gathered from a sample
    b. describe information obtained from empirical observation
    c. interpret descriptive statistics
    d. none of the above
86. The standard deviation of a sampling distribution is called a
    a. sampling error
    b. standard error
    c. variance parameter
    d. parameter
87. A major factor that affects the standard error of the mean is
    a. point estimation
    b. confidence limits
    c. sample size
    d. value of the mean
88. For which of the following levels of significance is the risk of making a Type I error greater?
    a. 0.10
    b. 0.05
    c. 0.01
    d. 0.001
89. A 95% confidence level is associated with how many standard deviation units?
    a. 1.96
    b. 2.36
    c. 2.58
    d. depends on sample size
90. If a researcher calculates a t-statistic to be -2.2 and the tabled t-value (for $df = 60$ and level of significance of .05) is 2.0, the researcher would
    a. conclude that an error in calculation had been made
    b. accept the null hypothesis
    c. reject the null hypothesis
    d. use a different level of significance
91. A statistical procedure that is used to determine whether a significant difference exists between any number of group means is the
    a. t-test
    b. analysis of variance
    c. correlation coefficient
    d. Mann-Whitney U-test

92. How many null hypotheses would there be for a study with 40 subjects using a two-way ANOVA?
    a. 2
    b. 3
    c. 5
    d. 10
93. If a researcher wanted to determine whether observed proportions differ significantly from expected proportions, the statistic would be a(n)
    a. *t*-test
    b. correlation coefficient
    c. analysis of variance
    d. chi-square
94. When both the independent and dependent variables are measured on a ratio scale, the appropriate test statistic is a(n)
    a. *t*-test
    b. ANOVA
    c. chi-square
    d. Pearson's *r*
95. Suppose a researcher hypothesized that a relationship existed between nurses' leadership behavior and job satisfaction. Correlational analysis revealed an *r* = .60 that had a *p* value beyond the .001 level. The researcher may conclude all of the following *except:*
    a. the greater the leadership behavior of the nurse, the higher the degree of job satisfaction
    b. the data analysis demonstrated that the research hypothesis was correct
    c. a statistically significant relationship exists between nurses' leadership and job satisfaction
    d. high levels of leadership behavior caused high job satisfaction
96. The answer to whether the researcher went "beyond the data" in a study would be found in which section of the research report?
    a. introduction
    b. methods
    c. results
    d. discussion
97. The medium through which the findings of research would be communicated to the broadest audience is the
    a. dissertation
    b. journal article
    c. results
    d. discussion

98. The person who critiques a published research report should strive to
    a. consider that all flaws have equivalent value
    b. focus only on the inadequacies inherent in the study
    c. judge the merits of the study based on the researcher's background
    d. remain as objective as possible

99. All of the following aspects of a study would be evaluated in the methods section *except*
    a. underlying assumptions
    b. subject selection
    c. description of instruments
    d. rationale for research design

100. "Does the research control for threats to the internal and external validity of the study?" would be asked in which section of a research report?
    a. introduction
    b. methods
    c. results
    d. discussion

101. Which of the following journals would most likely contain the highest number of primary sources for a research literature review?
    a. *American Journal of Nursing*
    b. *Nursing '82*
    c. *Nursing Outlook*
    d. *Nursing Research*

102. In a dissertation or technical report, a copy of the data collection instrument would be included in which of the following sections?
    a. introduction
    b. methods section
    c. appendix
    d. bibliography

Note. All items in Part I of this instrument are from *Instructor's manual for nursing research: Principles and methods* (2nd ed.) (pp. 1–150), by D. Polit and B. Hungler, 1983, Philadelphia: J. B. Lippincott. Reprinted with permission. All abstracts and items in Part II were developed by C. Stetler and A. Sheridan.

Part II

*Abstract 1***
The Effect of Relaxation Training on Postoperative Pain and Vomiting

Relaxation training has been theorized to decrease abdominal tension (a cause of postoperation pain) as well as to reduce anxiety (a correlate of postoperative vomiting). A two-group, post-test only design, with random assignment, was used to determine if postoperative pain and vomiting differ in adult cholecystectomy patients in two treatment conditions.

All cholecystectomy patients in a small community hospital operated on in July and who agreed to participate were included. Data were collected on pain, through the use of a self-report scale, and on vomiting. Information regarding the latter was retrieved from the patient's chart and measured in terms of quantity of vomitus. Seven patients received relaxation training and seven other patients received the unit's standard preoperative teaching, which did not include relaxation.

The mean scores were analyzed through analysis of variance. Results indicated statistically significant, positive effects ($p = .01$) for pain but not for vomiting.

103. The independent variable in this study was
    a. pain
    b. vomiting
    c. relaxation training
    d. standard pre-operative teaching
104. The type of research design utilized was
    a. nonexperimental
    b. pre-experimental
    c. experimental
    d. ex post facto
105. The type of sample selected was
    a. probability
    b. nonprobability
    c. stratified
    d. randomized
106. The use of random assignment increased the study's
    a. generalizability
    b. internal validity
    c. variance
    d. reliability

**Fictitious study.

107. The operational definition of vomiting can be considered weak
     due to a question of
     a. intervening variables
     b. true definition of vomiting
     c. reliability of charts
     d. reliability of vomitus
108. Analysis of variance enables the researcher to
     a. randomize to a complete population
     b. describe characteristics of subjects
     c. draw inferences for a hypothetical population
     d. randomize for a hypothetical population
109. The results of this study should be generalized to
     a. all postoperative patients
     b. all cholecystectomy patients
     c. all patients with relaxation training
     d. no other group of patients

Abstract 2**
Bereavement Crisis Intervention for Mothers Upon the Loss of a Child

It has been suggested that grief or bereavement is an acute stage of anxiety caused by the precipitating factor of the death of a person with whom one is emotionally involved.

This grief in turn causes specific behavior and feelings in affected individuals. These reactions can be lessened by the presence of a strong support system or exacerbated by the presence of psychiatric illness.

In order to test a nursing intervention designed to facilitate coping, the following hypothesis was tested: There is no difference in the change of self-report of depression by mothers who received crisis intervention and mothers who received no such treatment.

Fifty mothers whose children died in a large teaching center in the midwest were enrolled in the study. The first 25 mothers whose children died after the study was initiated were placed in the treatment group; the second 25 were merely interviewed to obtain the needed data.

An Adjective Scale for Depression (ASD) was used at two points in time. With the ASD, subjects were asked to indicate their current level of depression on a series of 5-point scales. Split-half reliability coefficients for this tool are .35 for males and .29 for females.

The crisis treatment consisted of a series of support group sessions conducted by a psychiatric nurse clinician according to a standardized pro-

---

**Fictitious study.

tocol. In addition, individual follow-up sessions were held with each mother, again according to a recommended protocol.

A *t*-test was used to analyze the difference in change scores between the two groups. The results indicated no significant differences but there was a trend (p = .08) in the expected direction. No significant differences were found between the two groups for age, education, or marital status. However, past psychiatric illness was found to be significantly related to the level of depression across the total sample.

110. The variables of depression and crisis intervention can be considered which of the following?
    a. a model of bereavement intervention
    b. an example of critical thinking
    c. concepts relevant to a theory of bereavement
    d. a framework for probability testing
111. Of potential concern to a reviewer of this study would be which of the following?
    a. relevance of the bereavement theory to patient care
    b. consent process used to obtain subjects
    c. qualifications of the bereavement group leader
    d. focus of the study on death of children
112. What type of hypothesis was used?
    a. null
    b. research
    c. alternative
    d. retrospective
113. Past psychiatric illness was measured as a means of
    a. testing the stated hypothesis
    b. manipulating the independent variable
    c. providing a control group
    d. controlling an intervening variable
114. The reliability coefficient of .29 indicates
    a. an acceptable level of consistency for the tool
    b. an unacceptable level of consistency for the tool
    c. an acceptable level of relevancy for the tool
    d. an unacceptable level of relevance for the tool
115. The statement that "there was a trend (p = .08) in the expected direction" should be interpreted as indicating
    a. that crisis intervention most probably does decrease depression
    b. that crisis intervention most probably does not decrease depression
    c. that the researcher has accepted the results of inferential testing
    d. that the researcher has not accepted the results of inferential testing

116. A standardized protocol was utilized by the psychiatric nurse
     clinician in order to control for
     a. the precise definition of the independent variable
     b. randomization
     c. the subject's extraneous characteristics
     d. the subject's relevant characteristics
117. An alternative method of measuring depression that would control
     for a socially desirable response would be
     a. a checklist for subjects with only yes/no response alternatives
     b. use of a galvanic skin response
     c. observation and rating of subject behavior by a nonparticipant
        observer
     d. observation and rating of subjects by a fellow subject
118. This is an example of what type of research design?
     a. experimental
     b. quasi-experimental
     c. ex post facto
     d. descriptive correlational
119. What level of measurement is the Adjective Depression Scale?
     a. nominal
     b. at least ordinal
     c. at least ratio
     d. Guttman

Abstract 3**
The Relationship of a Social Support Network to the Perception of Health Status

A researcher hypothesized that clients with a strong support network would
describe themselves as being healthier than clients with a weak support
network. To test this hypothesis, the first 100 residents of a housing complex for the elderly, who were attendees at a mobile health clinic held
each week, were asked to rate themselves on a 7-point scale regarding
their current health physical health status (1 = very poor health and 7 =
excellent health) and their system of support. (A 10-item Likert-like scale
was used to measure the quality of individual support networks.)

The self-ratings of descriptions of physical health were normally distributed for the sample as a whole: 3% excellent, 14% very good, 23%
good, 21% neither good nor poor, 14% very poor, and 4% extremely poor.
These were then classified into three categories: 17 (17%) of these clients

_____

**Fictitious study.

were classified as having a high level of health, 44 (44%) with a moderate level, and 39 (39%) with a low level of health. When the data were reviewed, it was also found that the clients ranged in age from 65 to 75 years; there were 45 females and 55 males.

The groups were compared according to health ratings and support systems. The means and standard deviations are as follows:

Level of Support

Health Status	Mean	Standard Deviation
Low	7.1	7.4
Moderate	11.9	4.5
High	23.3	3.2

In this sample, a Pearson r was used to describe the relationship of the ratings on health status and intensity of support network: $r = .76$, $p < .05$.

120. The type of sample selected for this study is referred to as
    a. stratified sample
    b. random sample
    c. convenience sample
    d. cluster sample
121. The Pearson r of .76 is best interpreted as
    a. a measure of the differences between the responses of men and women
    b. a significant relationship between the intensity of support net work and health status rating
    c. a relatively weak relationship between a self-report of health status and assessment of support network
    d. an indication that the hypothesis is poorly supported by the data collected
122. The study is best described as
    a. descriptive-correlational
    b. ex post facto
    c. quasi-experimental
    d. experimental
123. In which category of level of health status was the highest degree of variability in the scores on social support found?
    a. high
    b. medium
    c. low
    d. not reported

124. What type of instrument is the health status measurement?
     a. structured interview schedule
     b. summated rating scale
     c. graphic rating scale
     d. critical incident
125. The hypothesis in this study is best described as
     a. statistical hypothesis
     b. directional hypothesis
     c. null hypothesis
     d. not a hypothesis as stated
126. If this study were to be read and considered for inclusion in a review of literature, which of the following is most appropriate?
     a. State: "It was found that clients with strong support networks are healthier than their counterparts with weak support networks."
     b. State: "This study found a positive relationship between the health status of elderly clients and support networks."
     c. State: "A difference was observed between men and women in their reports of health status and support networks."
     d. The findings are so inconclusive that the study should not be included in the review.

32

A Program Evaluation Model for Continuing Education Programs

Angeline M. Jacobs, DeAnn M. Young,
and Felicitas A. dela Cruz

PURPOSE

This chapter describes the development of a Program Evaluation Model, designed to assess outcomes of continuing education programs in nursing. The model was applied to two certified continuing education offerings: a hospice nursing program (240 hours); and an end-stage renal disease program, with emphasis on hemodialysis (200 hours).

DESCRIPTION OF THE MODEL

The emphasis on continuing education as a major vehicle for ensuring the development and maintenance of competent practitioners has resulted in increased emphasis on the need for models for assessing the outcomes of continuing education (Dickerson, 2000; Hawkins & Sherwood, 1999).

Development of an evaluation model that could be shared within the nursing community was a primary focus of two continuing education programs (Jacobs, Young, & dela Cruz, 1990). The model that evolved, illustrated in Figure 32.1, has both formative and summative aspects; it is built on a model developed by Jacobs and Larsen (1976) at the American Institutes for Research.

The relationship of process and outcome to ultimate program impact is found in the model. The components are described as follows:

- *Program input* includes curriculum objectives, behaviorally stated terminal objectives, and overall project objectives; the student's demographic and experiential characteristics; and the curriculum itself.

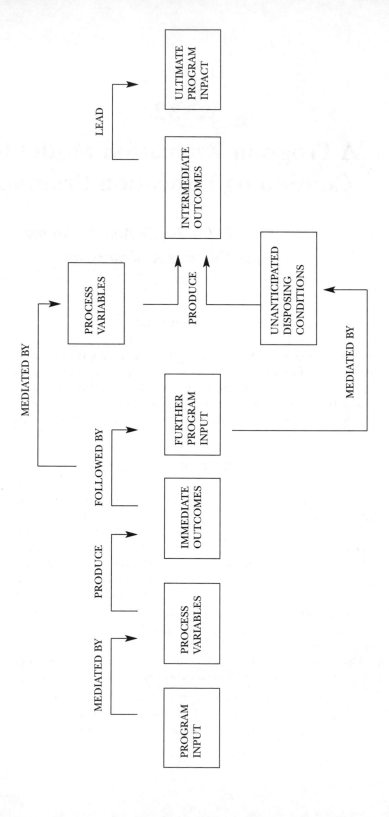

FIGURE 32.1 Program evaluation model.

- *Process variables* are the activities planned to bring about the curriculum and program objectives, such as recruiting, selection of students, selection of faculty, and instructional strategies.
- *Immediate outcomes* occur as the activities of the program are implemented. For example, course A is completed by n students, n dropped out, and n students expressed satisfaction or dissatisfaction with the course.
- *Further program input* refers to interventions that are applied as a result of process assessment. For example, in the hospice program, rap sessions were instituted for the first group of students, who were experiencing stress because of the workload, especially the clinical experiences. As a result of the feedback from the first group (who experienced high attrition), the clinical practicum for subsequent groups of students was modified, and retention of students was improved.
- *Unanticipated disposing or intervening variables* are those events that influence program outcome either positively or negatively. Examples are unanticipated absences of project staff because of illness or unexpected changes in faculty. These events are recorded on process evaluation instruments and are incorporated into the data analysis.
- *Intermediate outcomes* are those that occur relatively close in time and can be measured within the scope of the project; for example, total number of graduates and dropouts, application of learning in employment situations, "ripple effect" on other staff in employing agencies, and benefits or detriments to the graduates.
- *Ultimate program impact* includes those outcomes that are more global and later maturing; for example, improvement in patient care, and long-term collaborative relationships or other resultant programs. Some of these occur and can be measured within a project's time frame, but most require a longer maturation time.

The model is decision oriented, with data collected while the program is in progress; this allows for decision making about program modification as well as program replication. The model is based on a program rationale that makes explicit the dynamics of cause-and-effect relationships. This makes it possible to identify individual program components needing modification. The model emphasizes *impact-referenced* indicators of accomplishment, meaning that benefits of a program should be observable and offer strong evidence of meaningful improvement.

APPLICATION OF THE MODEL

The model described above was applied to two continuing education programs, each consisting of multiple courses and composed of both didactic and clinical experiences. During the formative evaluation phase, activities included:

- A milestone and task audit conducted monthly at the beginning of each project and quarterly toward the end of the project periods.
- Review of teaching strategies for acceptability by students and effectiveness of instruction.
- Collection of anonymous critical-incident reports of unanticipated events from students, faculty, clinical facility personnel, and project staff.
- Assessment of student progress in each of the courses of the curriculum and comparison of student grades among cohorts of students in each program.
- End-of-course evaluations by students for each course.
- End-of-course evaluations by faculty for each course.
- End-of-course evaluations by the students at the time of their graduation.
- End-of-course evaluations at the end of the project by faculty and participating clinical agencies.

Summative evaluation was conducted using a quasi-experimental design (Isaac & Michael, 1995) with follow-up 6 months after graduation from the program. The control group consisted partly of students who withdrew from the program. These students had the same three data collection points as students in the program (pre, intermediate, and 6-month follow-up). The control group also included applicants who were not accepted. Their data set was not complete. Six months after graduation from the program, graduates, drop-outs, and those not accepted were interviewed, as well as personnel from agencies employing graduates. Variables considered in the postgraduation data collection included: postprogram employment in the field studied, job promotions, salary increases, job satisfaction, extent of implementation of learning, retrospective assessment of satisfaction with the program, professional and personal benefits (or detriments) resulting, supervisor ratings, and agency characteristics that might mediate outcome.

Several instruments were developed for use in pre- and post-testing within the evaluation model. Common approaches to instrument development included input from content experts, formating for computer entry, pilot testing on 20 to 30 respondents (nonprogram participants), revision of the first version based on results from piloting, administration of the revised version on 5 to 10 respondents, and estimation of reliability and validity.

Knowledge tests were developed for each program, with the hospice program version consisting of 120 items and the hemodialysis version having 100 items. Estimates of internal consistency were .90 and .72, respectively.

Attitudes were measured by a 100-item measure in the hospice program. The response format was a 6-point, Likert-type scale used to indicate extent of agreement with item statements. The reliability coefficient was .97. In the hemodialysis program, two measures of attitude were used. One contained 78 items and had an alpha value of .91; the other was a behavioral intentions scale that had an alpha value of .78.

Performance ratings were included in the evaluation model. For the hospice program, 14 competencies were measured, including pain management, symptom management, making referrals, providing nutrition, patient/family support, and providing bereavement support. In the performance assessment for the nephrology program, 69 competencies were addressed in 14 categories, including administering hemodialysis, administering peritoneal dialysis, patient teaching, performing physical assessment, interviewing and counseling patient/family, providing emotional and spiritual support, providing crisis intervention, making referrals, applying research, and documenting patient care. A sample of items from this measure is found in Figure 32.2. Interrater reliability on these two performance measures ranged from $r = .80$ to .90.

A videotaped test was used for pre- and post-assessment in the hospice program. Using a standardized script, a two-track cueing system allowed for different tracks to be used for appropriate and inappropriate student responses. A segment of the script is found in Figure 32.3.

FIGURE 32.2 Sample items from performance assessment, end-stage renal disease.

	Circle the number that best fits your opinion of the individual's competence					
	5	4	3	2	1	0
	Out-Standing		Competent		Not Competent	Not Observed
A. Administer hemodialysis						
1. Prepares equipment, materials, and dialysis baths	5	4	3	2	1	0
2. Computes trans-membrane pressure	5	4	3	2	1	0

FIGURE 32.3 Excerpt from patient interviewing test: script and observation checklist.

> I've lost so much weight.
> I looked at myself in a picture the
> other day and now . . .
> Shake head, quiet, sad expression

Observation IX:

_____Neutral Response

Observation IX: Positive Response	Observation IX: Negative Response
____ 7. Reinforces verbalization through words or sounds.	Makes statement 14 ____ that avoids feelings.
AND	OR
	Asks question that elicits yes/no. 15 ____
____ 8. Uses silence with position of attending.	OR
	Extinguishes 16 ____ verbalization through absence
OR	or reinforcement.
____ 9. Reaches out to touch.	AND
	Uses silence without 17 ____ attending.
OR	OR
____ 12. Leans toward person.	Turns body away or 21 ____ folds arms.

An actor portrayed the patient as indicated in the box in Figure 32.3. The student's response was videotaped and later was scored independently by two mental health nursing instructors. A segment of the scoring criteria used by the two raters is shown in Figure 32.4.

Interrater reliability calculated from the two independent ratings was .61.

An inventory of 11 skills was used in the hospice program. The skills were pain management, cardiopulmonary assessment, gastrointestinal assessment, urinary catheter insertion, ostomy care, wound care, IV therapy, parental feedings, tracheostomy care, symptom assessment, and family assessment. Students and their supervisors rated students' level of competency on a 3-point scale (1 = I have done this activity and I feel competent, to 3 = I have not done this activity). The percentage agreement

FIGURE 32.4 Excerpt from videotaped patient interviewing test: scoring criteria.

Positive	Score	Negative	Score
Verbal			
1. Paraphrases accurately with question	____	13. Paraphrases inaccurately or without a question	____
Nonverbal			
12. Leans toward person	____	21. Turns body away from person or folds arms	____

between students and supervisor ratings was .80. In the nephrology program, a performance test containing 10 behaviors was used. This instrument was also used as a challenge examination for the program.

Results from application of the evaluation of the model in these two continuing education programs were favorable (Jacobs, dela Cruz, & Young, 1986; Young & Jacobs, 1984). This evaluation model is adaptable to other types of nursing education. The general methodology and evaluation tools are easily modified for programs in many content areas.

REFERENCES

Dickerson, P. S. (2000). A CQI approach to evaluating continuing education: process and outcomes. *Journal of Nursing Staff Development, 16*(1), 34–40.

Hawkins, V. E., & Sherwood, G. D. (1999). The pyramid model: An integrated approach for evaluating continuing education programs and outcomes. *Journal of Continuing Education in Nursing, 30*(5), 203–212.

Isaac, S., & Michael, W. B. (1995). *Handbook in Research and Evaluation (3rd ed.). San Diego, CA: EdITS.*

Jacobs, A. M., dela Cruz, F. A., & Young, D. (1986). Model curriculum for continuing education in nephrology nursing: Final report. *Los Angeles: California State University.*

Jacobs, A. M., & Larsen, J. K. (1976). Evaluation of WICHE's regional program for research development. *Palo Alto, CA: American Institutes for Research.*

Jacobs, A. M., Young, D. M., & dela Cruz, F. A. (1990). *Evaluating prototype continuing education programs. In C. F. Waltz & O. L. Strickland (Eds.),* Measurement of nursing outcomes: Vol. 3. Measuring clinical skills and professional development in education and practice *(pp. 349–363). New York: Springer Publishing Company.*

Young, D., & Jacobs, A. M. (1984). Model curriculum for continuing education in hospice nursing: Final report. *Los Angeles: California State University.*

33

Opinionnaire:
Computing in Nursing

Barbara S. Thomas

PURPOSE

This chapter describes the **Opinionnaire: Computing in Nursing,** which is used to measure attitudes of nurses and nursing students toward the use of computers in nursing.

INSTRUMENT DESCRIPTION

Despite the ever-increasing use of computers in everyday life, student nurses may have surprisingly little awareness of the use of computers in hospitals (Abbott, 1993). There continues to be a need for assessing and teaching computer skills (Graveley, Lust, & Fullerton, 1999). Considering favorable attitudes as antecedent to developing and using skills (Fishbein & Ajzen, 1975), there is an ongoing need to measure attitudes toward computers in nursing students and nurses.

Identifying beliefs and feelings of nurses and nursing student respondents about computing as well as quantifying willingness to develop and use computer skills were the objectives that guided the process of instrument development. Two forms of the Q-CN were developed (Thomas, 1990). Attitudes were conceptualized as "a learned predisposition to respond in a consistently favorable or unfavorable manner with respect to a given object" (Fishbein & Ajzen, 1975, p. 6).

A matrix of topic areas by beliefs was developed. The topic areas were drawn from a review of all indexed material related to computing in nursing in Medline or ERIC from 1984 through 1987; five categories, plus an unspecified class were produced using content analysis. Beliefs were identified from comments of nurses ($n = 34$) and nursing students ($n = 36$) regarding computing in nursing. Again, content analysis was used.

This matrix was refined with five columns of topics: general or unspecified, research, administration, practice, and education. The six rows identified were effectiveness (increase or decrease accuracy, time, or effort), comprehensible/incomprehensible, flexible/inflexible, dependable/undependable, positive or negative affect (e.g., pleasant/unpleasant or comfortable/uncomfortable, and appropriate/inappropriate. Six experts confirmed that cells were unique and appropriately labeled and that nothing had been omitted.

A pool of 80 items was developed from this matrix drawing on suggestions from reviewers, the literature, and comments of nurses and nursing students. Experts were asked to place each item in its respective category (rows and columns named above). The extent of agreement was 99%; all items were retained. Each item was also rated on a 4-point rating scale as good (3) to impossible (0) on parameters of relevance, clarity, accuracy, and simplicity. All but three items were rated good or fair; thus, 77 items were retained. Two remaining items were revised and another replaced. The total number of items was 80. Form I was comprised of the first 40 items and Form II of the last 40 items.

The Q-CN is a paper-and-pencil, self-administered measure. The two forms each contain randomly ordered, positively and negatively worded items.

The response format is a 5-point, Likert-type scale with 1 = strongly disagree and 5 – strongly agree. Reverse scored items are the opposite of this with 5 = strongly disagree and 1 = strongly agree. Item scores are summed to produce a total score. For each form of the instrument, the possible range of scores is stated as 30 to 150. For handling of missing item scores, the z score for the unadjusted scale score for that person after transforming that z score with the unadjusted item mean and standard deviation should be substituted. In pilot testing, scannable forms were used for responses. A copy of the Q-CN is included at the end of the chapter.

RELIABILITY AND VALIDITY ASSESSMENT

Internal consistency reliability was estimated at .90 and .89 in a pilot test of the two forms, using 109 graduate and undergraduate nursing students at a university in the midwestern United States. Because of the interest in estimating whether the two forms of the instrument were parallel, scores were carefully examined. For the first form, the mean score was 139.52 (*SD* 15.97); for the second form it was 135.67 (*SD* 14.88). Item correlations were positive or negative as expected, depending upon whether the item was positively or negatively worded. Items with correlations equal to or greater than .35 were eliminated from the instrument. A total of 20 items were eliminated (10 from each form), leaving 30 items on each form. To further enhance the similarity of the scores obtained on the two forms, some switching of items was done to make the mean and standard deviations closer. Eleven pairs of items were exchanged across forms. The re-scored forms of the instrument had means of 105.50 (*SD* 13.77) and 105.25 (*SD* 14.03). On this basis, and a correlation of .86 between scores on the two revised forms, sufficient evidence was obtained to claim the two forms as parallel. The estimates of internal consistency on the two revised two forms were .91 and .92.

Test-retest reliability was estimated from scores of 24 students who took both of the original forms of the instrument 2 weeks apart. The resulting correlation coefficient was .88.

Evidence for face and content validity was claimed from statements from nurses and nursing students about computing, the grounding of items in the literature, and the expert panel review used in the process of instrument development. Evidence for concurrent criterion validity was gathered. Respondents in the pilot test who answered "daily" or "some-time during every week" ($n = 15$) to a demographic question on how frequently they used computers, scored significantly ($p = .015$) higher than the 76 respondents who replied "less than monthly" or "not at all."

Results of the reliability and validity testing suggest that there is sufficient evidence to support continued use of the instrument. It is recommended that it be administered and tested with larger samples more representative of nursing students and nurses.

REFERENCES

Abbott, K. (1993). Student nurses' conceptions of computer use in hospitals. *Computers in Nursing, 11*(2), 78–89.

Fishbein, M., & Ajzen, I. (1975). *Belief, attitude, intention, and behavior.* Reading, MA: Addison-Wesley.

Graveley, E. A., Lust, B. L., & Fullerton, J. T. (1999). Untergraduate computer literacy: Evaluation and intervention. *Computers in Nursing, 17*(4), 166–170.

Thomas, B. S. (1990). Attitudes toward computing in nursing. In C. F. Waltz & O. L. Strickland (Eds.), *Measurement of nursing outcomes: Vol. 3. Measuring clinical skills and professional development in education and practice* (pp. 192–202). New York: Springer Publishing Company.

Opinionnaire: Computing in Nursing

Form A

This measure consists of 30 items to be answered using the scale below. There are no right or wrong answers. Please be candid and report your true reaction to each item.

    A or 1 = Strongly Disagree
    B or 2 = Disagree
    C or 3 = Neither Disagree nor Agree (neutral)
    D or 4 = Agree
    E or 5 = Strongly Agree

1. Nurses should stick to patient care and leave computing to computer scientists.
2. Computers malfunction easily.
3. Computers can be programmed to do many nursing tasks.
4. When nurses I know discuss the effectiveness of computers, I feel out of place.
5. Upon completion of my nursing program I (did) plan to use computing to study nursing care problems.
6. Using computers is boring.
7. Computers can be programmed to do only one kind of task, limiting their usefulness.
8. Statistical programs for computers are very difficult to understand.
9. Nurses can use their own time more efficiently by using computers for data analysis problems they have.
10. Computer-assisted instruction (CAI) programs should be developed for simulations of complex nursing decisions, such as those during a patient's cardiac arrest.
11. Computer literacy should be a part of all nursing education programs.
12. Barring human error, I can depend on statistical analyses from package programs like SAS, BMDP, or SPSSX to be correct.
13. Computers make nursing tasks more interesting.
14. I like the flexibility of computers.
15. One cannot use computers without a good background in computer science.
16. Since research often depends on quantifying results by using sophisticated mathematical techniques, computers can save time.
17. Computer-based staffing is the best approach for the hospital's director of nursing.
18. For nursing research, I will not use computer-based statistical packages.

19. I feel threatened by nursing's move toward more use of computers.
20. Computer printouts of staffing and other personnel matters could save nursing service administrators a lot of time.
21. It's not worth the effort for a nursing student who types to learn word processing.
22. Confidentiality is nearly impossible if computers are used for patient records.
23. The use of computers improves patient care by giving the nurse more time with the patients.
24. Learning about computers must be the worst part of nursing education today.
25. I expect to expand my knowledge about computers.
26. Nursing service directors and their staffs can and should be active in the design of hospital information systems.
27. Computers make nursing tasks more fun.
28. It takes as much effort to maintain patient records by computer as it does by hand.
29. Nurses should use computers for programs of care.
30. Entry and retrieval of patient records in a computerized hospital information system takes much more time than traditional charting and maintenance of files.

Form B

This measure consists of 30 items to be answered on the scale below. There are no right or wrong answers. Please be candid and report your true reaction to each item.

    A or 1 = Strongly Disagree
    B or 2 = Disagree
    C or 3 = Neither Disagree nor Agree (neutral)
    D or 4 = Agree
    E or 5 = Strongly Agree

1. Use of the computer would save me time in my research.
2. Statistical computer programs can perform analyses that would require too much effort without computers.
3. Staffing in a large hospital via computers is much easier than non-computer approaches.
4. If I had a choice, I wouldn't learn more about computers.
5. A single computer program can provide nurse scientists with both descriptive and inferential statistics.
6. Computer systems can be adapted to assist nurses in many aspects of care.

7. The most sensible use for computers in hospitals is for billing and staffing rather than more complex administrative tasks.
8. Maintenance of nurses' continuing education credits by computer has been a real time saver.
9. Most CAI programs are so difficult to use that they result in frustration rather than learning.
10. CAI can take many forms—drill and practice, tutorials, simulations, and even games.
11. There is little job satisfaction in nursing management using computer-based information systems.
12. Scheduling courses by computer for nursing students produces more dependable, accessible information.
13. Most computer skills have no application to nursing.
14. Computers are down so often that they're not there when you need them the most.
15. I am comfortable using computers.
16. Generally, computers are inflexible.
17. I would like to use the computer more to save time in my work.
18. I feel that computers create more problems than they solve in nursing practice.
19. I'm afraid to depend on computer output where patient records are concerned.
20. Micrcomputers have too little power and storage to do anything except the most simple tasks.
21. Acronyms for computer terms like JCL or SPSSX make computing very hard to understand.
22. Computers can be very time consuming to work with.
23. I dislike the inflexibility of computers.
24. Reliance on computerized patient records is likely to cause serious problems.
25. I feel pleased by nursing's move toward computers.
26. The use of word processing instead of typing is exhausting.
27. Statistical programs provide accurate analyses with all the tests displayed and summarized.
28. The use of computers dehumanizes patient care.
29. Confidentiality of patient records must be sacrificed if they are to be computerized.
30. Patients must hate receiving computer-generated clinic appointment information.

34

Software Evaluation Tool

Sandra Millon Underwood

PURPOSE

The purpose of the **Software Evaluation Tool for Nursing** (SET-N) is to assess computer-based instructional programs for nursing education. In addition, the SET-N allows for evaluation of the cognitive skills employed by the learner using the simulation (Underwood, 1988).

INSTRUMENT DESCRIPTION

Computer-based instructional programs are widely used. They range broadly in purpose to include such as activities as: (a) clinical simulation (Bauer, 1998); (b) computerized test development (Kirkpatrick et al., 1996); (c) computerized testing (Bloom, 1997); (d) computerized academic advisement (Bingham, 1997); and (e) multimedia courseware (Goodman & Blake, 1996). Systematic evaluation of such software is critical before purchase and utilization.

While no specific conceptual framework guided the development of the SET-N, several educational theorists ranging from Dewey (1938) forward were identified in forming the context for instrument development. The criterion-referenced measurement framework was used (Waltz, Strickland, & Lenz, 1991).

Specific objectives of the process included development of an instrument that would provide the user with a mechanism to allow for: (a) assessment of the instructional characteristics of selected computerized nursing simulations; (b) critical evaluation of contextual design and constant presentation of selected computerized simulations; (c) description of cognitive, affective, and psychomotor nursing behaviors required for the completion of selected computerized nursing simulations; and (d) identification of technical characteristics that aid or impede utilization. Four conceptual domains are included: nursing content, pedagogy, technical quality of the media, and policy (i.e., degree of appropriateness) (Underwood, 1988).

Literature review served as a source of information for instrument development, particularly the work of Klopfer (1983), who developed an instrument for evaluating a software designed for science content. In addition, a group of 30 authors, editors, and nursing software distributors completed a questionnaire asking them to identify the most critical characteristics of computerized instructional media for nursing that should be assessed in formal evaluation. The most critical variables identified included application to nursing, program purpose, program objectives, program clarity, effectiveness of the simulation, instructional design, adequacy of documentation, content accuracy, clinical correlates, effective utilization of the technology, and hardware and software requirements.

Item development proceeded with Weaver's (1982) work serving as a model. Items were tailored to meet standards expected for nursing media. Items are pairs of short statements that serve as bipolar descriptors. Respondents use a 7-point, Likert-type scale to rate the computer program being evaluated from –3 to +3. These ratings may be summed to produce a numerical score. If desired, this score can be compared to minimal standards set by the rater or institution. This comparison can be used in decision making related to purchase and/or use of the software being evaluated.

The initial instrument contained 45 items. It has been revised to the current number as seen at the end of this chapter.

RELIABILITY AND VALIDITY ASSESSMENT

Reliability of the SET-N was estimated from usage of the instrument by five nurse educators who rated two computer-assisted instructional programs. Two hours after completing the SET-N, they were asked to review the programs and complete the instrument again. The correlation between ratings was .892. Using another approach to estimating test-retest reliability, P_o was .834, P_c was 0.62, K was 0.56, and K_{max} was 0.71. These calculations resulted in $K/K_{max} = 0.79$. A Cronbach alpha value of .834 was also calculated.

Estimates of content validity were conducted with the initial 45-item instrument. Five content specialists (a computer media specialist, and well-qualified nurse educators) each completed ratings. Item-objective congruence was rated using a 3-point scale. The index value was 1.0 for 21 of the 45 items, and greater than .75 for another 15 items. The nine items receiving index values of less than .75 were eliminated.

Content validity was further estimated on the 36 items calculated from the ratings of two reviewers. The content validity index (Waltz, Strickland,

& Lenz, 1991) computed from these ratings was .805. Interrater agreement was also estimated with a P_o of .861, P_c of .78, and K of .368.

REFERENCES

Bauer, M. D. (1998). Nursing students' blood pressure measurement following CD-ROM and conventional classroom instruction: A pilot study. *International Journal of Medical Informatics 50*(1–3), 103–109.
Bingham, R. M. (1997). Increasing the effectiveness and efficiency of academic advising through computerization. *Computers in Nursing, 15*(3), 137.140.
Bloom, K. C. (1997). The efficacy of individualized computerized testing in nursing education. *Computers in Nursing, 15*(2), 82–89.
Dewey, J. (1938). *Experience in education.* New York: Macmillan.
Goodman, J., & Blake, J. (1996). Multimedia courseware: Transforming the classroom. *Computers in Nursing, 14*(5), 287–296.
Kirkpatrick, J. M., Billings, D. M., Carlton, K. H., Cummings, R. B., Hanson, C., Malone, J., Miller, A., Robinson, L., & Zwirn, E. E. (1996). Computerized test development software: a comparative review. *Computers in Nursing, 14*(2), 113–115.
Klopfer, L. (1983). *Microcomputer software evaluation instrument.* Washington, DC: National Science Teachers' Association.
Underwood, S. M. (1988). Measuring the validity of computer-assisted instructional media. In O. L. Strickland & C. F. Waltz (Eds.), *Measurement of nursing outcomes: Vol. 2. Measuring nursing performance: Practice, education and research* (pp. 294–313). New York: Springer Publishing Company.
Waltz, C. F., Strickland, O. L., & Lenz, E. R. (1991). *Measurement in nursing research* (2nd ed.). Philadelphia: F. A. Davis.
Weaver, P. (1982). *The evaluator's guide for microcomputer-based instructional packages.* Eugene, OR: International Council for Computers in Education.

SOFTWARE EVALUATION TOOL FOR NURSING
(SET-N, 1985)
Softwre Evaluation Tool for Evaluation
of Computer-Based Instructional Media
for Nursing Education (SET-N)

Given the apparent lack of valid and reliable means for evaluating computer-based instructional media for use within nursing education, the following software evaluation tool (SET-N) has been developed. Adapted from the 1983 Micro-Software Evaluation Instrument (Task Force on Assessing Computer Augmented Science Instructional Materials—National Science Teachers Association), this SET-N purports to evaluate computer-based instructional materials for nursing.

Following the preview/review of any computer-based instructional program for nursing, evaluators may use this tool to assess the software package in four specific areas: Nursing Content, Pedagogy, Technical Quality, and Policy Issues — appropriateness of use of the media.

This program allows the evaluator to numerically describe any software program related to nursing. Using multiple sets of bipolar descriptors, the evaluators rate the program using a 7-point, Likert-type scale. Following the evaluation, the scores may then be compiled and compared with an established profile of minimal standards for nursing educational media.

Each section of this tool contains a sct of bipolar descriptors. Carefully consider the descriptors at both ends of each scale and then assign a value on the −3 to +3 scale according to how well the left or right descriptor applies to the software package you are judging.

Definitely True	Partly True	Slightly True	Neither Description Applies	Slightly True	Partly True	Definitely True
−3	−2	−1	0	+1	+2	+3
____	____	____	____	____	____	____

Consider for a moment the following bipolar descriptor:

The program makes the computer act as a little more than a page turner or workbook.	The program exploits the computer's special capabilities (e.g., graphic animation, simulation) to provide a learning experience not easily possible through other media.

If you believe that the left descriptor is definitely true about the program you just reviewed, you should rate that item as −3.

Definitely True -3	Partly True -2	Slightly True -1	Description Applies 0	Slightly True +1	Partly True +2	Definitely True +3
X	___	___	___	___	___	___

If you believe that the right descriptor is definitely true about the program you have just reviewed, you should rate the item +3.

Definitely True -3	Partly True -2	Slightly True -1	Description Applies 0	Slightly True +1	Partly True +2	Definitely True +3
___	___	___	___	___	___	X

If you cannot make a decision about a particular scale, mark the zero (0) point for the item.

Definitely True -3	Partly True -2	Slightly True -1	Description Applies 0	Slightly True +1	Partly True +2	Definitely True +3
___	___	___	X	___	___	___

To obtain the rating for each section, find the arithmetic sum of the values you assigned to all the scales in the section. A comparison of the obtained ratings within each category (Nursing Content, Pedagogy, Technical Quality, and Policy Issues) with the "established" minimums can lead to a recommendation concerning the suitability of the software package. (Please note that the established minimum may be set by yourself, your faculty, or through peer review.)

Characteristics of the Computer-assisted Instruction Software

Title
Author
Topics/Subjects
Level of the learner
Instructional purpose and techniques

Remediation/development _____

Standard instruction _____

Enrichment _____

Data analysis _____

Drill and practice _____

Word processing _____

Tutorial _____

Information retrieval _____

Programming _____

Educational game _____

Laboratory device _____

Simulation _____

Teaching aid _____

Problem solving _____

Testing _____

Computer-managed instruction _____

Test construction _____

Program development _____

Nursing Content Standards

The package presents topics that are irrelevant to the educational needs of the intended student users.

The topics included in the package are very significant in the education of the intended student/user population.

Definitely True -3	Partly True -2	Slightly True -1	Description Applies 0	Slightly True +1	Partly True +2	Definitely True +3
____	____	____	____	____	____	____

The nursing content is very inaccurate.

The nursing content is free from errors.

Definitely True -3	Partly True -2	Slightly True -1	Description Applies 0	Slightly True +1	Partly True +2	Definitely True +3
____	____	____	____	____	____	____

Racial, ethnic, or sex-role
stereotypes are displayed.

The presentation is free
from any objectionable
stereotyping.

Definitely True -3	Partly True -2	Slightly True -1	Description Applies 0	Slightly True $+1$	Partly True $+2$	Definitely True $+3$
____	____	____	____	____	____	____

Biased or distorted information
is paraded as factual information.

Well-balanced and
representative information
is presented.

Definitely True -3	Partly True -2	Slightly True -1	Description Applies 0	Slightly True $+1$	Partly True $+2$	Definitely True $+3$
____	____	____	____	____	____	____

The package includes nursing
information that is greatly
outdated.

The nursing content
presented in the package
represents current nursing
theory and knowledge.

Definitely True -3	Partly True -2	Slightly True -1	Description Applies 0	Slightly True $+1$	Partly True $+2$	Definitely True $+3$
____	____	____	____	____	____	____

The presentation of the nursing
content is confusing.

The nursing content is very
clearly presented.

Definitely True -3	Partly True -2	Slightly True -1	Description Applies 0	Slightly True $+1$	Partly True $+2$	Definitely True $+3$
____	____	____	____	____	____	____

The package gives no attention to the utilization of the nursing process.

The application of the nursing process is well integrated into this software package.

Definitely True −3	Partly True −2	Slightly True −1	Description Applies 0	Slightly True +1	Partly True +2	Definitely True +3
_____	_____	_____	_____	_____	_____	_____

Attention is primarily given to the utilization of lower-level cognitive processes.

Utilization of higher-level cognitive processes are encouraged throughout the software program.

Definitely True −3	Partly True −2	Slightly True −1	Description Applies 0	Slightly True +1	Partly True +2	Definitely True +3
_____	_____	_____	_____	_____	_____	_____

The software offers limited exposure to the development of affective behaviors related to the subject matter

Multiple opportunities are provided for the application of higher-order processes within the affective domain.

Definitely True −3	Partly True −2	Slightly True −1	Description Applies 0	Slightly True +1	Partly True +2	Definitely True +3
_____	_____	_____	_____	_____	_____	_____

No attempt is made to integrate processes related to psychomotor skills within the software package.

The program challenges the student to "demonstrate" proficiency in the psychomotor domain throughout the program.

Definitely True −3	Partly True −2	Slightly True −1	Description Applies 0	Slightly True +1	Partly True +2	Definitely True +3
_____	_____	_____	_____	_____	_____	_____

| There is limited opportunity for the user to become actively involved in the process of making clinical nursing decisions. | Clinical decision making by the student/user is encouraged throughout the software package. |

Definitely True −3	Partly True −2	Slightly True −1	Description Applies 0	Slightly True +1	Partly True +2	Definitely True +3
____	____	____	____	____	____	____

Comments (Nursing Content Standards):

Software Program Profile

	Policy	*Nursing content*	*Pedagogy*	*Technical quality*
Ratings				
Minimal Standards				

35

Trends and Implications for Measurement

Carolyn F. Waltz and Louise S. Jenkins

In this rapidly changing health care landscape, nursing educators and administrators are faced with constant challenges to develop and implement new strategies for assuring quality outcomes. One factor, however, remains stable, the salient need for the development and use of reliable and valid methods for measuring nursing performance outcomes. The Pew Health Commission (O'Neil and The Pew Health Professions Commission, 1991; 1998) in delineating practitioner outcomes for 2005 included among the expected core competencies: to develop outcomes measurement to assure continuity and comprehensiveness of care across sites, levels, and episodes of care; active management of clinical quality; accountability; client satisfaction; health status; costs; and management of interactions between and among components of the integrated network of services and efficiency. Thus, it is imperative that nurses remain cognizant of trends and issues having impact on the future of nursing practice, education, and research; implications for the measurement of nursing performance; and resources available for keeping abreast of new developments in measuring nursing outcomes.

TRENDS AND ISSUES IN NURSING PRACTICE, EDUCATION AND RESEARCH

Time does not permit an extensive discussion of trends and issues, but a few that are likely to have the greatest impact on the measurement of nursing performance in practice, education, and research are discussed here.

Nursing Shortage

While employment opportunities for registered nurses are expected to grow faster than the average for all U.S. occupations through 2008, nation-wide schools of nursing have been challenged to increase applications and enrollments that have been declining at the baccalaureate, masters and doctoral levels during the last five years (AACN, 1996a; 2000a; 1997–2000). The acute shortage of nurses in both practice and education has been attributed to many factors including an aging workforce, increased and varied career opportunities for women, and a longstanding less than favorable image of nursing as a career. This shortage, expected to result in 114,500 job vacancies by 2015 (National Advisory Council on Nurse Education and Practice, 1996), is projected to be longer and more diffi-cult to resolve than previous ones (Buerhaus, 2000). As a result, it has heightened awareness on the part of nursing educators and administra-tors of the need to work together to devise both long- and short-term strategies to increase the nursing workforce.

Outcomes to Measure:

- Effectiveness of recruitment, and retention strategies designed to increase the supply of practicing nurses, nursing faculty, and nurse researchers;
- Outcomes of efforts to market nursing as a career option and for improving/reinventing the image of nursing.

Changes in Nursing Practice Environment

The environments in which nurses practice are more variable, and there is greater diversity in nursing roles, especially for advanced practice nurses including the emergence of careers in case management, biotechnology, clinical trials management, and as entrepreneurs and independent prac-titioners, than ever before. More nurses are employed in community-based and nontraditional settings such as in industry, information technology, and pharmaceutical companies. Practice in the community requires nurses to be skillful in working with other disciplines, to provide care along a continuum across diverse health care settings, to diverse populations in terms of age, gender, ethnicity, health, illness, acute, and chronic states (AACN, 1999b, p. ii). Shifting population demographics that result in increased diversity necessitate that nurses have the requisite knowledge and experience to provide care for diverse populations in a variety of envi-ronments (Stanley, 2000). Increased incidence of chronic and infectious diseases requires nurses to have a broader background in the biological, social, and behavioral sciences. Further, nurses practicing in a managed care environment are expected to demonstrate a high level of productivity, and provide high quality care while working with limited resources. For these reasons the practice environment presents challenges more than ever before for nurses who are faced with ethical dilemmas and the need to compromise.

Outcomes to measure:

- Nurses knowledge and skill relative to new content and performance required to effect quality care within the changing nursing practice environment, including:
  - working with other disciplines, with diverse populations, especially those from other cultures and ethnic backgrounds, within diverse settings;
  - management of clinical quality within integrated network services, accountability, financial management, shaping health policy;
  - scientific background and experience relevant to increased incidence of infections, chronic illness;
  - productivity within clinical environments with limited resources, managed care;
  - ability to respond to ethical dilemmas and make decisions without compromising quality of care.
- Outcomes of interdisciplinary/collaborative practice;
- Evaluation of consumer satisfaction.

Changes in the Clinical Learning Environment

AACN's Essentials of Master's Education for Advanced Practice Nurses (1996c) clearly state, "When preparing a graduate who will provide direct client care . . . the educational program should provide the student with the opportunity to master knowledge and skills in extensive clinical practice." The National Organization of Nurse Practitioner Faculty (NONPF) in their criteria for evaluation of nurse practitioner programs (1997, 1995) include the expectation that clinical resources support the educational program and that the student has experience with patient populations specific to the area of practice and in sufficient number and variability. Enrollment in nurse practitioner programs represents 60.8% of all Master's degree students (AACN, 1999). On the other hand, 53.7% of schools are unable to admit qualified applicants due to lack of clinical sites and 31.7% of schools have too few clinical staff to serve as preceptors. Similarly, a limited supply of clinical training sites has been cited as one of the primary reasons for intentional cutbacks in baccalaureate nursing program enrollments (AACN, 2000b).

In a 1998 AACN survey of members regarding clinical training issues, 84% of the schools stated they were having problems related to a decline in the number of clinical education sites or in placing students at clinical sites (AACN, 1998b). Reasons for this problem are the direct result of the changes in the practice environment where there are fewer nurses with the prerequisite baccalaureate and higher degrees necessary to precept students (Moses, 1997); where nurses with the necessary credentials to do so have little time to teach, mentor, and precept students; and where there are greater numbers of requests from the increasing numbers of nurse practitioner programs seeking more extensive clinical placements and/or preceptorships. In response to this growing concern, the document Essential Clinical Resources for Nursing's Academic Mission was developed by AACN (1999b) in which they called for nursing educators to design new models of clinical learning that will afford nursing the opportunity to establish meaningful relationships between the clinical enterprise and schools of nursing, and to prepare highly qualified practitioners for the future health care system (p. i).

Outcomes to Measure:

- Impact of changes in the clinical environment on clinical learning outcomes relative to:
  - Adequacy of clinical resources,
  - Evaluation of new models of clinical learning,
  - Strategies designed to address clinical training issues, e.g. evaluation of clinical sites, evaluation of preceptors and faculty clinical competence.

Changes in Nursing Education

Nursing educators must address the concerns of consumers who are holding them accountable for evaluating the outcomes of their programs especially in regard to quality, relevance to societal needs, and cost-effectiveness. Nursing education programs must be carefully examined and modified, as necessary, to ensure that graduates are prepared with the content and skills necessary to function competently and confidently within a rapidly changing, largely unpredictable practice environment. Nursing faculty must work in concert with nurses in practice to assume responsibility for preparing expert practitioners who can participate as full partners in health care delivery and in shaping health policy (AACN, 1997). Accordingly, AACN (1997) in A Vision of Baccalaureate and Graduate Nursing Education: The Next Decade delineates the following priorities that nursing education programs at all levels must address: development of critical thinking and clinical judgment skills; preparation to practice across multiple traditional and nontraditional settings; emphasis on primary health care, patient education, health promotion, rehabilitation, self-care, alternative methods of acute care and tertiary care; attainment of racial and ethnic diversity among students and faculty that mirrors society; curricula that focus on case management, health policy, and economics; research on quality indicators, outcome measures, financial management, legislative advocacy, privatization, data management, and technology.

To be successful in this regard requires faculty to be current, clinically competent, and versed in the art and science of teaching; to base their teaching in active clinical practice, and to embrace practice as integral to their teaching, research, and service (AACN, 1996b, 1997). Faculty must employ new ways of delivering instruction, such as problem based learning, case studies, grand rounds, and other student centered learning methods. To enable students to develop the necessary skills and confidence to provide care in less than optimal clinical learning environments, faculty need to increase the use of technologies such as interactive computer programs, preclinical simulations with intelligent computerized manikins, and standardized patients (live actors) prior to working with actual patients. Students should be afforded increased opportunities to learn and practice side by side with students in other disciplines and as members of teams of health care providers working with individuals, groups, and communities across the continuum of care. Changing student demographics and increased diversity of nursing student bodies also need to be taken into account when designing educational programs. Students typically are older, more varied in race, country of origin, previous educational background, and experience. Increasing numbers of students enter the nursing program with degrees in another field; with English as their second language; with commitments and responsibilities that preclude their attending school full-time; and/or live and work in areas geographically distant from where the program is located. To meet the needs of this diverse student body requires flexible scheduling with classes offered during the day, evenings, and on weekends, within the traditional semester or quarter hour system and in condensed time frames; increased use of technology to deliver courses using distance learning methods such as interactive video, CDs, web-based courses, and other methods that allow students to learn wherever they live and work. In addition, the internet affords students at distance sites the opportunity to maintain contact and continuous interaction with faculty and each other via e-mail, bulletin boards, and chat rooms.

The increased emphasis on accountability, and requirements to comply with a wide variety of standards and regulations requires the development and implementation of a systematic evaluation plan designed to collect data necessary to make informed decisions regarding program processes, outcomes, and to serve as the basis for program modifications.

Outcomes to Measure:

- Quality, cost-effectiveness, social relevance of nursing education programs;
- Employer satisfaction with nursing performance of students and graduates;
- Outcomes of interdisciplinary learning experiences;
- Student outcomes relative to critical thinking abilities, clinical judgment, ability to practice across diverse clinical sites, clinical competence;
- Determination of the ethnic, racial, and/or cultural sensitivity and relevance of existing measures of student performance;
- Quality of curricular outcomes in terms of standards, quality indicators, inclusion of necessary content and practice experiences;
- Evaluation of faculty performance, teaching skills, clinical competence, research productivity;
- Adequacy of new instructional models, outcomes of student centered learning strategies and their impact on critical thinking, and other important student outcomes;
- Student knowledge, practice skills and clinical confidence;
- Quality of outcomes resulting from implementation of new models of clinical learning;
- Impact of the use of technology on program, student, and graduate outcomes;
- Differences in outcomes resulting from varied approaches to delivery of nursing education programs, including patterns of sequencing, part-time/full-time study, flexible/traditional scheduling;
- Impact of use of distance technology on educational outcomes, student satisfaction with distance learning methods;
- Quality of student performance resulting from distance learning as compared with traditional learning methods;
- Faculty knowledge, skills, and attitudes toward use of internet as a teaching tool.

Faculty Shortage

There are inadequate numbers of doctorally prepared faculty and with the average age of full-time faculty 49 years, retirements are expected to peak within the next ten years (AACN, 1998c, 1999c). This shortage of faculty has given rise to serious concern regarding how to maintain a quality program when the numbers of faculty are inadequate. Factors adversely affecting the recruitment of nursing faculty include: declining enrollments in doctoral programs; faculty salaries that are lower than those of nurses employed in nonacademic settings; lack of sufficient numbers of faculty with the requisite teaching, clinical, and/or research skills; and difficult working conditions resulting from increased workload demands on existing faculty who must take on additional responsibility including the mentoring of greater numbers of part-time master's-prepared faculty employed to fill the void. Thus, there is an acute need to develop nurses to provide leadership in nursing education.

Research, Scholarship, and Evidence-Based Practice

An important aspect of the nursing faculty role is research and scholarship (AACN, 1998d, 199a; Boyer, 1990; Brown, et al., 1995). Within nursing the goal is to undertake research that advances nursing science and produces findings that can serve as the basis for practice. Resources necessary to produce a research intensive environment likely to result in this outcome include Centers of Excellence defined by faculty, ongoing programs of research, and a strong research infrastructure with a comprehensive set of services necessary to support their research efforts (Hinshaw and Berlin, 1997).

Essentials for Baccalaureate Education, (1998b, 1998e), Essentials for Master's Education for Advanced Practice Nursing (1996c), and The Indicators of Quality in Doctoral Programs in Nursing (1993) provide for the inclusion of research content at all program levels and for students to have opportunities to participate in the research endeavor. Criteria that serve as the basis for decisions regarding faculty appointment, promotion, and tenure reflect the expectation that faculty have well established programs of research in important substantive areas; serve as mentors for junior faculty and students; and disseminate their research results in peer-reviewed journals in nursing and other fields.

Changes in nursing education and practice present challenges to faculty who find it progressively more difficult to implement this important aspect of their role. Challenges to the research mission include competing demands for faculty time and major financial pressures to deliver educational and health services in a more cost-effective manner, leading to difficult decisions regarding how to spend limited time and money. To address complex clinical questions requires interdisciplinary across-site studies. Most nurse researchers, having only conducted primarily single-site studies within nursing have little background and experience with such studies, diminishing their ability to successfully compete for funding. Post doctoral training has not been the norm in nursing as it has been for most other professions. The next generation of researchers must be encouraged to seek post doctoral training if research-intensive environments are to be sustained, and funding for post-doctoral education must be increased. Concern regarding research integrity, potential conflicts of interest, and academic freedom is increasing as a result of the growing emphasis on research partnerships between schools of nursing and private and public industries. The limited access to professional, public, and private funding sources is exacerbated by the growing number of doctoral programs, and by the number of new doctorally prepared researchers and senior researchers who have major programs of research. The increased recognition of the importance of evidence-based practice and innovation require a long term commitment to conducting health services research studies to examine the impact of nursing processes and structures on the health care outcomes of patients and populations and the concomitant need to develop more nurses with basic and advanced degrees who have the ability to employ research findings skillfully in their practice (AACN, 1998d, pp. 5–6).

Outcomes to Measure:

- Quality and intensity of the research environment, faculty and student research productivity, quality of research reports, mentorship efforts;
- Faculty and student knowledge and skill in conducting interdisciplinary, across site research studies;
- Quality of post doctoral training programs, participant outcomes;
- Evaluation of the research environment relative to quality, cost, productivity, and intensity;
- Effectiveness of strategies for addressing issues of research integrity, academic freedom, and conflicts of interest, especially in regard to research partnerships between schools of nursing and both public and private organizations.

Increased Need for Educational Mobility, Continuing Education, and Use of Distance Learning Technologies

Inherent in the preceding discussion is the need for additional learning opportunities, both credit and noncredit, to prepare nurses to deal in creative ways with the emerging trends and issues in practice, education, and research. Educational mobility, a process by which individuals complete formal and/or informal educational offerings to acquire additional knowledge and skills, should build on previous learning without unnecessary duplication of learning and be focused on outcomes (AACN, 1998f, p. 1). Educational mobility opportunities at the undergraduate and graduate levels is an important means for addressing the shortage of nurses, especially advanced practice nurses, and for increasing the number of nurses able to provide leadership in nursing education and practice (AACN, 1998a, 1998f). Continuing education is a means for updating the knowledge and skills of practicing nurses and faculty with undergraduate and graduate degrees, who find themselves with deficits in knowledge and skills necessary to meet the expectations imposed by changes in nursing practice, education, and research. Distance learning technologies are a vehicle for increasing access to both credit and noncredit educational experiences for nurses who are unable to take advantage of traditional on-site delivery methods (AACN 2000b; Reinert & Fryback, 1997).

As technology further permeates the health care system and educational settings nurses must keep pace with new developments. Areas of focus for continuing education for practicing nurses include, but are not limited to: increased skill development to enable nurses to practice in settings where there is managed care; diverse patient populations; ethical dilemmas resulting from the need to balance care with cost; changes in regulations, standards, and expectations for quality care; new, emerging expanded nursing roles; and evidence-based practice and outcomes assessment.

Students entering nursing education programs have been coined the digital generation, because of their dependence on technology, a tool they have used effectively for most of their educational experiences and have come to take for granted. Unfortunately, nursing faculty, many of whom are nearing the end of their professional career, have not kept pace and there is thus a gap in background and experience between a large number of faculty and students. Other continuing education needs for nursing faculty include, but are not limited to: learning new ways to teach that are more student centered; increasing clinical skills and competence; developing new models of clinical learning; assessing program and student learning outcomes; mastering specific content areas such as population-based care, research content and methods, financial management, and policy development and analysis; meeting the needs of more diverse, nontraditional student bodies; and delivering courses via distance methods such as interactive video, CDs, and web-based courses.

Outcomes to Measure:

- Effectiveness of continuing education programs in preparing nurses to function in practice, education, and research within the changing environment;
- Participant satisfaction with educational mobility, credit and non-credit programs;
- Evaluation of existing outcome measures for use in different cultures and languages;
- Effectiveness of translation strategies;
- Effectiveness of technology as a vehicle for communication and dissemination of information and collaboration in education and research across continents.

Increased Focus on Globalization and International Partnerships

A higher number of international students are entering nursing education programs in the U.S. Study abroad opportunities for U.S. nursing
students are increasing. As shared health problems and educational issues
are identified worldwide, partnerships between practicing nurses, nurse
educators, and researchers are growing in numbers aided by technological advances that enable rapid communication and dissemination of information across continents. Distance learning technologies have enabled
students here and abroad to study and learn together and as a result educational programs here and in other countries are seeking common standards and criteria to define quality education. Thus, there is a salient need
to give attention to developing a global perspective among nurses, nursing faculty, and students; to increase the emphasis on culture and language and awareness of their impact on nursing practice, education, and
research. Outcome assessment has become a universal requirement and
the need for development and modification of measurement methods
across cultures and for translating well-established tools into other languages for use in cross continent research has become imperative.

Outcomes to Measure:

- Outcomes of study-abroad programs;
- Performance of students with English as a second language relative to student outcome measures including NCLEX RN;
- Relevance of U.S. educational programs for preparing international
  students to achieve expected outcomes necessary to practice, education, and research in their country.

RESOURCES FOR ACCESSING NEW DEVELOPMENTS
IN MEASURING NURSING PERFORMANCE

To address the measurement needs discussed in the preceding sections,
it is essential to remain up-to-date regarding new developments in measuring nursing performance outcomes in practice, education, and research.
Resources available to accomplish this purpose include the internet where
a number of electronic resources are available including online journals,
discussion groups, LISTSERVs, bulletin boards, newsgroups, and search
engines. Other sources include professional and government organizations that make current information available in print and on web pages,
and publications like the *Journal of Nursing Measurement, Outcomes
Management for Nursing Practice*, and *Evaluation and the Health Professions*
that are specifically focused on measurement in nursing and the health
field. The following selected internet resources are presented as a start-

ing point for those seeking to keep abreast of developments in measuring outcomes salient to nursing.

Online Resources

The following general nursing web sites can help orient you to what is available online to nurses:

www.greatnurse.com
This site offers an international message board, chat room, and links to a comprehensive list of professional organization and foundation home pages, graduate research online journals, and schools of nursing home pages. A particularly valuable link is to PubMed, the National Library of Medicine search service that provides access to over 11 million citations in MEDLINE, Pre-MEDLINE, and other related databases with links to online journals.

www.nursesworld.com
Information provided here includes nursing/health news, education (with an assessment section that includes tools), a comprehensive list of professional organizations, and links to other important resources on the World Wide Web. Of particular significance are links to a number of nursing journals including but not limited to *Advances in Nursing Science, American Journal of Nursing, Applied Nursing Research, Computers in Nursing, International Journal of Nursing Practice, Journal for Nurses in Staff Development, Journal of Nursing Administration, Nurse Educator, Australian Online Journal of Nursing Education, Online Journal of Nursing Informatics,* and *Online Journal of Issues in Nursing.*

In addition to the discussion groups/LISTSERVs available at the greatnurse and nursesworld websites, other resources for identifying discussion lists and news groups include: CataList from L-Soft International, the catalog of LISTSERV lists and Tile.Net from Lyris Technologies, Inc.

The following online resources are more specific to outcomes research:

Agency for Health Care Research and Quality *www.ahrq.gov*
    This U.S. government agency site has a section on Outcomes and Effectiveness and a Center for Outcomes and Effectiveness Research.
International Society of Quality in Health Care (ISQHC) *www.isqua.org.au*
    This is an international membership organization dedicated to quality practice and performance improvement in Health Care. One of its objectives is to promote research in quality improvement through measures of quality of life and consumer satisfaction.

National Institute of Nursing Research *www.nih.gov/ninr*
The nursing research institute of the U.S. National Institutes of Health
funds nursing research and provides information on ongoing research
and how to obtain funding.

In summary, while not inclusive, this chapter presented an overview of
the trends and issues impacting on nursing practice, education, and
research, explicated the implications for measuring outcomes that derive
from them, and identified resources available for keeping current regarding future developments in measuring nursing outcomes.

REFERENCES

American Association of Colleges of Nursing. (October, 1993). *Indicators of quality in doctoral programs in nursing.* Washington, DC: Author.

American Association of Colleges of Nursing. (1996a). *1995–1996 Enrollment and Graduations in Baccalaureate and Graduate Programs in Nursing* (p. 13). Washington, DC: Author.

American Association of Colleges of Nursing. (June, 1996b). *Nursing schools seek balance of teaching and research skills in an effort to boost the PhD supply.* Washington, DC: Author.

American Association of Colleges of Nursing. (1996c). *The Essentials of Master's Education for Advanced Practice Nursing.* Washington, DC: Author.

American Association of Colleges of Nursing. (1997). *A vision of baccalaureate and graduate nursing education: The next decade.* Washington, DC: Author.

American Association of Colleges of Nursing. (1997–2000). *Enrollment and graduations in baccalaureate and graduate programs in nursing* (1999–2000, p. 2, 6; 1998–1999, p. 2, 5; 1997–1998, p. 1–2, 5; 1996–1997, p. 2, 10). Washington, DC: Author.

American Association of Colleges of Nursing. (1998a). *Educational Mobility,* Revised March, 1998. Washington, DC: Author.

American Association of Colleges of Nursing. (April, 1998b). *New AACN "Essentials" defines core standards for bachelor's degree nursing education.* Washington, DC: Author.

American Association of Colleges of Nursing. (1998c). *Issue bulletin: As RNs age, nursing schools seek to expand the pool of younger faculty.* Washington, DC: Author.

American Association of Colleges of Nursing. (1998d). *Position statement on nursing research.* Washington, DC: Author.

American Association of Colleges of Nursing. (1998e). *The essentials of baccalaureate education for professional nursing practice.* Washington, DC: Author.

American Association of Colleges of Nursing. (1998f). *Educational mobility.* Washington, DC: Author.

American Association of Colleges of Nursing. (1999a). *Position statement on defining scholarship for the discipline of nursing.* Washington, DC: Author.

American Association of Colleges of Nursing. (1999b). *Essential clinical resources for nursing's academic mission.* Washington, DC: Author.

American Association of Colleges of Nursing. (1999c). *Faculty shortages intensify nation's nursing deficit.* Washington, DC: Author.

American Association of Colleges of Nursing. (2000a). *Issue Bulletin: Amid nursing shortages, schools employ strategies to boost enrollment.* Washington, DC: Author.

American Association of Colleges of Nursing. (2000b). Distance technology in nursing education: Assessing a new frontier. *Journal of Professional Nursing, 16*(2), 116–122.

Boyer, E. (1990). *Scholarship reconsidered: Priorities for the professoriate.* Princeton, NJ: The Carnegie Foundation for the Advancement of Teaching.

Brown, S. A., Cohen, S. M., Kaeser, L., Leane, C. D., Littleton, L. Y., Otto, D. A., & Rickman, K. J. (1995). Nursing perspective on Boyer's scholarship paradigm. *Nurse Educator, 20*(5), 26–30.

Buerhaus, P. (2000). A nursing shortage with a fundamental difference. *Syllabus,* Sept–Oct, 2000, pp. 3–10. Washington, DC: American Association of Colleges of Nursing Newsletter.

Hinshaw, A. S., & Berlin, L. E. (1997). *The future for quality doctoral nursing programs: Are the resources there?* Sanibel Island, FL: Paper presented at the American Association of Colleges of Nursing 1997 Doctoral Conference.

Moses, Evelyn B. (1997). *The registered nurse population, March 1996: Findings from the National Sample Survey of Registered Nurses.* Rockville, MD: US Department of Health & Human Services, Health Resources & Services Administration, Bureau of Health Professions, Division of Nursing.

National Advisory Council on Nurse Education and Practice. (1996). *Report to the Secretary of the Department of Health and Human Services on the basic registered nurse workforce.* Rockville, MD: US Department of Health & Human Services, Health Resources & Services Administration, Bureau of Health Professions, Division of Nursing.

National Organization of Nurse Practitioner Faculty (1995). *Advanced nursing practice: Curriculum guidelines and program standards for nurse practitioner education.* Washington, DC: Author.

National Organization of Nurse Practitioner Faculty (1997). *Criteria for evaluation of nurse practitioner programs.* Report of the National Taskforce on Quality Nurse Practitioner Education. Washington, DC: Author.

O'Neil, E.H. and the Pew Health Professions Commission (1991). *Healthy America: Practitioners for 2005. An Agenda for Action for U.S. Health*

Professional Schools. San Francisco, CA: Pew Health Professions Commission.

O'Neil, E.H. and the Pew Health Professions Commission (1998). *Recreating Health Professional Practice for a New Century.* San Francisco, CA: Pew Health Professions Commission.

Reinert, B., & Fryback, P. (1997). Distance learning and nursing education. *Journal of Nursing Education, 36*(9), 421.

Stanley, J. (2000). *Introduction in implementing community-based education in the undergraduate nursing curriculum proceedings of the 1997 Faculty Development Workshops in Community-Based Care for Undergraduate Education.* Sponsored by the American Association of Colleges of Nursing and the Helene Fuld Health Trust, 2000.

INDEX